D0908143

Cancer in Pregnancy and Lactation: The Motherisk Guide

Cancer in Pregnancy and Lactation: The Motherisk Guide

Edited by

Gideon Koren
Founder and Director, Motherisk Program and Professor of Pediatrics,
Pharmacology, Pharmacy and Medical Genetics, University of Toronto, Canada.

Michael Lishner
Professor of Medicine, Sackler Faculty of Medicine,
Tel Aviv University and Head of Department of Medicine A, Meir Hospital, Kfar Saba, Israel.

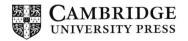
CAMBRIDGE
UNIVERSITY PRESS

CAMBRIDGE UNIVERSITY PRESS
Cambridge, New York, Melbourne, Madrid, Cape Town,
Singapore, São Paulo, Delhi, Tokyo, Mexico City

Cambridge University Press
The Edinburgh Building, Cambridge CB2 8RU, UK

Published in the United States of America by
Cambridge University Press, New York

www.cambridge.org
Information on this title: www.cambridge.org/9781107006133

First published 2011

Printed in the United Kingdom at the University Press, Cambridge

A catalog record for this publication is available from the British Library

Library of Congress Cataloging-in-Publication Data

Cancer in pregnancy and lactation : the Motherisk guide / edited by
Gideon Koren, Michael Lishner.
    p.   ;   cm.
  Includes bibliographical references and index.
  ISBN 978-1-107-00613-3 (Hardback)
  1. Cancer in pregnancy.   2. Pregnancy–Complications.   3. Fetus–
Effect of drugs on.   4. Lactation–Effect of drugs on.   I. Koren, Gideon,
1947– II. Lishner, M. (Michael)   III. Motherisk Program.
  [DNLM: 1. Pregnancy Complications, Neoplastic.   2. Fetus–drug
effects.   3. Fetus–radiation effects.   4. Lactation–drug effects.
5. Lactation–radiation effects.   6. Prenatal Exposure Delayed Effects.
WQ 240]
  RG580.C3C354 2011
  618.3′268–dc23

                                                          2011015544

ISBN 978-1-107-00613-3 Hardback

Contents

Preface

Cancer in pregnancy, the tragic collusion of the best time in a woman's life with her worst of times, creates a serious clinical and ethical challenge. The very drugs that can eradicate rapidly growing cancer may damage the rapidly growing embryo.

Cancer is the second leading cause of death among women during their reproductive years, yet sources of concise data and guidance for the management of cancer in pregnancy are scarce. *Cancer in Pregnancy and Lactation: The Motherisk Guide* fills that resource gap as it contains updated data published over the past 5 years.

Written by a dedicated group of experts in the fields of clinical pharmacology, maternal–fetal toxicology, and hemato-oncology, this *Guide* contains the evidence-based information physicians need to address complex issues of maternal diagnosis, treatment, prognosis, and long-term impact on the unborn child.

This book is complemented by the Motherisk On-line Cancer in Pregnancy Consultative Forum. The Forum provides clinicians with ready access to expert guidance and a place to share their clinical experiences. Operational since 2000, the on-line Consultative Forum is receiving questions from individuals throughout the world. Questions and comments to the Forum are reviewed and answered by Consortium of Cancer in Pregnancy Evidence (CCoPE) members.

We invite you to visit the Forum at www.motherisk.org/cforum, review past questions and answers, and submit your own queries and comments. For as more and more clinicians engage in the informed dialog that this *Guide* and the Consultative Forum promote, their shared insights will help to generate new knowledge. We can think of no more effective way to advance the cause of science while also addressing immediate, life-threatening clinical issues.

Gideon Koren, MD
Michael Lishner, MD

Acknowledgement

Supported by an unrestricted grant by Shoppers Drug Mart, Canada

Contributors

Liat Drucker, MD
Oncogenetic Laboratory, Meir Medical
Center, Kfar Saba, Israel

Eyal Fenig, MD
Professor of Oncology, Head of
Radiotherapy, Davidoff Center, Rabbin
Medical Center, Petha Tikva, Israel

Hisaki Fujii, MD, PhD
Clinical Fellow, Division of Clinical
Pharmacology and Toxicology, The
Hospital for Sick Children, Toronto,
Ontario, Canada

Rinat Hackmon, MD
High Pregnancy Risk Fellow, University of
Toronto, Saint Michael's Hospital,
Toronto, Ontario, Canada

Shinya Ito, MD, FRCPC
Professor and Division Head, Division of
Clinical Pharmacology and Toxicology,
The Hospital for Sick Children, Toronto,
Ontario, Canada

Geert W. 't Jong, MD, PhD
Fellow in Clinical Pharmacology, Division
of Pharmacology and Toxicology, The
Hospital for Sick Children, Toronto,
Ontario, Canada

Taro Kamiya, MD
Division of Clinical Pharmacology and
Toxicology, The Hospital for Sick Children,
Toronto, Ontario, Canada

Deborah A. Kennedy, MBA, ND
Graduate Student, Leslie Dan Faculty of
Pharmacology, University of Toronto, The
Hospital for Sick Children, Toronto,
Ontario, Canada

Avi Leader, MD
Resident, Department of Medicine A, Meir
Medical Center, Kfar Saba, Israel

Michael Lishner, MD
Professor of Medicine,
Sackler Faculty of Medicine,
Tel Aviv University and Head of
Department of Medicine A,
Meir Hospital, Kfar Saba, Israel

Ronen Loebstein, MD
Director, Institute of Clinical
Pharmacology and Toxicology, Sheba
Medical Center, Tel Hashomer, Israel

Angela Mallozzi, MD
Maternal Fetal Medicine, Department of
Obstetrics and Gynecology, Royal Victoria
Hospital, Montreal, Quebec, Canada

Caroline Maltepe, BA
Coordinator, Motherisk NVP Helpline,
The Motherisk Program, The Hospital for
Sick Children, Toronto, Ontario, Canada

Israel Mazin, MD
Department of Medicine, Meir Medical
Center, Kfar Saba, Israel

Liat Mlynarsky, MD
Meir Medical Center, Kfar Saba, Israel

Irena Nulman, MD, FRCPC Neurology, PhD
Associate Director, Motherisk
Program, Division of Clinical
Pharmacology and Toxicology, The
Hospital for Sick Children, Toronto;
Associate Professor of Pediatrics, and
Program Director, Fellowship Training
Program in Clinical Pharmacology,
University of Toronto, Ontario, Canada

Alla Osadchy, MD
Clinical Fellow, Division of Clinical
Pharmacology and Toxicology, The
Hospital for Sick Children, Toronto,
Ontario, Canada

David Pereg, MD
Doctor of Internal Medicine and
Cardiology, Meir Medical Center, Kfar
Saba, Israel

Tal Schechter, MD
Assistant Professor of Pediatrics, Staff
Physician, Division of Hematology-
Oncology, The Hospital for Sick Children,
Toronto, Ontario, Canada

Tal Shapira-Rotenberg, MD
Department of Internal Medicine A, Meir
Medical Center, Kfar Saba, Israel

Alon Shrim, MD
The Motherisk Program, Division of
Clinical Pharmacology and Toxicology,
The Hospital for Sick Children, Toronto,
Ontario, Canada

Nava Siegelmann-Danieli, MD
Maccabi Health Services, Tel-Aviv, Israel

Michael P. Tan, MD, MSc
Motherisk Counselor, Division of
Pharmacology and Toxicology, The

Hospital for Sick Children, Toronto,
Ontario, Canada

Shelly Tartakover-Matalon, PhD
Researcher, Meir Medical Center, Kfar-
Saba and Tel-Aviv University, Tel-Aviv,
Israel

Claire Tobias, BA
Fetal Alcohol Syndrome Clinic
Coordinator, The Hospital for Sick
Children, Toronto, Ontario, Canada

Elizabeth Uleryk
Library Director, The Hospital for Sick
Children, Toronto, Ontario, Canada

Asnat Walfisch, MD
High Risk Pregnancy, Department of
Obstetrics and Gynecology, Hilil-Yafe
Medical Center, Hadera, Israel

Bi Lan Wo, MD
Fellow in Maternal-Fetal Medicine,
Department of Obstetrics and
Gynecology, Royal Victoria Hospital,
McGill University, Montreal, Quebec,
Canada

Parvaneh Yazdani-Brojeni, MD
Clinical Pharmacologist, Research Fellow,
The Hospital for Sick Children, Toronto,
Ontario, Canada

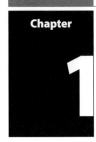

Chapter

1

Bone malignancies in pregnancy

Michael Lishner and Alla Osadchy

Introduction

Primary bone cancer is rarely associated with pregnancy [1,2]. The available information regarding its evaluation and management is very limited. A delay in diagnosis due to misinterpretation of tumor-related symptoms as those of normal pregnancy has been suggested [3].

Diagnosis

Although magnetic resonance imaging is the diagnostic method of choice [4] and can be repeated many times in pregnancy [5], ultrasound, biopsy to stage the tumor, and clinical examination remain equally safe and important in arriving at the diagnosis. Tests applying X-rays or gamma-rays (isotope scans) should be avoided [6]. Independence of bone tumors from hormonal regulation was shown [3]. The association of bone neoplasm with pregnancy may be fortuitous [7]. Rare cases of recurrent bone tumors diagnosed during pregnancy might be due to increased medical surveillance [8].

Treatment

Therapeutic considerations are complex, and a combined modality approach including surgery, radiation, and chemotherapy is often used and should be tailored to the individual patient. While surgical resections are generally regarded as safe during pregnancy, chemotherapy and radiation treatment are likely to be deferred until after delivery [6,9].

The decision-making analysis should include the type and site of the primary tumor, its growth rate and associated symptoms, the use of specific diagnostic tests, and appropriate treatment options [10]. Vaginal deliveries are possible [6,9]. In cases of bone malignances involving the pelvis, cesarean section delivery might be considered to increase fetal safety [11]. Nevertheless, spontaneous vaginal deliveries after hemipelvectomy due to malignant tumors of the pelvis have been reported [12].

Prognosis

Although based on very limited data, it was suggested that pregnancy does not appear to exacerbate tumor growth or affect the outcome of the patients [9,13]. Based on small series, reproductive outcomes of long-term survivors of malignant bone tumors appear to be favorable, with a high rate of success to conceive and no birth defects in offspring reported [14,15].

Cancer in Pregnancy and Lactation: The Motherisk Guide ed. Gideon Koren and Michael Lishner.
Published by Cambridge University Press. © Cambridge University Press 2011.

References

1. Dhillon MS, Singh DP, Gill SS, Sur R, Sarode VR, Nagi ON. Primary bone malignancies in pregnancy. A report of 4 cases. *Orthop Rev.* 1993;**22**:931–7.

2. Longhi A, Mercuri M, Bianchi G, Errani C, Bacci G. Maternal and neonatal outcomes in pregnancies complicated by bone and soft-tissue tumors. *Obstet Gynecol.* 2005;**105**:447; author reply 447–8.

3. Komiya S, Zenmyo M, Inoue A. Bone tumors in the pelvis presenting growth during pregnancy. *Arch Orthop Trauma Surg.* 1999;**119**:22–9.

4. Malawer MM, Link MP, Donaldson SS. Sarcomas of bone. In: DeVita VT, Hellman S, Rosenberg SA, editors. *Cancer. Principles and practice of oncology.* 5th ed. Philadelphia: Lippincott-Raven Publishers; 1997. p. 1789–852.

5. Campanacci M, Gasbarrini A, Campanacci L. The value of imaging in the diagnosis and treatment of bone tumors. *Eur J Radiol.* 1998;**27**(suppl 1):S116–22.

6. Molho RB, Kollender Y, Issakov J, et al. The complexity of management of pregnancy-associated malignant soft tissue and bone tumors. *Gynecol Obstet Invest.* 2008;**65**:89–95.

7. Lamovec J, Bracko M. Epithelioid hemangioma of small tubular bones: a report of three cases, two of them associated with pregnancy. *Modern Pathol.* 1996;**9**:821–7.

8. DuBois SG, Perez-Atayde AR, McLean TW, Grier HE. Late recurrence of Ewing sarcoma during pregnancy: a report of 2 cases. *J Pediatr Hematol Oncol.* 2008;**30**:716–8.

9. Maxwell C, Barzilay B, Shah V, Wunder JS, Bell R, Farine D. Maternal and neonatal outcomes in pregnancies complicated by bone and soft-tissue tumors. *Obstet Gynecol.* 2004;**104**:344–8.

10. Merimsky O, Le Cense A. Soft tissue and bone sarcomas in association with pregnancy. *Acta Oncol.* 1998;**37**:721–7.

11. Merimsky O, Le Chevalier T, Missenard G, et al. Management of cancer in pregnancy: a case of Ewing's sarcoma of the pelvis in the third trimester. *Ann Oncol.* 1999;**10**:345–50.

12. Heetkamp A, Feijen HW, Papatsonis DN. Spontaneous delivery after hemipelvectomy because of chondrosarcoma: a case report and review of the literature *Am J Perinatol.* 2008;**25**:255–8.

13. Simon MA, Philips WA, Bonfiglio M. Pregnancy and aggressive or malignant primary bone tumors. *Cancer.* 1984;**53**:2564–9.

14. Longhi A, Porcu E, Petracchi S, Versari M, Conticini L, Bacci G. Reproductive functions in female patients treated with adjuvant and neoadjuvant chemotherapy for localized osteosarcoma of the extremity. *Cancer.* 2000;**89**:1961–5.

15. Hosalkar HS, Henderson KM, Weiss A, Donthineni R, Lackman RD. Chemotherapy for bone sarcoma does not affect fertility rates or childbirth. *Clin Orthop Relat Res.* 2004;**428**:256–60.

Breast cancer and pregnancy

Liat Mlynarsky and Michael Lishner

Introduction

Breast cancer is the most commonly occurring malignancy among women of reproductive age and the second most common pregnancy-associated cancer, after cervical cancer [1,2]. Pregnancy-associated breast cancer (PABC) is defined as breast cancer diagnosed during pregnancy or within one year postpartum and it is estimated to account for up to 3% of all breast cancers. The prevalence of PABC is between 1 in 3,000 and 1 in 10,000 pregnancies.

Diagnosis

A high index of suspicion is required when evaluating a breast mass among pregnant and lactating women because of the substantial physiological changes of the female body during pregnancy. When a new breast mass is suspected, diagnostic evaluation must begin promptly.

Although mammography is the imaging of choice among nonpregnant women with a breast mass, its sensitivity declines among pregnant and lactating women due to the glandularity and the water content of the breast [1]. In one study, the false-negative mammography rate was significantly higher among pregnant women than among non-pregnant women (14% vs. 6%, respectively; $P < 0.0001$) [3]. Ultrasound is the modality of choice when PABC is suspected. It has been reported to distinguish solid from cystic lesions in 97% of cases [4], and with 100% sensitivity in a few studies [1,5,6].

There are insufficient evidence-based data regarding the efficacy of magnetic resonance imaging (MRI) and the safety of gadolinium during pregnancy. Thus, the international recommendations from an expert meeting summarized by Loibl et al. recommended against it [7].

When there is a palpable breast mass, the diagnostic procedure of choice is excisional biopsy under local anesthesia [8,9]. Fine needle aspiration can discriminate a cyst from a solid tumor, but the diagnostic value of cytology is diminished in pregnant or lactating women due to the presence of a hyperproliferative state which leads to a high false-positive rate.

Where there is a large mass, incisional biopsy should be considered. The yield of the biopsy is equivalent among pregnant and nonpregnant women, but the rate of complications is higher among pregnant or lactating women due to increased vascularity and the presence of breast milk as a culture medium. Another possible complication is milk fistula formation, more prevalent in central biopsies [8]. Some authors recommend emptying

Cancer in Pregnancy and Lactation: The Motherisk Guide ed. Gideon Koren and Michael Lishner.
Published by Cambridge University Press. © Cambridge University Press 2011.

the breast a week before the procedure by ceasing breast feeding, binding the breast, and placing ice packs. If it fails, bromocriptine can be used [4,10,11]. Nevertheless, there are no clear guidelines regarding prevention of biopsy-related complications.

Pathology

Invasive ductal carcinoma is the most commonly found histology in both pregnant and nonpregnant women of similar ages. It represents 75%–90% of the breast cancers in pregnant women [7,12,13]. The incidence of inflammatory breast cancer in pregnant women is 1.5%–4% [14]. However, as mentioned, pregnant women are more likely to present with larger, more poorly differentiated tumors, positive lymph nodes, and distant metastases than nonpregnant women [2,11,15]. Approximately 65%–90% of tumors diagnosed during pregnancy are at stage II or III, compared to 45%–66% diagnosed at these stages among nonpregnant women [2].

Estrogen receptor-negative and progesterone receptor-negative tumors, which correlate with poor prognoses, are more common among pregnant women than among age-matched controls, possibly due to receptor down-regulation in pregnancy [2,11,13,16]. The incidence of HER2 positivity was investigated in small studies; thus, it is not possible to conclude whether it is more common among pregnant women [17].

Metastases to the placenta and/or the fetus are very rare and account for 13% of all 81 known cases of maternal cancers with this type of distant metastasis [18]. Metastases to the fetus have been described only in cases of maternal metastatic melanoma, metastatic lung cancer, and hematologic malignancies [18]. A recent study published by our group demonstrated that the placenta impedes breast cancer cell growth in the area adjacent to it, probably through modifications of hormonal pathways and microenvironmental changes [19].

Therapeutic abortion

In the past, the belief was that hormonal changes during pregnancy endorse the growth of breast cancer. According to more recent literature, termination of pregnancy does not improve the prognosis of PABC [9]. Nevertheless, the decision should be made after multidisciplinary team discussion with the patient and her family.

Surgery

Surgical intervention during pregnancy is safe, but it should be postponed until after the 12th gestational week, because the risk for spontaneous abortion is higher in the first trimester [4,10]. Currently, the rate of mastectomy among pregnant women is higher than the rate of lumpectomy due to large tumor size and avoidance of adjuvant radiation, but breast-conserving surgery is becoming more frequent [20]. Kuerer and colleagues compared the outcomes of breast-conserving surgery and modified radical mastectomy in patients with stages I and II PABC and found no differences in disease-free and overall survival [21]. Lymphatic mapping (TC-99) to evaluate axillary involvement poses a low risk of radiation to the fetus, according to some studies [12]. On the other hand, isosulfan blue dye mapping is not recommended, because it is not FDA approved for the use in pregnant women and due to previous reports of anaphylaxis [7].

Radiotherapy

Radiation therapy administered either to complete breast-conserving surgery, as post-mastectomy adjuvant treatment in high-risk patients or as a palliative treatment for metastatic cancer, is contraindicated during pregnancy because of fetal exposure. As such, radiation must be postponed until after delivery [7].

Systemic therapy

All chemotherapeutic agents used to treat breast cancer are pregnancy category D, meaning teratogenicity was observed among humans. Nevertheless, when administered after the first trimester, standard protocols are safe and the rate of fetal malformations is not increased [22–25]. The incidence of fetal malformations from various cytotoxic drugs during the first trimester was reported to range from 14% to 19%, compared to only 1.3% in the second and third trimesters [26]. Other possible complications reported from the small prospective study by Berry *et al* [24]. were preterm labor, transient tachypnea of newborn, low birth weight, hyaline membrane disease, and transient leukopenia.

In the Royal Marsden retrospective series [27], 28 women were treated with different chemotherapy protocols such as FAC (fluorouracil, doxorubicin, cyclophosphamide), AC (doxorubicin, cyclophosphamide), EC (epirubicin, cyclophosphamide), and CMF (cyclophosphamide, methotrexate, fluorouracil). The use of these protocols in the second and third trimesters was considered safe. The median gestational age at delivery was 37 weeks (range, 30 to 40 weeks), and the median birth weight was 3.0 kg (range, 1.4 to 3.5 kg). None of the infants had a birth weight lower than the 10th percentile for gestational age, and no fetal abnormalities were recorded.

In the largest prospective study to date, from M.D. Anderson [25], 57 women were treated with FAC chemotherapy and followed for a median of 38.5 months. No significant complications were observed when chemotherapy was administered during the second and third trimesters. No stillbirths, miscarriages, or perinatal deaths occurred. However, 3 deliveries were before the 34th week and 1 was before the 29th week, due to preeclampsia. One child was born with Down's syndrome and 1, born in the 38th week, had subarachnoid hemorrhage 2 days after delivery due to pancytopenia. Long-term results were not reported. Chemotherapy should be avoided 4 weeks before the anticipated delivery date to reduce the risk for infection, or hemorrhage due to pancytopenia [8].

The use of methotrexate during pregnancy is contraindicated, and tamoxifen is not recommended due to evidence of genital tract malformations [7]. Taxane use has only been described in case reports and thus the information is not reliable. Data regarding the effects of trastuzumab are very scarce; thus, it should be used with caution and careful monitoring of fetal growth and kidney function [8].

Prognosis

Comparisons between pregnant and nonpregnant women of matched age, nodal status, estrogen receptor status, and tumor histopathology and size yielded no differences in prognosis [7,23]. However, while breast cancer is usually diagnosed approximately 1 month after detection of a nodule among nonpregnant women, the diagnosis among pregnant and lactating women can be delayed for 9 to 15 months [8]. Indeed, pregnant women have a 2.5-fold higher risk for metastases at presentation than do nonpregnant women [2].

However, the true biological effects of the hormonal changes associated with pregnancy have also been suggested to induce more aggressive clinical behaviors. Thus, higher TNM stages are observed among pregnant women and result in worse metastasis-free survival and overall survival.

We believe that a pregnant woman with a breast lump should be evaluated promptly, to avoid diagnostic delay. The effects of the pregnant state on breast cancer cells should be studied, as this may provide biological insights that can lead to new therapeutic interventions.

References

1. Liberman L, Giess CA, Dershaw DD, Deutch BM, Petreck JA. Imaging of pregnancy-associated breast cancer. *Radiology.* 1994;**191**:245–8.

2. Ishida T, Yokoe T, Kasumi F, et al. Clinicopathologic characteristics and prognosis of breast cancer patients associated with pregnancy and lactation: analysis of case-control study in Japan. *Jpn J Cancer Res.* 1992;**83**:1143–9.

3. Ibrahim EM, Ezzat AA, Baloush A, Hussain ZH, Mohammed GH. Pregnancy-associated breast cancer: a case-control study in a young population with a high-fertility rate. *Med Oncol.* 2000;**17**:293–300.

4. Woo JC, Yu T, Hurd TC. Breast cancer in pregnancy: a literature review. *Arch Surg.* 2003;**138**:91–8.

5. Yang WT, Dryden MJ, Gwyn K, Whitman GJ, Theriault R. Imaging of breast cancer diagnosed and treated with chemotherapy during pregnancy. *Radiology.* 2006;**239**:52–60.

6. Merezak S, Reusens B, Renard A, et al. Pregnancy- and lactation-associated breast cancer: mammographic and sonographic findings. *J Ultrasound Med.* 2003;**22**:491–7.

7. Loibl S, von Minckwitz G, Gwyn K, Ellis P, Blohmer JU, Schlegelberger B. Breast carcinoma during pregnancy. International recommendations from an expert meeting. *Cancer.* 2006;**106**:237–46.

8. Vinatier E, Merlot B, Poncelet E, Collinet P, Vinatier D. Breast cancer during pregnancy. *Eur J Obstet Gynecol Reprod Biol.* 2009;**147**:9–14.

9. Psyrri A, Burtness B. Pregnancy-associated breast cancer. *Cancer.* 2005;**11**:83–95.

10. Barnes DM, Newman LA. Pregnancy-associated breast cancer: a literature review. *Surg Clin North Am.* 2007;**87**:417–30.

11. Petrek JA. Breast cancer during pregnancy. *Cancer.* 1994;**74**:518–27.

12. Gentilini O, Masullo M, Rotmensz N, et al. Breast cancer diagnosed during pregnancy and lactation: biological features and treatment options. *Eur J Surg Oncol.* 2005;**31**:232–6.

13. Bonnier P, Romain S, Dilhuydy JM, et al. Influence of pregnancy on the outcome of breast cancer: a case control study. *Int J Cancer.* 1997;**72**:720–7.

14. Clark RM, Chua T. Breast cancer and pregnancy: the ultimate challenge. *Clin Oncol (R Coll Radiol).* 1989;**1**:8–11.

15. Bunker JP, Houghton J, Baum M. Putting the risk of breast cancer in perspective. *BMJ.* 1998;**317**:1307–9.

16. Rodriguez AO, Chew H, Cress R, et al. Evidence of poorer survival in pregnancy-associated breast cancer. *Obstet Gynecol.* 2008;**112**:71–8.

17. Elledge RM, Ciocca DR, Langone G, McGuire WL. Estrogen receptor, progesterone receptor, and HER-2/neu protein in breast cancers from pregnant patients. *Cancer.* 1993;**71**:2499–506.

18. Al-Adnani M, Kiho L, Scheimberg I. Maternal pancreatic carcinoma metastatic to the placenta: a case report and literature review. *Pediatr Dev Pathol.* 2007;**10**:61–5.

19. Tartakover-Matalon S, Mizrahi A, Epstein G, et al. Breast cancer characteristics are modified by first trimester human placenta: in vitro co-culture study. *Hum Reprod.* 2010;**25**:2441–54.

20. Lenhard MS, Bauerfeind I, Untch M. Breast cancer and pregnancy: challenges of

chemotherapy. *Crit Rev Oncol Hematol.* 2008;**67**:196–203.

21. Kuerer HM, Cunningham JD, Brower ST, Tartter PI. Breast carcinoma associated with pregnancy and lactation. *Surg Oncol.* 1997;**6**:93–8.

22. Pereg D, Lishner M. Maternal and fetal effects of systemic therapy in the pregnant woman with cancer. *Recent Results Cancer Res.* 2008;**178**:21–38.

23. Zemlickis D, Lishner M, Degendorfer P, et al. Maternal and fetal outcome after breast cancer in pregnancy. *Am J Obstet Gynecol.* 1992;**166**:781–7.

24. Berry DL, Theriault RL, Holmes FA, et al. Management of breast cancer during pregnancy using a standardized protocol. *J Clin Oncol.* 1999;**17**:855–61.

25. Hahn KM, Johnson PH, Gordon N, et al. Treatment of pregnant breast cancer patients and outcomes of children exposed to chemotherapy in utero. *Cancer.* 2006;**107**:1219–26.

26. Doll DC, Ringenberg QS, Yarbro JW. Antineoplastic agents and pregnancy. *Semin Oncol.* 1989;**16**:337–46.

27. Ring AE, Smith IA, Jones A, Shannon C, Galani E, Ellis PA. Chemotherapy for breast cancer during pregnancy: an 18-year experience from five London teaching hospitals. *Clin Oncol.* 2005;**23**:4192–7.

Chapter

3

Cervical cancer during pregnancy

Asnat Walfisch

Introduction

Cervical cancer is one of the most common cancers diagnosed during pregnancy, with an incidence of 1.5 to 12 per 100,000 pregnancies [1–3]. It is estimated that between 1% and 3% of patients with invasive cervical cancer are pregnant at the time of diagnosis [4,5].

The cervix plays an extremely important role in the continuation of a successful term pregnancy. This, together with the vulnerability of the fetus to common cancer treatment modalities, results in an exceedingly challenging dilemma for the physician and patient. Unfortunately, randomized controlled trials are almost impossible to perform due to the obvious ethical considerations and relative rarity of the disease. Thus, treatment guidelines are lacking. Most of the published data are composed of small series mainly focusing on evaluating treatment efficacy and safety. It is important to note that the progression of pre-invasive disease to cervical carcinoma during the course of a pregnancy is rare. In fact, the opposite process is more common. Nevertheless, it is imperative that a proper histologic diagnosis be made in situations of possible invasive disease.

Symptoms and signs

The majority of women with early cervical cancer are asymptomatic and are diagnosed by abnormal cytology [6,7]. Other patients may have symptoms similar to the nonpregnant population, that is, vaginal bleeding, discharge, and pain. Lee *et al* [8]. reported no symptoms in any of the patients diagnosed with a stage IA lesion, and Smutek *et al* [9]. reported vaginal discharge in 29% of patients and postcoital bleeding or spotting in 59% of patients with stage IB lesions during pregnancy. In another series, 63% of patients with stage I disease presented with an abnormal Papanicolaou (Pap) smear, whereas only 20% presented with postcoital bleeding [10]. Patients with advanced or disseminated disease can have a wide variety of symptoms including pelvic pain, flank pain, sciatica, chronic anemia, and even intestinal obstruction and/or respiratory distress. However, presentation at this late stage is increasingly less common [11].

Diagnosis

Pregnancy represents a unique opportunity for the early diagnosis of cervical cancer because visual inspection, cytologic examination of the cervix, and bimanual palpation are all considered part of routine antenatal care. Complete visualization of the transformation zone

Cancer in Pregnancy and Lactation: The Motherisk Guide ed. Gideon Koren and Michael Lishner.
Published by Cambridge University Press. © Cambridge University Press 2011.

is usually possible due to the eversion of the squamo-columnar junction that occurs as part of the normal physiologic changes associated with the pregnant state. Interpretation of Pap smears obtained during pregnancy is somewhat problematic because several common physiologic changes associated with the gravid state can lead to false-positive results. For example, eversion of the transformation zone and exposure of columnar cells to the acid pH of the vagina causes squamous metaplasia, which may be interpreted as dysplasia. The Arias-Stella reaction may resemble an adenocarcinoma [12,13]. Tropho-blast cells may be retrieved on the smear and resemble low grade dysplasia. It is essential that the cytopathologist be made aware that the smear has been obtained from a pregnant patient.

Evaluation of the cervix by Pap smear (including endocervical sampling) and biopsy of all suspicious lesions is mandatory in all pregnant patients. Cervical biopsy was not shown to be associated with excess bleeding or any pregnancy complications [14–17]. Thus, colposcopically directed biopsy should be performed in all indicated cases (suspected cervical intraepithelial neoplasia [CIN] $\geq$ III). Endocervical curettage has not been defini-tively proven to cause complications in pregnancy; however, it has only been evaluated in small, nonrandomized trials and should be avoided [18]. Large-loop electro excision procedure of the transformation zone (LLETZ) and other excisional procedures must be used with caution [19]. Conization during pregnancy should be viewed as diagnostic and not therapeutic due to a high rate of positive margins and residual disease as demonstrated by Hannigan et al [20]. Other limitations of this procedure include complications such as bleeding, spontaneous abortion, infection, and preterm labor. Hemorrhage and miscarriage occur in a minority of patients, and perinatal death rates range from 3% to 6% [21].

Staging

Cervical carcinoma is clinically staged using the International Federation of Gynecology and Obstetrics (FIGO) classification [22], which is a summary of information derived mainly from the clinical examination and biopsy or cone histology and is no different during pregnancy. However, for the pregnant patient, pelvic examination may be less sensitive in detecting both size and extension of a cervical cancer. The clinical staging may also include plain film radiographs, an intravenous pyelogram (IVP), or a barium enema, but not findings at the time of surgery, computerized tomography (CT), or magnetic resonance imaging (MRI). During pregnancy, decisions regarding the use of radiological investigations must take into account the gestational age and the estimated dose of radiation delivered with the respective imaging study. CT scanning can be per-formed with minimal risk in the pregnant patient [23] and is helpful in determining the presence of lymphadenopathy or hydronephrosis. With an estimated fetal dose of 30 milligray (mGy), multiple scans should be avoided, particularly in the first trimester. In the pregnant patient, ultrasound and MRI should be considered as alternatives to CT scans because both are noninvasive and do not subject the fetus to ionizing radiation. Choi et al. [24,25] evaluated 115 patients with cervical cancer using MRI before undergoing radical hysterectomy. They reported a negative predictive value of 95%, 96%, and 93% for predicting invasion into the parametria, vagina, and pelvic lymph nodes, respectively.

Other authors have also advocated the increasing role that MRI plays in cervical cancer staging [26]. The effects of positron emission tomography (PET) and the radioactive isotopes it uses on the developing fetus are unknown, and as such, the test is contraindicated in pregnancy.

Pathology and biology

Similar to the nonpregnant population, the majority of invasive cervical cancer cases have a squamous histology (>80%). Of the remaining cases, the majority are adenocarcinomas [27]. Other, less common, histologies such as neuroendocrine tumor of the cervix have been described [28]. There is no conclusive evidence that the pregnant state alters the biology of cervical cancer. However, some authors have found a higher proportion of early stage tumors in pregnant patients, which is likely a consequence of the increased cervical cancer screening performed during routine antenatal care [4,29]. In a series of 28 pregnant patients with invasive disease, Takushi et al. found 22 patients (79%) presenting with stage I disease and 6 (21%) with stage II or III [30].

Treatment

The initial evaluation of the pregnant patient with cervical cancer must include a thorough and complete assessment of the fetus, including accurate gestational age, a thorough ultrasound examination of the fetus for presence of anomalies and growth, as well as, obtaining results of serum markers for aneuploidy, if possible. Once the diagnosis, stage, and extent of invasive cervical cancer have been established, a multidisciplinary team should discuss appropriate treatment strategies. This team should, ideally, include specialists in maternal–fetal medicine, gynecologic oncology, neonatology, social work, and radiation oncology.

Whereas in the nonpregnant patient population the decision to proceed with either surgical excision or radiation with chemotherapy is based almost exclusively on the stage, in the pregnant patient, other considerations are involved. The decision to initiate or delay treatment has ethical, moral, cultural, and religious implications that need to be carefully addressed. The patient should decide whether the present pregnancy, and future fertility, are desired. At times, a decision must be made of whether to terminate the pregnancy or depart from standard treatment modalities. An alternative treatment path can be cautiously decided upon, based on a lower level of evidence.

Noninvasive cervical carcinoma

Treatment of noninvasive carcinoma can safely be deferred to the postpartum period, provided that a careful colposcopic evaluation is performed in addition to cytology [4,31].

Invasive cervical carcinoma
FIGO stage IA

Controversy persists regarding the management of patients with IA1 squamous cell carcinoma of the cervix. In the nonpregnant population, excisional procedures are reserved for patients in whom occult malignancy cannot be ruled out. Extra-fascial hysterectomy remains the treatment of choice for the nonpregnant patient with no desire for future fertility. Fertility-sparing alternatives to hysterectomy have been explored and debated [32].

For the pregnant patient who desires immediate treatment of a IA1 lesion, with the intent on ending the pregnancy, choices include termination followed by hysterectomy or removal of the uterus with the fetus in situ. Delaying the treatment of an occult lesion during pregnancy may have no impact on survival. Thus, excisional procedures are not recommended during a desired pregnancy due to associated morbidities (significant blood loss and other pregnancy complications).

Patients who are diagnosed with stage IA2 are not eligible for the same fertility-sparing excisional procedures and, outside pregnancy, are generally treated with radical hysterectomy.

Options for a pregnant patient include a purposeful delay in treatment or a termination of the pregnancy followed by immediate treatment. These patients may also be candidates for the fertility-sparing radical trachelectomy. The first case of a successful vaginal radical trachelectomy during pregnancy was reported in 2008 by van Niewenhol *et al* [33].

FIGO stage IB1

Before fetal viability, and in the presence of invasive cervical cancer, a common approach is to treat the pregnant woman without fetal-sparing intentions. However, this approach does not include multiple nonmedical factors that largely influence the final decision. In general, treatment options for a patient with stage IB1 (or IIA disease- with a lesion of less than 4 cm) include external beam irradiation and brachytherapy with concomitant systemic cisplatin or radical hysterectomy with bilateral pelvic lymphadenectomy followed by postoperative therapy, depending on the pathological findings [34]. The survival with both approaches is similar. For young patients, surgical management has the added benefits of ovarian and sexual function preservation and is therefore considered the treatment of choice [35]. Postoperative chemoradiotherapy is recommended in patients with high-risk disease (positive margins, positive lymph nodes, or parametrial extension) [36]. Several publications describing treatment delay, in stage I disease, of up to 282 days showed favorable outcome without an obvious compromise in maternal overall survival [37,38]. Cell type, depth of penetration, and tumor size should all be considered in the decision to recommend treatment delay. If treatment is delayed, close tumor surveillance is warranted. A repeat pelvic examination every 6–8 weeks (including visual inspection and colposcopy) is recommended. The use of serial MRI in this setting is also a possibility. Although treatment delay is a possibility in early stage invasive cervical cancer, for advanced stage disease, i.e., IB2 and IIA, treatment delay is usually not advised [39].

Radical hysterectomy can be performed either following an elective termination or while the fetus remains *in utero*. Several published case series of this surgical approach in pregnant patients have demonstrated no increase in major complication rates and generally good outcome [35,40].

FIGO stage IB2 to stage IVA

Surgical treatment in stages IB2 and IIA disease was shown to have a limited role in recent years [41]. Although pelvic radiation was considered the standard of care in advanced cervical cancer, an improved survival was shown with the addition of platinum-based radiosensitizing chemotherapy, and this has become the standard of care [42]. The use of radiation in late pregnancy and in the postpartum period was reported by several authors, demonstrating no difference in maternal survival when compared to matched controls [43]. Radiation in early pregnancy usually results with a rapid spontaneous abortion at a cumulative dose of 30–50 Gy [43]. Treatment in the second-trimester results in abortion at a higher cumulative dose and less reliably. Thus, some advocate the use of misoprostol to promote expulsion of the fetus that does not spontaneously abort following radiotherapy [44]. There are no published data comparing maternal outcome in spontaneous miscarriage versus hysterotomy for fetus removal in the first and second trimester. Hysterotomy in this setting may result in significant blood loss and thus should not be routinely undertaken [39].

When advanced cervical cancer is diagnosed in the third trimester delaying treatment by 2–4 weeks may result in significantly improved neonatal outcome without a significant impact on maternal prognosis. This is mainly true for pregnancies of less than 32 weeks. There is probably no need to delay treatment beyond 32–34 weeks, and delivery can safely be ensued [45]. On the other hand, for the severely premature neonate, even a brief increase in the length of the gestation can have a profound effect on morbidity and mortality rates.

Metastatic disease and chemotherapy in pregnancy

Treatment for cervical cancer that has spread to distant organs is palliative. Various chemotherapeutic agents have been used with varying success. In these patients, no planned delay in treatment is recommended because reports of patients insisting on delays have shown less than optimal outcomes [11]. Neoadjuvant chemotherapy is an option for pregnant patients with stage IV B disease who insist on treatment delay.

In general chemotherapeutic drugs are very potent teratogens. Data regarding the use of chemotherapy in pregnancy have been largely limited to case studies [46–48]. Chemotherapeutic agents more commonly associated with fetal malformations include methotrexate, 5-fluorouracil, cyclophosphamide, and chlorambucil [49]. The risk of malformations when chemotherapy is administered in the first trimester has been estimated to be roughly 10% for single agent and 25% for a combination of agents. Therefore, chemotherapy should be avoided during the first trimester, when fetal cells are actively dividing. Use of these agents in the second and third trimesters has been associated with an increased risk of prematurity, fetal death, intrauterine growth retardation, and low birth weight but not with fetal deformities. Long-term neurodevelopmental complications of *in utero* chemotherapy exposure have not been extensively studied. When chemotherapy is administered during pregnancy, delivery timing should take into account the expected fetal bone marrow depression and other potential complications such as bleeding or infections, and the pediatric team should be well prepared for such possibilities.

Mode of delivery

Few data exist examining the safety of cesarean section versus vaginal delivery. Sood *et al* [50]. showed higher rates of recurrence in patients delivered vaginally. Other authors have confirmed these observations [6], whereas still others have found no difference [8]. However, the risks of obstructed labor, hemorrhage, and episiotomy site recurrence with vaginal delivery have led to the recommendation of cesarean delivery as the preferred method [27,39,50]. During a cesarean section, a high vertical uterine incision should be performed, to allow optimal pathologic review of the lower uterine segment. Recurrence in an episiotomy site following a vaginal delivery carries an unfavorable prognosis [51,52]. Patients in whom radical hysterectomy is the treatment of choice should be delivered by cesarean section concomitant with their cancer surgery.

Prognosis

Due to limitations of the existing literature, the effect of pregnancy on prognosis is controversial, especially in the higher stages of the disease [4]. It appears that pregnancy-associated cervical carcinoma has an overall better prognosis than in the nonpregnant population due to the higher proportion of patients diagnosed at the early stage disease. After stratifying for stage, survival analyses do not differ between the two groups [30]. As in the nonpregnant population, FIGO staging is the most important factor in determining the overall prognosis.

Conclusion

Pregnancy poses a unique opportunity for cervical cancer screening. Thus, the coincident diagnosis of pregnancy and cervical cancer is not uncommon and possesses a great therapeutic and emotional dilemma. Due to the uniqueness of these circumstances and the large patient background diversity, no specific treatment algorithm should be considered as inflexible. Furthermore, lack of available concrete scientific data makes these proposed treatment algorithms suggestions only. The primary goal of treatment should be to balance the health and safety of both the mother and the fetus, with a close adherence to nonpregnant, evidence-based approaches [53].

References

1. Smith LH, Dalrymple JL, Leiserowitz GS, Danielsen B, Gilbert WM. Obstetrical deliveries associated with maternal malignancy in California, 1992 through 1997. *Am J Obstet Gynecol.* 2001;**184**: 1504–12.

2. Smith LH, Danielsen B, Allen ME, Cress R. Cancer associated with obstetric delivery: results of linkage with the California cancer registry. *Am J Obstet Gynecol.* 2003;**189**:1128–35.

3. Demeter A, Sziller I, Csapo Z, Szantho A, Papp Z. Outcome of pregnancies after coldknife conization of the uterine cervix during pregnancy. *Eur J Gynaecol Oncol.* 2002;**23**:207–10.

4. Hacker NF, Berek JS, Lagasse LD, Charles EH, Savage EW, Moore JG. Carcinoma of the cervix associated with pregnancy. *Obstet Gynecol.* 1982;**59**:735.

5. Donegan WL. Cancer and pregnancy. *CA Cancer J Clin.* 1983;**33**:194.

6. Mikuta JJ. Invasive carcinoma of the cervix in pregnancy. *South Med J.* 1967;**60**:843.

7. Dudan RC, Yon JL, Ford JH, et al. Carcinoma of the cervix and pregnancy. *Gynecol Oncol.* 1973;**1**:283.

8. Lee RB, Neglia W, Park RC. Cervical carcinoma in pregnancy. *Obstet Gynecol.* 1981;**58**:584–9.

9. Smutek J, Mielnik J, Jurczak M, Kadylak B, Sobol A. [Cervical cancer Ib associated with pregnancy]. *Ginekol Pol.* 1997;**68**:464–7.

10. Sood AK, Sorosky JI, Krogman S, Anderson B, Benda J, Buller RE. Surgical management of cervical cancer complicating pregnancy: a case-control study. *Gynecol Oncol.* 1996;**63**:294–8.

11. Liro M, Olszewski J, Kobierski J, Emerich J, Lukaszuk K. [An advanced cervical carcinoma coexisting with pregnancy in 19-years old primipara – a case report and review of current literature]. *Ginekol Pol.* 2002;**73**:325–30.

12. Rhatigan RM. Endocervical gland atypia secondary to Arias-Stella change. *Arch Pathol Lab Med.* 1992;**116**:943.

13. Pisharodi L, Jovanoska S. Spectrum of cytologic changes in pregnancy. *Acta Cytol.* 1995;**39**:905.

14. Economos K, Perez Veridiano N, Delke I, Collado ML, Tancer ML. Abnormal cervical cytology in pregnancy: a 17-year experience. *Obstet Gynecol.* 1993;**81**: 915–8.

15. Basta A, Szczudrawa A, Pitynski K, Kolawa W. [The value of colposcopy and computerised colposcopy in diagnosis and therapeutic management of CIN and early invasive cervical cancer in pregnant women]. *Ginekol Pol.* 2002;**73**:307–13.

16. Jain AG, Higgins RV, Boyle MJ. Management of low-grade squamous

intraepithelial lesions during pregnancy. *Am J Obstet Gynecol.* 1997;**177**:298–302.

17. Baldauf JJ, Dreyfus M, Gao J, Ritter J, Philippe E. [Management of pregnant women with abnormal cervical smears. A series of 146 patients]. *J Gynecol Obstet Biol Reprod (Paris).* 1996;**25**: 582–7.

18. El-Bastawissi AY, Becker TM, Daling JR. Effect of cervical carcinoma in situ and its management on pregnancy outcome. *Obstet Gynecol.* 1999;**93**:207–12.

19. Jemal A, Siegel R, Ward E, et al. Cancer statistics, 2008. *CA Cancer J Clin.* 2008;**58**:71–96.

20. Hannigan EV, Whitehouse HH III, Atkinson WD, Becker SN. Cone biopsy during pregnancy. *Obstet Gynecol.* 1982;**60**:450.

21. Shivvers SA, Miller DS. Preinvasive and invasive breast and cervical cancer prior to or during pregnancy. *Clin Perinatol.* 1997;**24**:369–89.

22. International Federation of Gynecology and Obstetrics. Staging announcement: FIGO staging of gynecologic cancers: cervical and vulva. *Int J Gynecol Cancer.* 1995;**5**:319.

23. Ratnapalan S, Bona N, Chandra K, Koren G. Physicians' perceptions of teratogenic risk associated with radiography and CT during early pregnancy. *AJR Am J Roentgenol.* 2004;**182**:1107–9.

24. Choi SH, Kim SH, Choi HJ, Park BK, Lee HJ. Preoperative magnetic resonance imaging staging of uterine cervical carcinoma: results of prospective study. *J Comput Assist Tomogr.* 2004;**28**:620–7.

25. Choi HJ, Roh JW, Seo SS, et al. Comparison of the accuracy of magnetic resonance imaging and positron emission tomography/computed tomography in the presurgical detection of lymph node metastases in patients with uterine cervical carcinoma: a prospective study. *Cancer.* 2006;**106**:914–22.

26. Menell JH, Chi DS, Hann LE, Hricak H. The use of MRI in the diagnosis and management of a bulky cervical carcinoma. *Gynecol Oncol.* 2003;**89**:517–21.

27. Jones WB, Shingleton HM, Russell A, et al. Cervical carcinoma and pregnancy: a national patterns of care study of the American College of Surgeons. *Cancer.* 1996;**77**:1479–88.

28. Turner WA, Gallup DG, Talledo OE, Otken LB Jr, Guthrie TH. Neuroendocrine carcinoma of the uterine cervix complicated by pregnancy: case report and review of the literature. *Obstet Gynecol.* 1986;**67**:80S.

29. Nevin J, Soeters R, Dehaeck K, Bloch B, van Wyk L. Cervical carcinoma associated with pregnancy. *Obstet Gynecol Surv.* 1995;**50**:228.

30. Takushi M, Moromizato H, Sakumoto K, Kanazawa K. Management of invasive carcinoma of the uterine cervix associated with pregnancy: outcome of intentional delay in treatment. *Gynecol Oncol.* 2002;**87**:185–9.

31. Baldauf JJ, Dreyfus M, Ritter J, Philippe E. Colposcopy and directed biopsy reliability during pregnancy: a cohort study. *Eur J Obstet Gynecol Reprod Biol.* 1995;**62**:31.

32. SEER*Stat Software based on SEER-9. Database: incidence – SEER 9 Regs Public-Use, Nov 2003 Sub (1973–2001). 2004. Available from: www.seer.cancer.gov

33. Van De Nieuwenhof HP, Van Ham MA, Lotgering FK, Massuger LF. First case of vaginal radical trachelectomy in a pregnant patient. *Int J Gynecol Cancer.* 2008;**18**:1381–5.

34. Im SS, Monk BJ. New developments in the treatment of invasive cervical cancer. *Obstet Gynecol Clin North Am.* 2002;**29**:659–72.

35. Monk BJ, Montz FJ. Invasive cervical cancer complicating intrauterine pregnancy: treatment with radical hysterectomy. *Obstet Gynecol.* 1992;**80**:199–203.

36. Peters W. Concurrent chemotherapy and pelvic radiation therapy compared with pelvic radiation therapy alone as adjuvant therapy after radical surgery in high-risk early-stage cancer of the cervix. *J Clin Oncol.* 2000;**18**:1606–13.

37. Sorosky JI, Squatrito R, Ndubisi BU, et al. Stage I squamous cell cervical carcinoma in

pregnancy: planned delay in therapy awaiting fetal maturity. *Gynecol Oncol.* 1995;**59**:207–10.

38. Duggan B, Muderspach LI, Roman LD, Curtin JP, d'Ablaing G III, Morrow CP. Cervical cancer in pregnancy: reporting on planned delay in therapy. *Obstet Gynecol.* 1993;**82**:598–602.

39. Sood AK, Sorosky JI. Invasive cervical cancer complicating pregnancy. How to manage the dilemma. *Obstet Gynecol Clin North Am.* 1998;**25**:343–52.

40. Sivanesaratnam V, Jayalakshmi P, Loo C. Surgical management of early invasive cancer of the cervix associated with pregnancy. *Gynecol Oncol.* 1993;**48**:68–75.

41. Yessaian A, Magistris A, Burger RA, Monk BJ. Radical hysterectomy followed by tailored postoperative therapy in the treatment of stage IB2 cervical cancer: feasibility and indications for adjuvant therapy. *Gynecol Oncol.* 2004;**94**:61–6.

42. Grigsby PW, Herzog TJ. Current management of patients with invasive cervical carcinoma. *Clin Obstet Gynecol.* 2001;**44**:531–7.

43. Sood AK, Sorosky JI, Mayr N, et al. Radiotherapeutic management of cervical carcinoma that complicates pregnancy. *Cancer.* 1997;**80**:1073–8.

44. Ostrom K, Ben-Arie A, Edwards C, Gregg A, Chiu JK, Kaplan AL. Uterine evacuation with misoprostol during radiotherapy for cervical cancer in pregnancy. *Int J Gynecol Cancer.* 2003;**13**:340–3.

45. Coles CE, Burgess L, Tan LT. An audit of delays before and during radical radiotherapy for cervical cancer – effect on

tumour cure probability. *Clin Oncol (R Coll Radiol).* 2003;**15**:47–54.

46. Marana HR, de Andrade JM, da Silva Mathes AC, Duarte G, da Cunha SP, Bighetti S. Chemotherapy in the treatment of locally advanced cervical cancer and pregnancy. *Gynecol Oncol.* 2001;**80**:272–4.

47. Sood AK, Shahin MS, Soroski JI. Paclitaxel and platinum chemotherapy for ovarian carcinoma during pregnancy. *Gynecol Oncol.* 2001;**83**:599–600.

48. Mendez LE, Mueller A, Salom E, Gonzalez-Quintero VH. Paclitaxel and carboplatin chemotherapy administered during pregnancy for advanced epithelial ovarian cancer. *Obstet Gynecol.* 2003;**5**:1200–2.

49. Pavlidis NA. Coexistence of pregnancy and malignancy. *Oncologist.* 2002;**7**:279–87.

50. Sood AK, Sorosky JI, Mayr N, Anderson B, Buller RE, Miebyl J. Cervical cancer diagnosed shortly after pregnancy: prognostic variables and delivery routes. *Obstet Gynecol.* 2000;**95**:832–8.

51. Cliby WA, Dodson MK, Podratz KC. Cervical cancer complicated by pregnancy: episiotomy site recurrences following vaginal delivery. *Obstet Gynecol.* 1994;**84**:179–82.

52. Gordon AN, Jensen R, Jones HW III. Squamous carcinoma of the cervix complicating pregnancy: recurrence in episiotomy after vaginal delivery. *Obstet Gynecol.* 1989;**73**:850–2.

53. Monk BJ, Tewari KS, Koh WJ. Multimodality therapy for locally advanced cervical carcinoma: state of the art and future directions. *J Clin Oncol.* 2007;**25**:2952–65.

Chapter

Hepatocellular carcinoma in pregnancy

Parvaneh Yazdani-Brojeni and Michael Lishner

Introduction

In nonpregnant women, the majority of neoplastic liver masses are malignant. On the contrary, liver masses identified during pregnancy are more commonly benign. Hepatocellular carcinoma (HCC) in pregnancy is very rare. There are only 37 reported cases of (HCC) in pregnancy [1–3].

Risk factors for HCC include hepatitis B virus (HBV) or HCV infections, aflatoxin exposure, cirrhosis, alcohol abuse, metabolic liver disease, carcinogen exposure, steroids, and male gender [4].

Relevant for this chapter, there is a report of association between high parity, HBsAg carriers, oral contraceptives, and HCC. Detailed medical history and the level of serum a-fetoprotein (AFP) may be helpful as screening tools [5–7].

Diagnosis

Most patients complain of right upper quadrant pain or distention and weight loss. An irregular liver mass together with excessively high serum AFP levels are suggestive of HCC [8]. AFP may also be used for screening HCC in high-risk pregnant women. Liver sonography and/or magnetic resonance imaging together with fine liver aspiration are used for definitive diagnosis during pregnancy [5,9].

Treatment

These imaging methods and measures (liver sonography and/or magnetic resonance imaging together with fine liver aspiration) are also used for staging. Partial hepatectomy is the treatment of choice [6]. The choice of aggressive approach is based on anatomical and surgical considerations, and tumor spread.

Prognosis

Although a shorter median survival for pregnant women with HCC has been suggested, the small number of published cases precludes any firm conclusions. Two case reports of HCC diagnosed in the second trimester reported favorable outcomes for both mother and child [6,10].

Cancer in Pregnancy and Lactation: The Motherisk Guide ed. Gideon Koren and Michael Lishner.
Published by Cambridge University Press. © Cambridge University Press 2011.

References

1. Athanassiou AM, Craigo SD. Liver masses in pregnancy. *Semin Perinatol.* 1998;**22**:166–77.

2. Alvarez de la Rosa M, Nicolas-Perez D, Muniz-Montes JR, Trujillo-Crrillo JL. Evolution and management of hepatocellular carcinoma during pregnancy. *J Obstet Gynaecol Res.* 2006;**32**:437–9.

3. Garko SB, David OS, Mohammed T, et al. Hepatocellular carcinoma in pregnancy. *Ann Afr Med.* 2009;**8**:284–6.

4. De Maria N, Manno M, Villa E. Sex hormones and liver cancer. *Mol Cell Endocrinol.* 2002;**193**:59–63.

5. Lau WY, Leung WT, Ho S, et al. Hepatocellular carcinoma during pregnancy and its comparison with other pregnancy associated malignancies. *Cancer.* 1995;**75**:2669–75.

6. Gisi P, Floyd R. Hepatocellular carcinoma in pregnancy. A case report. *J Reprod Med.* 1999;**44**:65–7.

7. Hsieh TT, Hou HC, Hsu JJ, Hsieh CC, Jeng LB. Term delivery after hepatocellular carcinoma resection in previous pregnancy. *Acta Obstet Gynecol Scand.* 1996;**75**:77–8.

8. To WK, Ghosh A. Primary liver carcinoma complicating pregnancy. *Aust N Z J Obstet Gynecol.* 1993;**33**:325–6.

9. Entezami M, Becker R, Ebert A, Pritze W, Weitzel H. Case report: hepatocellular carcinoma as a rare case of an excessive increase of a-fetoprotein during pregnancy. *Gyncol Oncol.* 1996;**62**:405–7.

10. To WK, Ghosh A. Primary liver carcinoma complicating pregnancy. *Aust N Z J Ostet Gynecol.* 1993;**33**:325–6.

Chapter

5

Hodgkin's lymphoma in pregnancy

David Pereg and Michael Lishner

Introduction

The early peak of Hodgkin's lymphoma (HL) is usually between 20 and 40 years of age and therefore overlaps the child-bearing years. HL is the most common type of lymphoma and the second most common malignancy diagnosed during pregnancy, occurring in 1:1,000 to 1:6,000 pregnancies [1]. Clinically, HL is characterized by painless lymph node enlargement, most commonly in the cervical area and is often detected at an early stage. With current treatment protocols, the disease is associated with long-term survival rates of up to 90%, especially in young patients without significant co-morbidities.

Diagnosis and staging

The diagnosis of lymphoma requires a lymph node biopsy for pathological examination. Such a biopsy can be safely performed under local anesthesia during pregnancy without harming either the mother or the fetus [2]. When there are no superficial lymph nodes available for excision, biopsy should be performed under general anesthesia. In general, it appears that, with modern surgical and anesthetic techniques, elective surgery is safe throughout pregnancy, without an increase in the risk for spontaneous abortion. Furthermore, there is no significant increase in the risk for maternal death, birth defects, or late neurodevelopmental delays [3].

The histological subtypes of HL in pregnancy are the same as in nonpregnant young women, with nodular sclerosis being the most prevalent [1].

Because the vast majority of lymphoma patients are initially treated with chemotherapy independent of disease stage, staging of a pregnant patient with lymphoma should be limited and include history, physical examination, routine blood tests, and bone marrow biopsies. The routine staging process for all lymphomas requires radiological evaluation usually with chest and abdominal computed tomography (CT). Abdominal and pelvic CT are associated with relatively high fetal radiation exposure of up to 0.02 Gy. This level of radiation exposure is below the threshold dose for severe congenital malformation and should not harm the fetus [4]. However, in many cases other types of examinations such as ultrasonography or magnetic resonance imaging (MRI), may provide the desired diagnostic information without any radiation exposure [5,6]. Concerns have been raised regarding the use of gadolinium-based contrast agents for MRI during pregnancy because their long-term effects on the fetus are unknown [7]. Nevertheless, because gadolinium is mainly distrib-

Cancer in Pregnancy and Lactation: The Motherisk Guide ed. Gideon Koren and Michael Lishner.
Published by Cambridge University Press. © Cambridge University Press 2011.

uted in the extracellular fluid and has negligible binding to plasma protein, gadolinium-based contrast agents are eliminated by the kidneys very rapidly and excessive quantities are not expected to cross the placenta [7]. Animal and human studies have reported no adverse fetal outcomes following exposure to gadolinium throughout pregnancy [7,8]. Therefore, according to the European Society of Radiology guidelines, gadolinium-based contrast agents are considered safe during pregnancy [8].

Therefore, abdominal and pelvic CT should be avoided during pregnancy. When MRI is available, it should be the modality of choice for the staging of lymphoma during pregnancy. Alternatively, abdominal ultrasonography or chest x-ray with abdominal shielding may be used.

Recently, positron emission tomography (PET)-CT has been increasingly used for both staging and treatment follow-up in patients with lymphoma. However, because ^{18}F-fludeoxyglucose can cross the placenta and reach the fetus, it may involve higher radiation exposure than conventional CT and should not be used during pregnancy.

Treatment

Although chemotherapy is currently recommended for the treatment of HL at all stages, radiotherapy can still be considered an appropriate treatment for stage 1. The latter is especially relevant in pregnant women with isolated involvement of cervical lymph nodes [9]. Generally, conventional doses of radiotherapy administered for the treatment of HL confined to the cervical region yields a total exposure of the fetus to only 4–20 cGy, which is far below the threshold dose for congenital malformations.

Data regarding the administration of chemotherapy to pregnant patients with HL are limited and are derived mainly from small studies and case reports [10–12]. The most popular chemotherapy regimen for the treatment of HL is ABVD (adriamycin, bleomycin, vinblastine, dacarbazine). Among those four drugs, dacarbazine is the least investigated. The literature describes 26 HL patients who were treated with ABVD during pregnancy [10–12]. Of these, chemotherapy was administered during the first trimester to only 3 patients, with a single report of thumb malformation. Among the 23 patients who were treated with ABVD during the second and third trimesters, no congenital malformations were reported, with a single case of intrauterine fetal death. Experience regarding treatment with the MOPP (mechlorethamine, vincristine, procarbazine, and prednisone) regimen during pregnancy is even more limited, and therefore, its administration to pregnant women cannot be recommended. There are no reports about treatment of pregnant patients with the Stanford V protocol, or with the high-dose BEACOPP regimen, which have become increasingly popular for treating high-risk patients.

For women with advanced disease at early stage of pregnancy, a delay in treatment might adversely affect maternal survival. Therefore, an appropriate chemotherapy protocol should be given promptly. This should follow a therapeutic abortion due to the potential teratogenic effects of chemotherapy in the first trimester.

Patients with early stage HL diagnosed during the first trimester may be followed-up at short intervals for signs of disease progression without any treatment until the second trimester. Another option that has been suggested is treatment with single-agent chemo-therapy (preferably a vinca alkaloid). Such treatment appears to be safe even during the first trimester. However, data regarding its efficacy are lacking. This option may also be considered in patients diagnosed with HL during the first trimester who reject therapeutic abortion as an option. In any case, adequate treatment with ABVD should be administered immediately at the beginning of the second trimester. Based on the limited data available, patients presenting in the second or third trimesters can be safely treated with chemotherapy similarly to nonpregnant women, and full treatment with ABVD may be given.

Prognosis and outcome

For many years, it was believed that pregnancy increased relapse and mortality rates in patients with HL. However, a case-control study of 48 women with pregnancy-associated HL has shown a 20-year survival rate similar to that of nonpregnant controls matched for age, stage, and treatment protocol [13]. Infants born to women with HL during pregnancy did not have a higher risk for prematurity or intrauterine growth retardation [13]. There are no reports of HL metastases to the placenta or the fetus. Long-term follow up of 84 children born to mothers with hematological malignancies, including 26 patients with HL reported normal physical, neurological, and psychological development [10].

References

1. Pereg D, Koren G, Lishner M. The treatment of Hodgkin's and non-Hodgkin's lymphoma in pregnancy. *Haematologica.* 2007;**92**:1230–7.

2. Weisz B, Meirow D, Schiff E, Lishner M. Impact and treatment of cancer during pregnancy. *Expert Rev Anticancer Ther.* 2004;**4**:889–902.

3. Cohen-Kerem R, Railton C, Oren D, Lishner M, Koren G. Pregnancy outcome following non-obstetric surgical intervention. *Am J Surg.* 2005;**190**:467–73.

4. Cohen-Kerem R, Nulman I, Abramow-Newerly M, et al. Diagnostic radiation in pregnancy: perception versus true risks. *J Obstet Gynaecol Can.* 2006;**28**:43–8.

5. Chen MM, Coakley FV, Kaimal A, Laros RK Jr. Guidelines for computed tomography and magnetic resonance imaging use during pregnancy and lactation. *Obstet Gynecol.* 2008;**112**:333–40.

6. Levine D. Obstetric MRI. *J Magn Reson Imaging.* 2006;**24**:1–15.

7. Garcia-Bournissen F, Shrim A, Koren G. Safety of gadolinium during pregnancy. *Can Fam Physician.* 2006;**52**:309–10.

8. Webb JA, Thomsen HS, Morcos SK. The use of iodinated and gadolinium contrast media during pregnancy and lactation. *Eur Radiol.* 2005;**15**:1234–40.

9. Fenig E, Mishaeli M, Kalish Y, Lishner M. Pregnancy and radiation. *Cancer Treat Rev.* 2001;**27**:1–7.

10. Aviles A, Neri N. Hematological malignancies and pregnancy: a final report of 84 children who received chemotherapy in utero. *Clin Lymphoma.* 2001;**2**:173–7.

11. Cardonick E, Iacobucci A. Use of chemotherapy during human pregnancy. *Lancet Oncol.* 2004;**5**:283–91.

12. Azim HA, Pavlidis N, Peccatori FA. Treatment of the pregnant mother with cancer: a systematic review on the use of cytotoxic, endocrine, targeted agents and immunotherapy during pregnancy. Part 2: Hematological malignancies. *Cancer Treat Rev.* 2010;**36**:110–21.

13. Lishner M, Zemlickis D, Degendorfer P, Panzarella T, Sutcliffe SB, Koren G. Maternal and foetal outcome following Hodgkin's disease in pregnancy. *Br J Cancer.* 1992;**65**:114–7.

Chapter

6

Intracranial tumors in pregnancy

Michael Lishner and Geert W. 't Jong

Introduction

Brain tumors are the fifth leading cause of cancer-related death in women ages 20 to 39 years. Although the presentation of intracranial tumors during pregnancy is relatively uncommon, neurosurgeons and obstetricians will undoubtedly encounter these patients in their everyday practices [1]. Symptoms and physical findings are not different from those of the nonpregnant population, although pregnancy may occasionally delay diagnosis.

There is some evidence to suggest that the different types of brain tumors seen in pregnant women occur with the same relative frequency as those seen in age-matched nonpregnant counterparts [2]. Gliomas represent the majority of symptomatic intracranial neoplasms, followed closely by meningiomas and then acoustic neuromas.

Clinical features

All primary as well as metastatic brain tumors share common clinical features that range from headache, nausea & vomiting, and other nonspecific symptoms to focal neurologic deficits such as hemiparesis and visual field defects. Pregnancy can exacerbate neurology, with the patient presenting acutely with impending or actual cerebral herniation: worsening headache, deteriorating Glasgow Coma Scale score, dilating ipsilateral pupil, hypertension, bradycardia, and respiratory irregularity [3]. Common symptoms of increased intracranial pressure, including nausea & vomiting, can potentially be confused with routine pregnancy-related conditions such as hyperemesis gravidarum, thereby posing specific diagnostic challenges for physicians. Physicians should in general have a low threshold to obtain a neuroimaging study in a patient in whom there is any concern for an intracranial mass lesion, and the onset of any new focal neurologic deficit during pregnancy warrants immediate evaluation with an imaging study.

Diagnosis

Although there seems to be no particular type of primary brain tumor specifically associated with pregnancy, the normal hormonal and physiologic alterations that accompany pregnancy can have profound effects on tumor growth and behavior, exacerbating neurologic symptoms and precipitating obstetric emergencies [2,4]. The association is especially true of meningiomas, which occur predominantly in females, and have accelerated growth during the luteal phase of the menstrual cycle, as well as during

Cancer in Pregnancy and Lactation: The Motherisk Guide ed. Gideon Koren and Michael Lishner. Published by Cambridge University Press. © Cambridge University Press 2011.

pregnancy [2]. A population-based evaluation did not find that intracranial tumors present more often during pregnancy [5].

Because brain tumors have the potential to seriously compromise the health of both mother and fetus if not properly managed, it is relevant to address the fundamental concepts of their diagnosis and clinical management. Careful history, physical examination, and imaging are essential diagnostic procedures [4]. MRI is probably the diagnostic imaging procedure of choice and should be performed when a brain tumor is suspected and when seizures appear during pregnancy [6]. Computed tomography however is the choice of many physicians for an initial neuroimaging test because of its low cost, widespread availability, and relative short procedure duration, and is considered safe during pregnancy [7].

Treatment

Management of brain tumors should be tailored to the individual patient. Surgery and radiotherapy are the main therapeutic procedures [3,8,9]. General principles of chemo- and radiotherapy during pregnancy are discussed elsewhere. Anticonvulsants and steroids should be used according to acceptable medical indications. Concerns for teratogenicity are considerable for several anticonvulsants [10]. Emergency delivery as a result of maternal deterioration should be anticipated.

Cerebral spinal fluid (CSF) pressure changes during normal labor have been well documented. Therefore, presence of increased intracranial pressure (ICP) has generally been considered a contraindication to labor and vaginal delivery. Epidural anesthesia is generally contraindicated in patients with an intracranial mass lesion as a "wet tap," or incidental lumbar puncture, can potentially lead to cerebral herniation and death. In patients in whom cesarean section is chosen, there are some special concerns in the intraoperative and immediate postpartum periods that should be addressed. For example, hypertension is a normal compensatory response in patients with increased ICP and is often necessary for those patients to maintain adequate cerebral perfusion pressures. Management of hypertension by lowering the blood pressure may inadvertently drop the patient's cerebral perfusion pressure and may exacerbate cerebral ischemia and neurologic decline [1].

If symptoms are amenable to pharmacological control, delivery is recommended in the early third trimester after documentation of fetal pulmonary maturity, which is sometimes already enhanced by corticosteroids used for decrease of ICP in the mother. In the case of nonendocrine pituitary tumor such as craniopharingeoma, vaginal delivery is a viable option for some patients with operative treatment being postponed until after delivery.

In prolactinoma, prolactine levels and MRI should not be routinely performed. Treatment should be decided on symptoms and signs, not on prolactine levels. Bromocriptine has been shown to be safe and remains the drug of choice during pregnancy, but should only be used for symptomatic treatment [11]. In case of bromocriptine intolerance, cabergoline and quinagolide (both dopamine agonists), were shown by some authors to be better tolerated and more effective. Treatment with cabergoline during pregnancy was not shown to cause structural abnormalities [12,13].

Prognosis

Most reported women delivered normal babies [4,14,15].

References

1. Stevenson CB, Thompson RC. The clinical management of intracranial neoplasms in pregnancy. *Clin Obstet Gynecol.* 2005;**48**:24–37.

2. Carroll RS, Zhan, J, Black PM. Expression of estrogen receptors alpha and beta in human meningiomas *J Neurooncol.* 1999;**42**:109–16.

3. Ng J, Kitchen N. Neurosurgery and pregnancy. *J Neurol Neurosurg Psychiatry.* 2008;**79**:745–52.

4. Isla A, Alvarez F, Gonzalez A, Garcia-Grande A, Perez-Alvarez M, Garcia-Blazquez M. Brain tumor and pregnancy. *Obstet Gynecol.* 1997;**89**:19–23.

5. Haas JF, Jänisch W, Staneczek W. Newly diagnosed primary intracranial neoplasms in pregnant women: a population-based assessment. *J Neurol Neurosurg Psychiatry.* 1986;**49**:874–80.

6. Awada A, Watson T, Obeid T. Cavernous angioma presenting as pregnancy-related seizures. *Epilepsia.* 1997;**38**:844–6.

7. Ratnapalan S, Bentur Y, Koren G. "Doctor, will that x-ray harm my unborn child?" *CMAJ.* 2008;**179**:1293–6.

8. Kal HB, Struikmans H. Radiotherapy during pregnancy: fact and fiction. *Lancet Oncol.* 2005;**6**:328–33.

9. Cohen-Gadol AA, Friedman JA, Friedman JD, Tubbs RS, Munis JR, Meyer FB. Neurosurgical management of intracranial lesions in the pregnant patient: a 36-year institutional experience and review of the literature. *J Neurosurg.* 2009;**111**:1150–7.

10. Jentink J, Loane MA, Dolk H, et al. Valproic acid monotherapy in pregnancy and major congenital malformations. *N Engl J Med.* 2010;**362**:2185–93.

11. Klibanski A. Clinical practice. Prolactinomas. *N Engl J Med.* 2010;**362**:1219–26.

12. Stalldecker G, Mallea-Gil MS, Guitelman M, et al. Effects of cabergoline on pregnancy and embryo-fetal development: retrospective study on 103 pregnancies and a review of the literature. *Pituitary.* 2010;**13**:345–50.

13. Lebbe M, Hubinont C, Bernard P, Maiter D. Outcome of 100 pregnancies initiated under treatment with cabergoline in hyperprolactinaemic women. *Clin Endocrinol (Oxf).* 2010;**73**:236–42.

14. Mazonakis M, Damilakis J, Theoharopoulos N, Varveris H, Gourtsoyiannis N. Brain radiotherapy during pregnancy: an analysis of conceptus dose using anthropomorphic phantoms. *Br J Radiol.* 1999;**72**:274–8.

15. Muratori M, Arosio M, Gambino G, Romano C, Biella O, Faqlia G. Use of cabergoline in the long-term treatment of hyperprolactinemic and acromegalic patients. *J Endocrinol Invest.* 1997;**20**:537–46.

Chapter

7

Treatment of acute and chronic leukemia during pregnancy

Tal Shapira-Rotenberg and Michael Lishner

Introduction

Leukemia occurs very rarely during pregnancy. Although the epidemiology of pregnancy-associated leukemia has never been studied, the estimated prevalence is approximately 1 in 100,000 pregnancies. The majority of cases are acute leukemia, of which two-thirds are myeloblastic (AML) and one-third are lymphoblastic (ALL). Chronic myeloid leukemia (CML) is found in less than 10% of leukemia cases during pregnancy, and chronic lymphocytic leukemia (CLL) is extremely rare [1].

Acute leukemia

Acute leukemia is a violent disease, but it is potentially curable with aggressive chemotherapy regardless of gestational stage. There are indications that postponing or modifying treatment is associated with increased maternal mortality [2–4]. Following a diagnosis of acute leukemia, decisions regarding management of the fetus and the mother must be made promptly and treatment should ensue as quickly as possible.

Acute leukemia may have adverse maternal and fetal effects. These include maternal anemia, disseminated intravascular coagulopathy, and decreased exchange of oxygen and nutrients. Only one case of vertical transmission of AML from a mother to a fetus has been reported in the literature [5].

Acute myeloid leukemia

The treatment of AML consists of high-dose combination therapy for induction, followed by consolidation therapy with lower doses of chemotherapy. When AML is diagnosed during pregnancy, treatment should not be delayed. The administration of induction chemotherapy during the first trimester must accompany a strong recommendation for pregnancy termination due to the teratogenic effects of chemotherapy.

The accepted protocol for induction therapy of AML consists of a combination of cytarabine and anthracycline. Cytarabine, an anti-metabolite, is teratogenic in animal models [6]. Five reports of pregnancies exposed to cytarabine during the first trimester are described in the English literature. Four of these five pregnancies ended with newborn limb malformations. Complications of cytarabine exposure during second and third trimesters include intrauterine fetal death (IUFD), intrauterine growth retardation (IUGR), transient neonatal cytopenia, and neonatal death due to severe infection.

Cancer in Pregnancy and Lactation: The Motherisk Guide ed. Gideon Koren and Michael Lishner.
Published by Cambridge University Press. © Cambridge University Press 2011.

Anthracyclines are a cornerstone of treatment for a variety of malignancies in addition to leukemia and are considered relatively safe during the second and third trimesters [7–10]. The use of anthracyclines during pregnancy is restricted mainly to doxorubicin and daunorubicin. Idarubicin is more lipophilic and has a higher affinity to DNA; hence, it should not be used during pregnancy.

Two reviews summarized the fetal cardiotoxic effect of anthracycline exposure during pregnancy. A long-term follow-up of 81 children, whose mothers were treated for various malignancies with chemotherapy regimens, including anthracyclines, revealed no myocardial damage based on fetal and post-natal echocardiography [11]. Germann *et al.* reviewed 160 pregnant women exposed to anthracyclines during pregnancy. There were 3 cases of fetal cardiotoxicity, of which 1 was lethal [12].

The limited data available suggest that cytarabine and anthracyclines may be administered safely after the first trimester. Close fetal follow-up is essential, and adequate supportive treatment, including anti-emetic and antibiotic therapy when indicated, is essential.

Acute promyelocytic leukemia

Induction therapy for patients with acute promyelocytic leukemia includes All-trans retinoic acid (ATRA) and chemotherapy (most commonly an anthracycline). Exposure to retinoic acid and its derivates during the first trimester is associated with an extremely high rate (up to 85%) of teratogenicity, including severe neurological and cardiovascular malformations. It is commonly accepted that administration of ATRA during the first trimester should be followed by pregnancy termination. The administration of ATRA alone or in combination with an anthracycline during the second and third trimesters is associated with relatively favorable fetal outcomes [13]. However, stringent fetal monitoring, with particular emphasis on cardiac function, is mandatory.

Acute promyelocytic leukemia is of special importance to the obstetrician because of its association with disseminated intravascular coagulopathy (DIC), which may severely complicate the management of pregnancy, labor, and delivery. Patients should be closely monitored for clinical and laboratory manifestations of DIC.

Acute lymphoblastic leukemia

ALL is relatively rare among adults [14–17]. Because ALL is highly aggressive, adequate chemotherapy must be administered immediately after diagnosis.

The scanty data regarding treatment of ALL during pregnancy do not allow firm recommendations. This issue is further complicated because methotrexate, which is a crucial component of most ALL intensification protocols, is extremely teratogenic. First-trimester methotrexate exposure is associated with an increased risk of miscarriage. Exposure to high-dose methotrexate (>10 mg/week) after the first trimester was associated with cranial dysostosis, delayed ossification, hypertelorism, wide nasal bridge, micrognatia, and ear anomalies (aminopterin syndrome) [18–26]. The risk for congenital malformations seems to diminish as pregnancy advances. However, methotrexate should not be used during pregnancy.

When the diagnosis is made before 20 weeks of gestation, termination of pregnancy should be strongly considered, followed by administration of an adequate anti-ALL regimen. ALL diagnosed after 20 weeks of gestation should be treated as in nonpregnant women. However, both the mother and the fetus should be kept under close observation, and delivery should be planned during a non-cytopenic period.

Several chemotherapeutic regimens that do not include methotrexate have been suggested for treating this group of patients [15,27,28]. However, the experience with these protocols, which are not often used for treating ALL patients, is extremely limited and therefore they may be used as a short "bridging treatment" for patients diagnosed during the first 20 weeks of gestation who refuse pregnancy termination.

Chronic leukemias

Chronic myeloid leukemia

CML accounts for 15% of all adult leukemias; only 10% of cases occur during the childbearing period [29]. It is a myeloproliferative disease characterized by the fusion gene *bcr-abl*. The product of this gene, Bcr-Abl protein, has constitutive tyrosine kinase activity and is the main driving force for the development and maintenance of the leukemic clone. The treatment of CML has evolved dramatically since the introduction of tyrosine kinase inhibitors (TKI). Currently, TKIs are the treatment of choice for newly diagnosed CML [30], while bone marrow transplantation is reserved for selected patients and is not a therapeutic option during pregnancy. The treatment of CML during pregnancy raises several important therapeutic questions.

Tyrosine kinase inhibitors

Imatinib mesylate, a TKI, entered clinical trials in 1998. For adult patients who present with CML in chronic phase, it is now generally agreed that initial treatment should be imatinib. After 5 years of imatinib treatment, approximately 60% of patients achieve and maintain complete cytogenetic response (CCyR). An appreciable proportion of them have a major molecular response [31,32].

Preclinical studies of fetal organogenesis in pregnant rats showed that imatinib is teratogenic, causing defects such as exencephaly, encephaloceles, and deformities of the skull bones. Female rats given doses greater than 45 mg/kg (approximately equivalent to a human dose of 400 mg/day based on body surface area) experienced significant postimplantation loss with increased fetal resorption, stillbirths, nonviable pups, and early pup mortality. Doses higher than 100 mg/kg resulted in total fetal loss. Consequently, contraception has been strongly recommended in all women with child-bearing potential during imatinib treatment.

Current practice is to continue imatinib treatment indefinitely, and the ability of the drug to eradicate the CML clone is uncertain. In the STIM trial [33], 100 CML patients in complete molecular response (CMR) for at least 2 years were followed after imatinib discontinuation. Molecular relapse occurred in 54 patients after a median follow up of 17 months. All patients responded to re-administration of imatinib. Factors predictive of durable CMR were low Sokal score, male sex, and duration of imatinib treatment. Other studies, mainly case reports, recorded higher rates of relapse after imatinib discontinuation and complete remission was regained in only a fraction of patients after re-administration of imatinib [34–36].

There are scanty data regarding the outcome of pregnant women who stopped imatinib during pregnancy. In all women but 1, the disease progressed following imatinib cessation and 11 women required treatment with different therapeutic measures, including interferon, hydroxyurea, and leukapheresis [37–39].

The decision regarding CML treatment during pregnancy depends on a combination of the patient, the pregnancy, and the stage of disease:

CML patients who conceive while on imatinib

Pye *et al.* [40] reported on 180 women treated with imatinib during pregnancy and the pregnancy outcomes. First-trimester exposure to imatinib occurred in 103 women. Of these, 8 pregnancies ended in spontaneous abortion, 21 in elective abortion (1 with fetal defect and 1 with stillbirth and meningocele). Of the 46 pregnancies that ended with a live birth, 40 were normal infants and 6 had different anomalies. Of concern are 3 cases with a combination of defects that were strikingly similar: all three had exomphalus and bony defects (2 hemivertebra, 1 scoliosis, and 1 a right shoulder anomaly). Two had urinary tract abnormalities (duplex left kidney, absent right kidney, right renal agenesis). One had hypoplastic lungs.

On the other hand, Azim *et al.* [41] reported 36 patients (38 pregnancies, 10 were reported by Pye *et al.*, as well) who were exposed to imatinib during the first trimester. Of these, 23 were exposed during first trimester only (treatment was stopped once pregnancy was diagnosed). Among these patients, 3 spontaneous abortions, 1 preterm delivery, 2 newborns with hypospadias, and 1 with a fatal meningocele were reported. Nine patients conceived while on imatinib, and continued pregnancy to term with no adverse events.

Due to these reports, it is prudent to avoid imatinib during the first trimester. If the patient prefers to continue treatment, the pregnancy should be closely monitored for significant abnormalities. In these circumstances, the couple should be made aware of potential risks, particularly from first-trimester exposure.

CML diagnosed during pregnancy

Of the 103 pregnancies reported by Pye *et al.*, fatal outcome and fetal defects were noted only among 16 women who were treated with imatinib during first trimester or throughout pregnancy (8/38). No malformations were reported among the 4 women treated after the first trimester.

A similar report by Azim *et al.* found that women who started imatinib during the second (2 patients) or third (2 patients) trimester achieved control of the disease without affecting the course and outcome of pregnancy. Only 11 newborns were followed for a year or more. It is unknown whether *in utero* exposure to imatinib is associated with long-term adverse outcomes.

Male CML patients treated with imatinib

There is increasing evidence that children born to men who are taking imatinib at the time of conception do not have an increased risk of congenital malformations. Apperly [42] reported over 60 pregnancies in the partners of imatinib-treated men without evidence of increased risk of pregnancy-associated complications or congenital abnormalities.

Second-generation TKIs: dasatinib, nilotinib

Dasatinib is an oral TKI that binds to active and inactive forms of *Bcr-Abl* kinase. It is a multi-targeted kinase inhibitor of Bcr-Abl and Src kinase, which have been developed to overcome intolerance or resistance to prior therapy. It has a 100- to 300-fold higher activity than imatinib [43]. Dasatinib is licensed for the treatment of adults with chronic, accelerated, or blast phase CML. Nilotinib was introduced in 2007 for the treatment of patients with chronic or blastic phase CML. Evidence from an *in vitro* study indicated that nilotinib was 20 times more potent than imatinib against cells expressing the wild-type *bcr-abl*.

Studies in rabbits showed that nilotinib is associated with increased rates of mortality, spontaneous abortion, and decreased gestational weights at lower doses than those used in humans [44]. There is 1 case report of a CML patient treated with nilotinib at the time of conception, while in complete cytogenetic remission and major molecular response. Pregnancy was diagnosed at 7 weeks of gestation, the treatment was stopped, and no further treatment was given until delivery. Preterm labor at 33 weeks of gestation resulted in a healthy baby. After delivery, the patient lost molecular, cytogenetic, and hematologic response. She received dasatinib therapy and regained complete hematologic response within 3 months [45].

Nine female patients were treated with dasatinib at some time during pregnancy. Three had a therapeutic abortion, 2 had spontaneous abortions, and 4 delivered. None of these women or their neonates experienced adverse outcomes [46,47].

There are still insufficient data on these newer medications to warrantee their safety in pregnant women with CML.

Interferon alpha

Interferon alpha (IFN-α) inhibits cell proliferation through its effect on protein synthesis, RNA degradation, and possibly by immune system modulation. It does not inhibit DNA synthesis. It is associated with cytogenetic responses in approximately 10% to 38% of CML patients. Due to the high molecular weight of IFN-α, it does not cross the placental barrier to a great extent [48]. Neither *in vitro* mutagenicity nor teratogenicity was observed in animal studies [49]. The 2 major reports regarding IFN therapy during pregnancy [50,51] described 40 cases, 8 of which were treated during the first trimester. There were no cases of fetal malformations when IFN was given as monotherapy. Hence, IFN-α is considered safe for pregnant CML patients.

Hydroxyurea

Hydroxyurea (HU) is a cytotoxic drug that inhibits DNA synthesis. It induces clinical and hematological remission in the majority of cases, but rarely results in cytogenetic response. Preclinical models have shown that HU is teratogenic in all animal species. Several cases of HU treatment during pregnancy have been reported. The main study [52] described a single center experience of 31 patients and a review of 19 additional women treated with HU during pregnancy. Of the 50 cases, there were 2 instances of IUFD in patients treated during the first trimester, 3 with minor malformations, and 9 cases of preterm delivery. Second- and third-trimester exposure was associated with an increased risk of pre-eclampsia.

Hydroxyurea should not be used during pregnancy due to a high rate of pregnancy complications during first-trimester exposure and better, safer treatment options during second and third trimesters.

Leukapheresis

Leukapheresis may be used in the management of acute and chronic leukemia for rapid cytoreduction in patients with impending vascular occlusion. There is limited information regarding the use of leukapheresis during pregnancy [53,54], but it was reported as being well tolerated in 2 cases. It may be used as an alternative for chemotherapy for patients until the end of the first trimester.

Chronic lymphocytic leukemia

CLL is the predominant leukemia among the elderly, and affects men twice as often as women. The median age at diagnosis is 60 years, with only 10%–15% of patients younger than 50 years. Therefore, it has been very rarely associated with pregnancy. It is an incurable disease, characterized by an indolent clinical course. Therefore, treatment can usually be delayed until post-partum unless the patient is symptomatic.

Only 4 cases of pregnancy-associated CLL have been reported [55–58]. In 1 patient with stage IV disease and severe leukocytosis (over 100,000/ml), treatment was indicated during pregnancy and she was successfully treated with 3 sessions of leukapheresis [52]. Another 2 patients had infections during pregnancy, 1 an episode of urinary tract infection, and the other recurrent respiratory tract infections. All patients gave birth to healthy infants without congenital malformations.

There are several options for the treatment of CLL. When treatment is indicated, cytoreduction may be accomplished mechanically with leukapheresis. The most popular drugs are: (1) chlorambucil, which is contraindicated during the first trimester of pregnancy because of its teratogenicity; (2) fludarabine, an anti-metabolite. There are no reports regarding the administration of fludarabine during pregnancy. Because anti-metabolites seem to be more teratogenic than other anticancer drugs, its use during pregnancy should be avoided if possible; and (3) corticosteroids may be used for the treatment of auto-immune complications, as in nonpregnant patients.

Hairy cell leukemia

Hairy cell leukemia (HCL) accounts for approximately 2%–3% of all adult leukemias in the Western world. Due to its median age at diagnosis and male predominance, HCL is very rare during pregnancy. The disease is characterized by an indolent course, which enables treatment delay. IFN-α was historically used in the treatment of this disease. To date, cladribine is considered the standard of care in managing HCL. However, use of this drug during pregnancy has not been reported. Six cases of pregnancy-associated HCL have been reported. In 2 cases, treatment was delayed until after delivery [59,60], 2 patients were treated with IFN-α [61] and 1 patient with splenectomy [62]. In another case, a medical abortion was performed.

Thus, when treatment for HCL is indicated during pregnancy, IFN-α is the drug of choice.

References

1. Pavlidis NA. Coexistence of pregnancy and malignancy. *Oncologist.* 2002;7: 279–87.

2. Kawamura S, Yoshike M, Shimoyama T, et al. Management of acute leukemia during pregnancy: from the results of a nationwide questionnaire survey and literature survey. *Tohoku J Exp Med.* 1994;174:167–75.

3. Greenlund LJ, Letendre L, Tefferi A. Acute leukemia during pregnancy: a single institutional experience with 17 cases. *Leuk Lymphoma.* 2001;41:571–7.

4. Iseminger KA, Lewis MA. Ethical challenges in treating mother and fetus when cancer complicates pregnancy. *Obstet Gynecol Clin North Am.* 1998;25:273–85.

5. Rizack R, Mega A, Legare R, Castillo J. Management of hematological malignancies during pregnancy. *Am J Hematol.* 2009;84:830–41.

6. Rahman ME, Ishikawa H, Watanabe Y, Endo A. Stage specificity of Ara-C induced

carpal and tarsal bone anomalies in mice. *Reprod Toxicol.* 1995;**9**:289–96.

7. Cardonick E, Iacobucci A. Use of chemotherapy during human pregnancy. *Lancet Oncol.* 2004;**5**:283–91.

8. Hahn KM, Johnson PH, Gordon N, et al. Treatment of pregnant breast cancer patients and outcomes of children exposed to chemotherapy in utero. *Cancer.* 2006;**107**:1219–26.

9. Lishner M, Zemlickis D, Degendorfer P, Panzarella T, Sutcliffe SB, Koren G. Maternal and foetal outcome following Hodgkin's disease in pregnancy. *Br J Cancer.* 1992;**65**:114–7.

10. Pereg D, Koren G, Lishner M. The treatment of Hodgkin's and non-Hodgkin's lymphoma in pregnancy. *Haematologica.* 2007;**92**:1230–7.

11. Aviles A, Neri N, Nambo MJ. Long term evaluation of cardiac function in children who received anthracyclines during pregnancy. *Ann Oncol.* 2006;**17**:286–8.

12. Germann N, Goffiner F, Godwasser F. Anthracyclines during pregnancy: embryo-fetal outcome in 160 patients. *Ann Oncol.* 2004;**15**:146–50

13. Yang D, Hladnik L. Treatment of acute promyelocytic leukemia during pregnancy. *Pharmacotherapy.* 2009;**29**:709–24.

14. Molkenboer JF, Vos AH, Schouten HC, Vos MC. Acute lymphoblastic leukaemia in pregnancy. *Neth J Med.* 2005;**63**:361–3.

15. Chelghoum Y, Vey N, Raffoux E, et al. Acute leukemia during pregnancy: a report on 37 patients and a review of the literature. *Cancer.* 2005;**104**:110–7.

16. Hansen WF, Fretz P, Hunter SK, Yankowitz J. Leukemia in pregnancy and fetal response to multiagent chemotherapy. *Obstet Gynecol.* 2001;**97**:809–12.

17. Bergstrom SK, Altman AJ. Pregnancy during therapy for childhood acute lymphoblastic leukemia: two case reports and a review of the literature. *J Pediatr Hematol Oncol.* 1998;**20**:154–9.

18. Milunsky A, Graef JW, Gaynor MF Jr. Methotrexate-induced congenital malformations. *J Pediatr.* 1968;**72**:790–5.

19. Powell HR, Ekert H. Methotrexate-induced congenital malformations. *Med J Aust.* 1971;**2**:1076–7.

20. Diniz EM, Corradini HB, Ramos JL, Brock R. Effect on the fetus of methotrexate (amethopterin) administered to the mother. Presentation of a case. *Rev Hosp Clin Fac Med Sao Paulo.* 1978;**33**:286–90.

21. Dara P, Slater LM, Armentrout SA. Successful pregnancy during chemotherapy for acute leukemia. *Cancer.* 1981;**47**:845–6.

22. Feliu J, Juarez S, Ordonez A, Garcia-Paredes ML, Gonzalez-Baron M, Montero JM. Acute leukemia and pregnancy. *Cancer.* 1988;**61**:580–4.

23. Kozlowski RD, Steinbrunner JV, MacKenzie AH, Clough JD, Wilke WS, Segal AM. Outcome of first-trimester exposure to low-dose methotrexate in eight patients with rheumatic disease. *Am J Med.* 1990;**88**:589–92.

24. Buckley LM, Bullaboy CA, Leichtman L, Marquez M. Multiple congenital anomalies associated with weekly low-dose methotrexate treatment of the mother. *Arthritis Rheum.* 1997;**40**:971–3.

25. Bawle EV, Conard JV, Weiss L. Adult and two children with fetal methotrexate syndrome. *Teratology.* 1998;**7**:51–5.

26. Addar MH. Methotrexate embryopathy in a surviving intrauterine fetus after presumed diagnosis of ectopic pregnancy: case report. *J Obstet Gynaecol Can.* 2004;**26**:1001–3.

27. Dara P, Slater LM, Armentrout SA. Successful pregnancy during chemotherapy for acute leukemia. *Cancer.* 1981;**47**:845–6.

28. Feliu J, Juarez S, Ordonez A, Garcia-Paredes ML, Gonzalez-Baron M, Montero JM. Acute leukemia and pregnancy. *Cancer.* 1988;**61**:580–4.

29. Kozlowski RD, Steinbrunner JV, MacKenzie AH, Clough Jd, Wilde WS, Segal AM. Outcome of first-trimester exposure to low-dose methotrexate in eight

patients with rheumatic disease. *Am J Med.* 1990;**88**:589–92.

30. Buckley LM, Bullaboy CA, Leichtman L, Marquez M. Multiple congenital anomalies associated with weekly low-dose methotrexate treatment of the mother. *Arthritis Rheum.* 1997;**40**:971–3.

31. Bawle EV, Conard JV, Weiss L. Adult and two children with fetal methotrexate syndrome. *Teratology.* 1998;**7**:51–5.

32. Addar MH. Methotrexate embryopathy in a surviving intrautine fetus after presumed diagnosis of ectopic pregnancy: case report. *J Obstet Gynaecol Can.* 2004;**26**:1001–3.

33. Mahon FX, Rea D, Guilhot J, et al. Discontinuation of imatinib in patients with chronic myeloid leukaemia who have maintained complete molecular remission for at least 2 years: the prospective, multicentre Stop Imatinib (STIM) trial. *Lancet Oncol.* 2010;**11**:1029–35.

34. Mauro MJ, Druker BJ, Maziarz RT. Divergent clinical outcome in two CML patients who discontinued imatinib therapy after achieving a molecular remission. *Leuk Res.* 2004;**28**S1:S71–3.

35. Cortes J, O'Brien S, Kantarjian H. Discontinuation of imatinib therapy after achieving a molecular response. *Blood.* 2004;**104**:2204–5.

36. Guastafierro S, Falcone U, Celenato M, Coppola M, Ferrara MG, Sica A. Is it possible to discontinue imatinib mesylate therapy in chronic myeloid leukemia patients with undetectable BCR/ABL? A case report and a review of the literature. *Leuk Res.* 2009;**33**:1079–81.

37. Garderet L, Santacruz R, Barbu V, van den Akker J, Carbonne B, Gorin NC. Two successful pregnancies in a chronic myeloid leukemia patient treated with imatinib. *Haematologica.* 2007;**92**:e9–10.

38. Ault P, Kantarjian H, O'Brien S, et al. Pregnancy among patients with chronic myeloid leukemia treated with imatinib. *J Clin Oncol.* 2006;**24**:1204–8.

39. Heartin E, Walkinshow S, Clark RE. Successful outcome of pregnancy in chronic myeloid leukaemia treated with imatinib. *Leuk Lymphoma.* 2004;**45**:1307–8.

40. Pye SM, Cortes J, Ault P, et al. The effects of imatinib on pregnancy outcome. *Blood.* 2008;**111**:5505–8.

41. Azim HA, Pavlidis N, Peccatori FA. Treatment of the pregnant mother with cancer: a systematic review on the use of cytotoxic, endocrine, targeted agents and immunotherapy during pregnancy. Part II: hematological tumors. *Cancer Treat Rev.* 2010;**36**:110–21.

42. Apperley J. CML in pregnancy and childhood. *Best Pract Res Clin Haematol.* 2009;**22**:455–74.

43. Shah NP, Tran C, Lee FY, Chen P, Norris D, Sawyers CL. Overriding imatinib resistance with a novel ABL kinase inhibitor. *Science.* 2004;**305**:399–401.

44. *Tasigna: (Nilotinib) [package insert]: East Hanover,* NJ: Novartis pharmaceuticals corporation. 2007.

45. Conchon M, Sanabani SS, Bendit I, Santos FN, Serpa M, Dorliac-Llacer PE. Two successful pregnancies in a woman with chronic myeloid leukemia exposed to nilotinib during the first trimester of her second pregnancy: case study. *J Hematol Oncol.* 2009;**2**:42–5.

46. Cortes-Franco J, O'Brien S, Ault P, et al. Pregnancy outcomes among patients with chronic myeloid leukemia treated with Dasatinib. Poster presentation, American Society of Hematology annual meeting, 2008. Available from: http://ash.confex.com/ash/2008/webprogram/Paper12602.html (Accessed January 12, 2011.)

47. Conchon M, Sanabani SS, Serpa M, et al. Successful pregnancy and delivery in a patient with chronic myeloid leukemia while on dasatinib therapy. *Adv Hematol.* 2010;**2010**:136252.

48. Roth MS, Foon KA. Alpha interferon in the treatment of hematologic malignancies. *Am J Med.* 1986;**81**:871–82.

49. Mubarak AAS, Kakil IR, Awidi A, et al. Normal outcome of pregnancy in chronic myeloid leukemia treated with interferon-alpha in 1st trimester: report of 3 cases and

review of the literature. *Am J Hematol.* 2002;**69**:115–8.

50. Hiratsuka M, Minakami H, Koshizuka S, Sato I. Administration of interferon-alpha during pregnancy: effects on fetus. *J Perinatol Med.* 2000;**28**:372–6.

51. Vantroyen B, Vanstraelen D. Management of essential thrombocythemia during pregnancy with aspirin, interferon alpha 2a and no treatment. A comprehensive analysis of the literature. *Acta Hematol.* 2002;**107**:158–69.

52. Thauvin-Robinet C, Maingueneau C, Robert E, et al. Exposure to hydroxyurea during pregnancy: a case series. *Leukemia.* 2001;**15**:1309–11.

53. Ali R, Ozkalemkas F, Ozkocaman V, et al. Successful pregnancy and delivery in patient with chronic myelogenous leukemia (CML) and management of CML with leukapheresis during pregnancy: a case report and review of the literature. *JPN J Clin Oncol.* 2004;**34**:215–7.

54. Klassen R, de Jong P, Wijermans PW. Successful management of chronic myeloid leukaemia with leukapheresis during a twin pregnancy. *Neth J Med.* 2007;**65**:147–9.

55. Gurman G. Pregnancy and successful labor in the course of chronic

56. Welsh TM, Thompson J, Lim S. Chronic lymphocytic leukemia in pregnancy. *Leukemia.* 2000;**14**:1155.

57. Chrisomalis L, Baxi LV, Heller D. Chronic lymphocytic leukemia in pregnancy. *Am J Obstet Gynecol.* 1996;**175**:1381–2.

58. Ali R, Ozkalemkaş F, Ozkocaman V, et al. Successful labor in the course of chronic lymphocytic leukemia (CLL) and management of CLL during pregnancy with leukapheresis. *Ann Hematol.* 2004;**83**:61–3.

59. Alothman A, Sparling TG. Managing hairy cell leukemia in pregnancy. *Ann Intern Med.* 1994;**120**:1048–9.

60. Williams JK. Hairy cell leukemia in pregnancy: a case report. *Am J Obstet Gynecol.* 1987;**156**:210–1.

61. Baer MR, Ozer H, Foon KA. Interferon alpha therapy during pregnancy in chronic myelogenous leukemia and hairy cell leukemia. *Br J Hematol.* 1992;**81**:167–9.

62. Stiles GM, Stanco LM, Saven A, Hoffmann KD. Splenectomy for hairy cell leukemia during pregnancy. *J Perinatol.* 1998;**18**:200–1.

lymphocytic leukemia. *Am J Hematol.* 2002;**71**:208–10.

Chapter

8

Lung cancer and pregnancy

Hisaki Fujii and Michael Lishner

Introduction

Lung cancer during pregnancy is rare. However, the number of cases may be growing due to the combined effects of increased cigarette consumption in young women and delayed child-bearing.

Diagnosis

The incidence of lung cancer complicating pregnancy is unknown. The presenting signs and symptoms associated with lung cancer and pregnancy are similar to the nonpregnant state and depend mainly on the stage of the lung cancer.

Symptoms related to the growth of the tumor, such as blood-streaked sputum, persistent cough or change in cough pattern, wheezing, decreased appetite with poor weight gain during pregnancy, along with other locoregional symptoms (with or without a detectable pleural effusion) are commonly seen. Delays in the diagnosis may occur due to reasons such as low index of suspicion, tendency to attribute symptoms such as fatigue and dyspnea on the pregnant state; and physician reluctance to order a chest radiograph during pregnancy.

A detailed history and accurate physical examination remain the most important steps in the evaluation of these patients, including assessment of risk factors. Plain anteroposterior and lateral chest radiographs are the most valuable tools in the diagnosis of lung cancer [1]. Ultrasound and MRI studies are probably appropriate for metastatic work-up, especially in subdiaphragmatic sites [2].

Diagnostic evaluation consists of histologic confirmation and staging. The former can be achieved by sputum cytology, percutaneous fine needle aspiration, bronchoscopy with biopsy or bronchoalveolar lavage. In patients with metastatic disease, biopsy of other readily accessible sites (i.e., palpable nodes) is also a reliable and relatively noninvasive procedure.

Preoperative staging

Lung cancer staging consists of physical examination in combination with surgical and radiologic investigations. Staging investigations must focus on the determination of the local extent of the disease if surgery is considered, and possible sites of metastatic disease. Decisions regarding the use of radiological investigations must take into account the age of the fetus and the estimated dose of radiation delivered with the respective imaging study.

Cancer in Pregnancy and Lactation: The Motherisk Guide ed. Gideon Koren and Michael Lishner.
Published by Cambridge University Press. © Cambridge University Press 2011.

The metastatic workup is determined by the presenting signs and symptoms as well as the histological subtype (small cell vs. non-small cell).

Therapeutic abortion

There is no evidence that therapeutic abortion offers a survival advantage. The need for chemotherapy or radiotherapy during the early stages of pregnancy for rapidly progressive disease (i.e., small cell lung cancer) may lead to consideration of termination of pregnancy.

Pathology and biology

Little is known about the effect of pregnancy on the course of lung cancer.

The prevalence of lung cancer in women has steadily increased over the past decades. Thirty-seven cases with non-small cell lung cancer during pregnancy have been reported [3–33]. The histologies recorded include the following: adenocarcinoma (22 cases), squamous cell (5 cases), large cell (3 cases), bronchoalveolar (1 case), and unknown (6 cases). The median age was 34.5 years (range, 17–45 years). With the exception of 3 patients, all the patients presented with metastatic disease.

Data on small cell lung cancer and pregnancy are also scarce. Nine case reports have been published [34–41]. All cases except 1 who received chemotherapy during pregnancy [41] had involvement of the placenta by the tumor, and 2 newborns had metastasis of maternal origin [39,40] suggesting extensive disease. Sixty percent of patients had a history of tobacco use.

Treatment

Non-small cell

Stage I and II (T1–2, N0–1, M0)

The treatment of choice in early stage non-small cell lung cancer is curative surgical resection. Despite primary control, combined-modality treatments are being investigated, because micrometastatic disease is probably present at the time of initial treatment. There is no contraindication to surgery during pregnancy, but appreciation of altered maternal physiology due to the pregnancy, teratogenicity of medications, and rates of fetal loss according to stage of pregnancy is mandatory for the anesthetist. Treatment delay until after delivery is an option in patients late in the pregnancy. There are 2 case reports dealing with early stage lung cancer [5,15]. A 34-year-old patient presented with a symptomatic left lower lobe mass in the seventh month of pregnancy. She delivered a healthy baby and postpartum underwent a left lower lobectomy. The pathology was consistent with squamous cell carcinoma; she died of metastatic disease 3.5 years later [5]. A 38-year-old patient with stage II adenocarcinoma had a therapeutic abortion at 18 weeks gestation. Complete resection by a left upper lobectomy was followed by radiotherapy. After a disease-free interval of 18 months, she suffered from headache, nausea, and vomiting, and MRI of the brain showed a brain metastasis when she was at 24 weeks gestation. Whole-brain irradiation was performed following complete resection of the metastasis. A full-term healthy male baby was delivered by cesarean section [15].

Stage III A (T1–3, N2, M0 or T3, N0–2, M0)

The treatment of patients with this stage of non-small cell lung cancer depends on the size and location of the primary tumor and the extent of nodal involvement. Treatment options in nonpregnant patients may include different combinations of surgery, chemotherapy, and radiotherapy.

Stage III B (any T, N3, M0 or T4, any N, M0)

Patients with this stage of lung cancer have a poor prognosis and generally receive radiation with or without chemotherapy.

Stage IV (any T, any N, M1)

This stage of lung cancer has a poor prognosis, and treatment is palliative. Treatment options include chemotherapy, radiotherapy to symptomatic areas, and palliative surgery for situations such as impending fracture of the femur. In light of the limited success of chemotherapy in treatment of metastatic non-small cell lung cancer, delay in treatment until after delivery is a reasonable option. Supportive care, to maximize maternal oxygenation and nutrition, is mandatory in all stages of lung cancer.

With respect to non-small cell lung cancer, experience with treatment during pregnancy is limited to 2 cases before 2000; both were in the later stages of pregnancy, and received radiation only [4,8]. After 2001, there were 9 cases reported. Three patients received radiation for brain metastasis [15,16,25]. Two patients accidentally received chemotherapy in the first trimester [25,27], and another 5 patients were planned to receive platinum-based systemic chemotherapy in the second or third trimester [14,24,28–30] (Table 1). There was no serious adverse reaction to fetus reported.

Small cell carcinoma

Small cell lung cancer is characterized by an aggressive clinical course and relatively good (although short lived) response to chemo/radiotherapy compared to other types of lung cancer. Treatment during pregnancy must balance the toxicity of treatment to mother and fetus against the morbidity of untreated disease. One patient with limited stage small cell lung carcinoma treated at 27 weeks gestation with 2 cycles of cisplatin and etoposide and subsequent delivery of a healthy child [41].

Chemotherapy

Most drugs have, at best, moderate activity in non-small cell lung cancer. Cisplatin is considered by many investigators to be the most active single agent [2]. Combination chemotherapy was investigated in an attempt to increase response rates.

To date, 8 patients were given platinum-based chemotherapy during pregnancy in combination with vinorelbine in 2 [14,24], taxane (docetaxel, paclitaxel) in 3 [25,28,30], gemcitabine in 2 [25,29], and etoposide in 1 [41].

Antineoplastic drugs are very potent teratogens. Currently, there is very little information on the effect of cancer chemotherapy on the fetus [33,42]. The risk of malformations when chemotherapy is administered in the first trimester has been estimated to be around 10% for single-agent chemotherapy [43] and 25% for combination chemotherapy [44]. It is generally suggested that chemotherapy be avoided during first trimester, when cells are

Table 1. Patients with NSCLC exposed to systemic chemotherapy during pregnancy

Reference	Stage	Maternal age	Exposure to chemotherapy (trimester)	Gestational age at delivery (week)	Metastasis	Treatment during pregnancy	Infant outcome	Maternal outcome (time after delivery)
4 Reiter (1985)	IV	35	2nd–3rd	30	+	Palliative radiation	Premature at delivery, mild RDS	Died (4 weeks)
8 Van Winter (1995)	IV	36	3rd	32	+	Palliative radiation	Healthy at 8 months	Died (7 months)
14 Janne (2001)	IV	31	3rd	27	+	Cisplatin + vinorelbine (26 weeks, 1 cycle)	Premature at delivery	Alive (9 months)
15 Magne (2001)	IV	40	2nd–3rd	40	+	Radiation (brain), surgery	Healthy at 3 years	Alive (3 years)
16 Mujaibel (2001)	IV	35	3rd	34	+	Radiation (brain)	Healthy at 2 weeks	Died (2 months)
24 Garrido (2008)	III	34	3rd	39	–	Cisplatin + vinorelbine (3 cycles by delivery)	Healthy at 16 months	Alive (16 months)
25 Kim (2008)	IV	35	1st–2nd	33	+	Radiation (brain; 1 week), cisplatin + docetaxel (9 weeks), cisplatin + gemcitabine (19–22 weeks)	Premature at delivery	Alive (10 months)
27 Zambelli (2008)	IV	30	1st	42	+	Erlotinib (2–10 weeks)	Healthy at delivery	Alive (1 month)
28 García-González (2008)	IV	39	2nd	30	+	Cisplatin + paclitaxel (21 weeks, 3 cycles)	Premature at delivery, RDS	Died (4 months)
29 Gurumurthy (2009)	IV	38	2nd–3rd	28	+	Carboplatin + gemcitabine (25 weeks, 1 cycle)	Premature at delivery, RDS	Died (2 weeks)
30 Azim (2009)	IV	33	2nd–3rd	30	+	Carboplatin + paclitaxel (19 weeks, weekly)	Healthy at delivery	Died (4 weeks)

RDS, respiratory distress syndrome.

actively dividing. Use of these agents in the second and third trimesters has been associated with an increased risk of stillbirth, intrauterine growth retardation, and low birth weight [42,45,46]. When chemotherapy is administered during pregnancy, timing of delivery of the infant should take into account the expected bone marrow depression and potential problems such as bleeding or infections. Self-limiting fetal hematopoietic depression has been described, and the neonate should be monitored for complications of this [47]. Long-term neurodevelopmental complications of *in utero* chemotherapy exposure have not been extensively studied [33,48]. Recent data suggested that exposure to chemotherapy after the first trimester does not increase the risk of preterm delivery and growth restriction compared with general populations [33].

Prognosis

There is no evidence that pregnancy alters the prognosis of lung cancer. Maternal outcome for both small cell and non-small cell lung cancer has been poor and is a reflection of the advanced stage at diagnosis. This may be due, in part, to misinterpretation of respiratory symptoms and physician's reluctance to perform radiologic imaging studies during pregnancy [49,50].

Fetal consequences

There is no evidence that fetal outcome is adversely affected by maternal lung cancer, provided that adequate supportive treatment is provided to the mother. Metastatic involvement of the placenta has been reported in the majority of the reported cases. In contrast, there were only 3 reports of fetal involvement [13,39,40].

Fertility

There is no evidence that fertility is adversely affected by lung cancer itself. However, some chemotherapeutic agents can cause sterility which may be age dependent.

References

1. Nicklas A, Baker M. Imaging strategies in the pregnant cancer patient. *Semin Oncol.* 2000;27:623–32.

2. Vincent T, Devita JR, Hellman S, Rosenberg SA. *Cancer. Principles & practice of oncology.* 5th ed. Philadelphia: Lippincott-Raven Publishers; 1997.

3. Read EJ Jr, Platzer PB. Placental metastasis from maternal carcinoma of the lung. *Obstet Gynaecol.* 1981;58:387–91.

4. Reiter AA, Carpenter RJ, Dudrick SJ, Hinkley CM. Pregnancy associated with advanced adenocarcinoma of the lung. *Int J Gynaecol Obstet.* 1985;23:75–8.

5. Stark P, Greene RE, Morgan G, Hildebrandt-Stark HE. Lung cancer and pregnancy. *Radiologe.* 1985;25:30–2.

6. Suda R, Repke JT, Steer R, Niebyl JR. Metastatic adenocarcinoma of the lung complicating pregnancy: a case report. *J Reprod Med.* 1986;31:1113–6.

7. Dildy GA III, Moise KJ Jr, Carpenter RJ Jr, Klima T. Maternal malignancy metastatic to the products of conception: a review. *Obstet Gynecol Surv.* 1989;44:535–40.

8. Van Winter JT, Wilkowske MA, Shaw EG, Ogburn L, Pritchard DJ. Lung cancer complicating pregnancy: case report and review of literature. *Mayo Clin Proc.* 1995;70:384–7.

9. Bitar RJ, Melillo N, Pesin JL. Lung cancer during pregnancy. [Letter]. *Mayo Clin Proc.* 1995;70:1130.

10. Cone LA, Dawson AC, Mata AM. Lung cancer during pregnancy. [Letter]. *Mayo Clin Proc.* 1995;70:1130.

11. Watanabe M, Tomita K, Burioka N, et al. Mucoepidermoid carcinoma of the trachea with airway hyperresponsiveness. *Anticancer Res.* 2000;**20**:1995–7.

12. Abul-Khoudoud R, Lwebuga-Mukasa JS. Primary lung cancer in a seventeen year old, twenty-seven-week pregnant woman. *Chest.* 1997;**112**(suppl 3):159S.

13. Harpold TL, Wang MY, McComb JG, Monforte HL, Levy ML, Reinisch JF. Maternal lung adenocarcinoma metastatic to the scalp of a fetus. *Pediatr Neurosurg.* 2001;**35**:39–42.

14. Jane PA, Rodriguez-Thompson D, Metcalf DR, et al. Chemotherapy for a patient with advanced non-small-cell lung cancer during pregnancy: a case report and a review of chemotherapy treatment during pregnancy. *Oncology.* 2001;**61**: 175–83.

15. Magne N, Marcie S, Pignol JP, Casagrande F, Lagrange JL. Radiotherapy for a solitary brain metastasis during pregnancy: a method for reducing fetal dose. *Br J Radiol.* 2001;**74**:638–41.

16. Mujaibel K, Benjamin A, Delisle MF, Williams K. Lung cancer in pregnancy: case reports and review of the literature. *J Matern Fetal Med.* 2001;**10**:426–32.

17. Jackisch C, Louwen F, Schwenkhagen A, et al. Lung cancer during pregnancy involving the products of conception and a review of the literature. *Arch Gynecol Obstet.* 2003;**268**:69–77.

18. Wong CM, Lim KH, Liam CK. Metastatic lung cancer in pregnancy. *Respirology.* 2003;**8**:107–9.

19. Adams FR, Levy DM, Reid MF, James D, Rubin PC. All that glisters. . .a generalised seizure at 31 weeks. *J Obstet Gynaecol.* 2004;**24**:174–5.

20. Folk JJ, Curioca J, Nosovitch JT, Silverman RK. Poorly differentiated large cell adenocarcinoma of the lung metastatic to the placenta. *J Reprod Med.* 2004;**49**: 395–7.

21. Innamaa A, Deering P, Powell MC. Advanced lung cancer presenting with a generalized seizure in pregnancy. *Acta Obstet Gynecol Scand.* 2006;**85**:1148–9.

22. Burlacu CL, Fitzpatrick C, Carey M. Anaesthesia for caesarean section in a woman with lung cancer: case report and review. *Int J Obstet Anesth.* 2007;**16**: 50–62.

23. But Hadzic J, Secerov A, Zwitter M. Metastatic adenocarcinoma of the lung in a 27-year-old pregnant woman. *J Thorac Oncol.* 2007;**2**:450–2.

24. Garrido M, Clavero J, Huete A, et al. Prolonged survival of a woman with lung cancer diagnosed and treated with chemotherapy during pregnancy. Review of cases reported. *Lung Cancer.* 2008;**60**:285–90.

25. Kim JH, Kim HS, Sung CW, Kim KJ, Kim CH, Lee KY. Docetaxel, gemcitabine, and cisplatin administered for non-small cell lung cancer during the first and second trimester of an unrecognized pregnancy. *Lung Cancer.* 2008;**59**:270–3.

26. Montilla F, Le Caer H, Boyer S, Digluelou JY, Amar P, Le Saux S. Pregnancy and lung cancer: a case report and review of the literature. *J Gynecol Obstet Biol Reprod (Paris).* 2008;**37**:808–10.

27. Zambelli A, Da Prada GA, Fregoni V, Ponchio L, Sagrada P, Pavesi L. Erlotinib administration for advanced non-small cell lung cancer during the first 2 months of unrecognized pregnancy. *Lung Cancer.* 2008;**60**:455–7.

28. García-González J, Cueva J, Lamas MJ, Curiel T, Graña B, López-López R. Paclitaxel and cisplatin in the treatment of metastatic non-small-cell lung cancer during pregnancy. *Clin Transl Oncol.* 2008;**10**:375–6.

29. Gurumurthy M, Koh P, Singh R, et al. Metastatic non-small-cell lung cancer and the use of gemcitabine during pregnancy. *J Perinatol.* 2009;**29**:63–5.

30. AzimJr HA, Scarfone G, Peccatori FA. Carboplatin and weekly paclitaxel for the treatment of advanced non-small cell lung cancer (NSCLC) during pregnancy. *J Thorac Oncol.* 2009;**4**:559–60.

31. Hata A, Harada Y, Seo R, et al. A case of lung cancer combined with pregnancy; dramatically deteriorating condition after

caesarean section. *Nihon Kokyuki Gakkai Zasshi.* 2009;**47**:585–90.

32. Thelmo MC, Shen EP, Shertukde S. Metastatic pulmonary adenocarcinoma to placenta and pleural fluid: clinicopathologic findings. *Fetal Pediatr Pathol.* 2010;**29**:45–56.

33. Cardonick E, Usmani A, Ghaffar S. Perinatal outcomes of a pregnancy complicated by cancer, including neonatal follow-up after in utero exposure to chemotherapy: results of an international registry. *Am J Clin Oncol.* 2010;**33**:221–8.

34. Barr JS. Placental metastases from a bronchial carcinoma. *J Obstet Gynaecol Br Emp.* 1953;**60**:895–7.

35. Hesketh J. A case of carcinoma of the lung with secondary deposits in the placenta. *J Obstet Gynaecol Br Commonw.* 1962;**69**:514.

36. Jones EM. Placental metastases from bronchial carcinoma. *BMJ.* 1969;**2**:491–2.

37. Delerive C, Locquet F, Mallart A, Janin A, Goselin B. Placental metastasis from maternal bronchial oat cell carcinoma. *Arch Pathol Lab Med.* 1989;**113**: 556–8.

38. Kochman AT, Rabczynski JK, Baranowski W, Palczynski B, Kowalski P. Metastases to the products of conception from a maternal bronchial carcinoma. A case report and review of literature. *Pol J Pathol.* 2001;**52**:137–40.

39. Tolar J, Coad JE, Neglia JP. Transplacental transfer of small cell carcinoma of the lung. *N Engl J Med.* 2002;**346**:1501–2.

40. Teksam M, McKinney A, Short J, Casey SO, Truwit CL. Intracranial metastasis via transplacental (vertical) transmission of maternal small cell lung cancer to fetus: CT and MRI findings. *Acta Radiol.* 2004;**45**:577–9.

41. Kluetz PG, Edelman MJ. Successful treatment of small cell lung cancer during pregnancy. *Lung Cancer.* 2008;**61**:129–30.

42. Zemlickis D, Lishner M, Koren G. Review of fetal effects of cancer chemotherapeutic agents. In: Koren G, Lishner M, Farine D, editors. *Cancer in pregnancy.* 1st ed. Cambridge: Press Syndicate of the University of Cambridge; 1996. p. 168.

43. Nicholson H. Cytotoxic drugs in pregnancy: review of reported cases. *J Obstet Gynecol Br Commonw.* 1968;**75**:307.

44. Doll DC, Ringenberg S, Yarbro DW. Management of cancer during pregnancy. *Arch Intern Med.* 1988;**148**:2058–64.

45. Zemlickis D, Lishner M, Degendorfer P, et al. Maternal and fetal outcome after breast cancer in pregnancy. *Am J Obstet Gynecol.* 1992;**166**:781–7.

46. Zemlickis D, Lishner M, Degendrofer P, Panzarella T, Sutcliffe SB, Koren G. Fetal outcome after in utero exposure to cancer chemotherapy. *Arch Intern Med.* 1992;**15**:573–6.

47. Blatt J, Milvihill JJ, Ziegler JL, Young RC, Poplack DG. Pregnancy outcome following cancer chemotherapy. *Am J Med.* 1980;**39**:828–32.

48. Aviles A, Diaz-Maqueo JC, Talavera A, Guzman R, Garcia EL. Growth and development of children of mothers treated with chemotherapy during pregnancy: current status of 43 children. *Am J Hematol.* 1991;**36**:243–8.

49. Chen KY, Wang HC, Shih JY, Yang PC. Lung cancer in pregnancy: report of two cases. *J Formos Med Assoc.* 1998;**97**:573–6.

50. Azim HA Jr, Peccatori FA, Pavlidis N. Lung cancer in the pregnant woman: to treat or not to treat, that is the question. *Lung Cancer.* 2010;**67**:251–6.

Malignant melanoma and pregnancy

Michael Lishner and Michael P. Tan

Introduction

Malignant melanoma is a serious health problem worldwide and is increasing at a rate that exceeds all other solid tumors [1]. The increasing incidence is accompanied by an associated decrease in age at presentation. It is the most common cancer in women ages 25–29 years and approximately 35% of women with melanoma are of child-bearing age [2]. Malignant melanoma during pregnancy has an estimated incidence between 0.14 and 2.8 cases per 1,000 births [3] and represents 8% of malignancies diagnosed during pregnancy [4].

Diagnosis

The signs and symptoms of melanoma are similar to the nonpregnant population and the anatomic location of the primary tumor does not differ between pregnant and nonpregnant women [5]. Changes in size, color, and configuration of any pigmented lesion suggest a malignant change and the need for further investigation [6]. Two-thirds of melanomas occur in pre-existing nevi [7]. However, some degree of hyperpigmentation during pregnancy is experienced by most women [8]. It has been suggested that this hyperpigmentation may lead to a delay in diagnosis of the disease [9]. A growing number of reports suggest minimal changes in size occur during pregnancy [10–12]. Bleeding and ulceration are more ominous signs and require immediate attention. Excisional biopsy is the recommended procedure for any suspicious lesions.

Staging

Clinical staging traditionally has included assessment of the local tumor site and adjacent skin, regional lymph node areas, and distant organs that are frequently the site of metastatic disease. The decision to perform radiological investigations in the pregnant patient should be based on the presence of symptoms, the stage of the pregnancy, the specific test needed, and the estimated dose of ionizing radiation and risks associated with that dose. In most cases, the doses involved in diagnostic radiology, including computed tomography scan of abdomen and pelvis, are lower than the threshold dose that may place the fetus at risk [13]. Intensive radiologic investigation(s) is not required for patients with early disease. Routine elective lymph node dissection (ELND) is not necessary for clinically node-negative patients since this procedure has not been shown

Cancer in Pregnancy and Lactation: The Motherisk Guide ed. Gideon Koren and Michael Lishner.
Published by Cambridge University Press. © Cambridge University Press 2011.

to have a consistent impact on survival with relatively significant morbidity [14,15]. The use of lymphatic mapping with blue dye or a radiolabeled tracer injected at the primary tumor site to identify the draining plus sentinel lymph node biopsy (SLNB) has been shown to have little morbidity (10.1%) with high accuracy (95%) [16,17]. This procedure has gained wider acceptance over the years and has largely replaced the need for routine ELND. During pregnancy, the radiolabeled technique used for lymphatic mapping delivers fetal doses of <5 mGy, which is far less than the threshold of 100 mGy that can cause teratogenic effect. The safety of isosulfan blue dye in pregnancy is not known. Due to the potential anaphylactic risk, rates as high as 0.7%–1.1%, some have chosen not to use the dye in pregnant women [2,18–20]. Ultrasound examination of the lymph node with fine needle biopsy has been used by others as an alternative for SLNB in clinically node-negative patients [21]. Ultrasound has several advantages: no radiation, noninvasive, highly portable, and low cost. Magnetic resonance imaging may be used at any stage in pregnancy [22] and usually preferred over CT scan.

Therapeutic abortion and contraception

There is no conclusive evidence that regression of melanoma occurs after therapeutic abortion [23,24]. Because the influence of pregnancy or hormones on melanoma has not been observed, the general consensus is that oral contraceptives are not contraindicated in patients with a prior history of melanoma, regardless of the duration of their use [24,25].

Pathology and biology

The role of the estrogen hormone is undetermined in the animal model. Feucht *et al.* showed inhibition of human melanoma cell line growth in athymic mice [26], whereas Lopez *et al.* demonstrated enhanced growth rate [27]. Several studies showed the absence of estrogen receptor alpha in melanoma [28–30]. Recently, a new estrogen receptor beta was discovered to be the prominent receptor type found in several types of nevi, including malignant melanoma. The clinical relevance of this finding remains unknown [31,32].

The effect of pregnancy on melanocytic nevi is unclear. Previous studies have suggested that patients may overestimate changes in melanocytic nevi [33,34]. Two prospective studies, 1 involving 22 patients following changes of nevi in pregnancy from first to third trimester using photographs and objective measurements while the other evaluated 47 patients at first trimester, third trimester, and 6 months postpartum using a digital surface microscopy video, failed to demonstrate any significant change in size of nevi [10,12]. Although there were changes in the feature of the nevi noted in pregnancy, the observers noted that these were transient and most changes recovered their pre-pregnancy appearance after delivery, presumably influenced by hormonal changes [11,12].

Another area of controversy exists regarding the effect of pregnancy on site of presentation. Some studies have suggested an increased risk in pregnancy of lesions in areas associated with a worse prognosis such as the head and neck and truncal regions [3,9], while others have not found this association [35,36].

Similarly, there is debate as to whether or not pregnancy is associated with increased tumor thickness [9,24,37]. Stage of the disease, especially tumor thickness and ulceration at diagnosis, and not pregnancy is the only consistent factor influencing the prognosis in terms of survival and disease-free interval [2,5,6,23].

Table 1. Comparison of surgical excision margins among different countries for primary cutaneous melanoma

Tumor thickness	Recommended surgical radial excision margins measured from the edge of the melanoma				
	US [38]	Australia and NZ [39]	Scotland [40]	UK [48]	Swiss [41]
In situ	0.5 cm	0.5 cm	0.2–0.5 cm	0.5 cm	0.5 cm
0.5–1 mm	0.5 cm	1 cm	1 cm	1 cm	1 cm
<1 mm	1 cm	1 cm	1 cm	1 cm	1 cm
1–2 mm	1–2 cm	1–2 cm	1–2 cm	1–2 cm	1 cm
1–4 mm	2 cm	1–2 cm	–	–	–
2–4 mm	2 cm	1–2 cm	2 cm	2–3 cm	2 cm
>4 mm	≥ 2 cm	2 cm	2 cm	3 cm	2 cm

Treatment

Early disease

Surgical removal of the melanoma with adequate margins remains the standard primary therapy for early melanoma. For thin melanomas (<1-mm thick) a 1-cm margin is considered adequate; for a Breslow intermediate thickness (1–4 mm), a 2-cm margin is used in most countries (see Table 1) [38–42]. The standard surgical margin for thick melanoma remains undefined [43,44], but a margin of at least 2 cm appears to be justified [42,45]. Elective lymph node dissection is not recommended [46]. Interim Multicenter Selective Lymphadenectomy Trial (MSLT-1) results revealed similar overall 5-year survival benefit between patients who had undergone wide excision and SLNB with immediate lymphadenectomy and those who had wide excision and postoperative observation of regional lymph node with lymphadenectomy if nodal relapse occurred [47]. Those who had undergone immediate lymphadenectomy after SLNB had prolonged disease-free survival and were spared from the trauma of recurrence. For most patients, surgical excision can be done with a local anesthetic with little risk to the fetus. Locally advanced disease requiring more extensive surgery or regional node dissection should be performed with a general anesthetic when needed.

Node-positive disease

The use of adjuvant interferon alpha-2b (IFN-α-2b) in patients with melanoma is controversial and remains experimental. Earlier pooled data from the Eastern Cooperative Oncology Group (ECOG) and intergroup trials showed no overall survival (OS) benefit with high-dose interferon therapy in stage IIb-III patients [49]. However, more recent meta-analysis suggested a small OS benefit [50,51]. The benefit was seen across all interferon regimens with better disease-free survival in the high-dose regimen but the overall survival was similar [51]. The benefit was greatest in those with ulcerated melanomas [50]. No optimal dose and/or duration of treatment were identified. Further prospective studies are required to identify which patient can derive the most benefit from this therapy.

The existing literature on use of IFN during pregnancy is restricted to case reports involving patients treated for various conditions such as hepatitis, myeloproliferative disorders (essential thrombocythemia and chronic myelogenous leukemia), multiple myeloma, and a case of melanoma. To date, there are a little more than 40 cases of first-trimester exposure reported, with no evidence of teratogenic or adverse effects on the fetus, regardless of timing of treatment during pregnancy [20,52–54]. This includes a mother with nodal malignant melanoma who underwent CT of the chest, abdomen, and pelvis, and SNLB and was treated with low-dose IFN-α-2b from 6 weeks until delivery at 36 weeks with normal healthy twins [20]. Doses used in the case reports have generally been in the range of 0.5–6.5 million units of subcutaneous interferon from weekly to daily regimens, significantly less than the recommended doses for the adjuvant treatment of melanoma. Lack of fetoplacental passage of IFN-α has been shown in one study of 2 HIV-seropositive patients before abortion [55]. Treatment with interferon does not appear to affect fertility [56,57]. No information regarding the safety of use of the much higher doses that may be used in the treatment of melanoma exists (i.e., 20 million units/m^2 intravenous 5 days per week for 4 weeks followed by 10 million units/m^2 subcutaneous 3 times weekly for 48 weeks). Toxicity of this therapy in the nonpregnant patient is significant. Nearly all patients experience flu-like symptoms to a moderate or severe degree. Other significant side effects include depression, cognitive changes, bone marrow suppression, and liver toxicity [58]. Delay of therapy until the postpartum period has been suggested [59]. The use of altered dosing of interferon in the adjuvant setting is under investigation [58].

Advanced or recurrent disease

Metastatic disease to lymph nodes, as well as isolated metastases to areas such as lung, breast, gastrointestinal tract, and brain may be palliated by surgical removal with a potential for long-term survival [60–62]. There is no contraindication to surgery during pregnancy, provided that the physiologic changes of pregnancy are understood.

Chemotherapy

Cancer chemotherapeutic drugs are potent teratogens. Currently, there is very little information on the effect of cancer chemotherapy on the fetus. The risk of malformations when chemotherapy is administered in the first trimester has been estimated to be around 7.5%–17% for single-agent chemotherapy and 25% for combination chemotherapy [63,64]. Excluding concomitant irradiation and anti-folate medications, the risk of malformation for single-agent chemotherapy exposure dropped to 6% [64]. It is generally suggested that chemotherapy be avoided during the first trimester, when cells are actively dividing. Use of these agents in the second and third trimesters has been associated with an increased risk of stillbirth, intrauterine growth retardation, and low birth weight [65]. When chemotherapy is administered during pregnancy, timing of delivery of the infant should take into account the expected bone marrow depression and potential problems such as bleeding or infections. Self-limiting fetal hematopoietic depression has been described, and the neonate should be monitored for this complication [66]. Long-term neurodevelopmental complications of *in utero* chemotherapy exposure have not been extensively studied. Limited data exist to suggest that this may be normal in the offspring of patients with hematologic malignancies treated during various stages of the pregnancy [67].

In the nonpregnant patient, chemotherapy and/or radiotherapy remain valid options for treatment of metastatic disease. Agents used in treatment include dacarbazine, the nitrosoureas (carmustine and lomustine), vinca alkaloids, platinum compounds, taxanes, and biologic agents such as interferon and interleukin. Use of dacarbazine with or without tamoxifen, carmustine, cisplatin, nimustine, vincristine, and IFN-β in pregnancy for malignant melanoma is limited to 5 case reports in which all 5 women were treated in the second and/or third trimester with 5 healthy babies, including 1 with intrauterine growth arrest [68–72]. In most cases, chemotherapy does not offer benefit to the pregnant woman to warrant the risk to the fetus [64].

Irradiation

The essentially palliative nature of therapy for advanced melanoma and the limited success rate(s) seen with existing therapies suggests that delay in therapy until the later stages of gestation or after delivery and aggressive use of supportive therapy during pregnancy (i.e., analgesics, steroids, oxygen) are reasonable options.

Prognosis

The effect of pregnancy on prognosis of melanoma has been a focus of interest in the medical literature for years. When matched for age, anatomic site, and stage, most studies have not demonstrated a difference in survival [5,9,36,73,74]. However, some studies have demonstrated a shorter disease-free interval in pregnant patients compared to controls [74]. It has been suggested that small patient numbers and variable follow-up time in these studies may have limited the ability to detect pregnancy-related changes in outcome [75,76]. Also, there is not sufficient data to establish the role of adjuvant chemotherapy or biological therapy during pregnancy [77].

Fetal outcome

Metastases to the placenta and fetus during pregnancy are rare but have been documented with hematologic as well as solid tumors. Malignant melanoma is the most frequent cancer that metastasizes to the placenta or fetus accounting for 31% (27/87 patient cases) of reported cases from 1918 to 2002 [78]. Therefore, the placenta should be thoroughly examined for metastasis. If present, the infant should be monitored for development of malignant disease. Currently, there are no guidelines on surveillance and therapy in this scenario given its rarity. Alexander et al. suggest skin inspection, liver enzymes including lactate dehydrogenase, baseline chest x-ray, abdominal ultrasound, and screening for melanogens in the infant's urine. The author reported approximately 22% (6/27) fetal affectation with placental involvement, 80% being male fetuses. It is postulated that this gender bias may be either due to the female fetuses being better at eliminating maternally derived melanoma or that male fetuses are more immunotolerant. Previously published reviews estimated a 20%–25% fetal mortality in cases of placental involvement [7,78].

Because the majority of recurrences occur in the first 3 years, some authors suggest delaying pregnancy during this interval after initial diagnosis and treatment [7,25].

Fertility

There is no evidence that a diagnosis of melanoma adversely affects fertility.

References

1. Kirkwood JM, Strawderman MH, Ernstoff MS, Smith TJ, Borden EC, Blum RH. Interferon alfa-2b adjuvant therapy of high-risk resected cutaneous melanoma: the Eastern Cooperative Oncology Group trial EST 1684. *J Clin Oncol.* 1996;**14**:7–17.

2. Schwartz JL, Mozurkewich EL, Johnson TM. Current management of patients with melanoma who are pregnant, want to get pregnant, or do not want to get pregnant. *Cancer.* 2003;**97**:2130–3.

3. Wong DJ, Strassner HT. Melanoma in pregnancy. *Clin Obstet Gynecol.* 1990;**33**:782–91.

4. Potter JF, Schoeneman M. Metastasis of maternal cancer to the placenta and fetus. *Cancer.* 1970;**25**:380–7.

5. O'Meara AT, Cress R, Xing G, Danielsen B, Smith LH. Malignant melanoma in pregnancy: a population-based evaluation. *Cancer.* 2005;**103**:1217–26.

6. Driscoll MS, Grant-Kels JM. Nevi and melanoma in the pregnant woman. *Clin Dermatol.* 2009;**27**:116–21.

7. Borden E. Melanoma and pregnancy. *Semin Oncol.* 2000;**27**:654–6.

8. Errickson CV, Matus NR. Skin disorders of pregnancy. *Am Fam Phys.* 1994;**49**:605–10.

9. MacKie RM, Bufalino R, Morabito A, Sutherland C, Cascinelli N. Lack of effect of pregnancy on outcome of melanoma. *Lancet.* 1991;**337**:653–5.

10. Pennoyer JW, Grin CM, Driscoll MS, et al. Changes in size of melanocytic nevi during pregnancy. *J Am Acad Dermatol.* 1997;**36**:378–82.

11. Gunduz K, Koltan S, Sahin MT, Filiz E. Analysis of melanocytic naevi by dermoscopy during pregnancy. *J Eur Acad Dermatol Venereol.* 2003;**17**:349–51.

12. Zampino MR, Corazza M, Costantino D, Mollica G, Virgili A. Are melanocytic nevi influenced by pregnancy? A dermatoscopic evaluation. *Dermatol Surg.* 2006;**32**:1497–504.

13. Kal HB, Struikmans H. Radiotherapy during pregnancy: fact and fiction. *Lancet Oncol.* 2005;**6**:328–33.

14. Sim FH, Taylor WF, Pritchard DJ, Soule EH. Lymphadenctomy in the management of stage 1 malignant melanoma: a prospective randomized study. *Mayo Clin Proc.* 1986;**61**:697–705.

15. Balch CM, Soong S, Ross MI, et al. Long-term results of a multi-institutional randomized trial comparing prognostic factors and surgical results for intermediate thickness melanomas (1.0 to 4.0 mm). Intergroup Melanoma Surgical Trial. *Ann Surg Oncol.* 2000;**7**:87–97.

16. Morton DL, Cochran AJ, Thompson JF, et al. Sentinel node biopsy for early stage melanoma: accuracy and morbidity in MSLT-1, an international multicenter trial. *Ann Surg.* 2005;**242**:302–11.

17. Essner R, Scheri R, Kavanagh M, Torisu-Itakura H, Wanek LA, Morton DL. Surgical management of the groin lymph nodes in melanoma in the era of sentinel lymph node dissection. *Arch Surg.* 2006;**141**:877–82.

18. Mondi MM, Cuena RE, Ollila DW, Stewart JH IV, Levine EA. Sentinel lymph node biopsy during pregnancy: initial clinical experience. *Ann Surg Oncol.* 2007;**14**:218–21.

19. Gentilini O, Cremonesi M, Toesca A, et al. Sentinel lymph node biopsy in pregnant patients with breast cancer. *Eur J Nucl Med Mol Imaging.* 2010;**37**:78–83.

20. Egberts F, Lischner S, Russo P, Kampen WU, Hauschild A. Diagnostic and therapeutic procedures for management of melanoma during pregnancy: risks for the fetus? *J Dtsch Dermatol Ges.* 2006;**4**:717–20.

21. Thomas JM. Prognostic false-positivity of the sentinel node in melanoma. *Nat Clin Pract Oncol.* 2008;**5**:18–23.

22. Kanal E, Barkovich AJ, Bell C, et al. ACR guidance document for safe MR practice:2007. *AJR Am J Roentgenol.* 2007;**188**:1447–74.

23. Slingluff CL, Seigler HF. Malignant melanoma and pregnancy. *Ann Plast Surg.* 1992;**28**:95–9.

24. Lens M, Bataille V. Melanoma in relation to reproductive and hormonal factors in women: current review on controversial issues. *Cancer Causes Control.* 2008;**19**:437–42.

25. Gupta A, Driscoll MS. Do hormones influence melanoma? Facts and controversies. *Clin Dermatol.* 2010; **28**:287–92.

26. Feucht KA, Walker MJ, DasGupta TK, Beattie CW. Effect of 17 beta-estradiol on the growth of estrogen receptor positive human melanoma in vitro and in athymic mice. *Cancer Res.* 1988;**48**:7093–101.

27. Lopez RE, Bhakoo H, Paolini NS, Rosen F, Holyoke ED, Goldrosen MH. Effect of estrogen on the growth of B-16 melanoma. *Surg Forum.* 1978;**29**:153–4.

28. Flowers JL, Seigler HF, McCarty KS Sr, Konrath J, McCarty KS Jr. Absence of estrogen receptor in human melanoma as evaluated by a monoclonal antiestrogen receptor antibody. *Arch Dermatol.* 1987;**123**:764–5.

29. Miller JG, Gee J, Price A, Garbe C, Wagner M, MacNeil S. Investigation of oestrogen receptors, sex steroids and soluble adhesion molecules in the progression of malignant melanoma. *Melanoma Res.* 1997;**7**: 197–208.

30. Duncan LM, Travers RL, Koerner FC, Mihm MC Jr, Sober AJ. Estrogen and progesterone receptor analysis in pregnancy-associated melanoma: absence of immunohistochemically detectable hormone receptors. *Hum Pathol.* 1994;**25**:36–41.

31. Ohata C, Tadokoro T, Itami S. Expression of estrogen receptor beta in normal skin, melanocytic nevi and malignant melanomas. *J Dermatol.* 2008;**35**:215–21.

32. de Giorgi V, Mavilia C, Massi D, et al. Estrogen receptor expression in cutaneous melanoma: a real-time reverse transcriptase-polymerase chain reaction and immunohistochemical study. *Arch Dermatol.* 2009;**145**:30–6.

33. Foucar E, Bentley TJ, Laube DW, Rosai J. A histopathologic evaluation of nevocellular nevi in pregnancy. *Arch Dermatol.* 1985;**121**:350–4.

34. Sanchez JL, Figueroa LD, Rodriguez E. Behaviour of melanocytic nevi during pregnancy. *Am J Dermatopathol.* 1984;**6** (suppl 1):89–91.

35. McManamny DS, Moss ALH, Pocock PV, Briggs. Melanoma and pregnancy: a long term follow-up. *Br J Obstet Gynaecol.* 1989;**96**:1419–23.

36. Slingnuff CL Jr, Reintgen D, Vollmer RT, Seigler HF. Malignant melanoma arising during pregnancy: a study of 100 patients. *Ann Surg.* 1990;**211**:552–7.

37. Travers RL, Sober AJ, Berwick M, Mihm MC Jr, Barnhill RL, Duncan LM. Increased thickness of pregnancy-associated melanoma. *Br J Dermatol.* 1995;**132**:876–83.

38. American Society of Plastic Surgeons. *Evidence-based clinical practice guideline: treatment of cutaneous melanoma.* Arlington Heights, IL: American Society of Plastic Surgeons; 2007.

39. Australian Cancer Network Melanoma Guidelines Revision Working Party. Clinical practice guidelines for the management of melanoma in Australia and New Zealand. *The Cancer Council Australia and Australian Cancer Network*, Sydney and New Zealand Guidelines Group, Wellington; 2008.

40. Scottish Intercollegiate Guidelines Network (SIGN). *Cutaneous melanoma. A national clinical guideline.* Edinburgh: SIGN; 2003.

41. Dummer R, Panizzon R, Bloch PH, Burg G; Task Force Skin Cancer. Updated Swiss guidelines for the treatment and follow-up of cutaneous melanoma. *Dermatology.* 2005;**210**:39–44.

42. Haigh PI, DiFronzo LA, McCready DR. Optimal excision margins for primary cutaneous melanoma: a systematic review and meta-analysis. *Can J Surg.* 2003;**46**:419–26.

43. Sladden MJ, Balch C. Barzilai DA, et al. Surgical excision margins for primary cutaneous melanoma. *Cochrane Database Syst Rev.* 2009;**4**:CD004835.

44. Lens MB, Nathan P, Bataille V. Excision margins for primary cutaneous melanoma: updated pooled analysis of randomized controlled trials. *Arch Surg.* 2007;**142**:885–91.

45. Balch CM, Soong SJ, Smith T, et al. Long-term results of a prospective surgical trial comparing 2 cm vs. 4 cm excision margins for 740 patients with 1–4 mm melanomas. *Ann Surg Oncol.* 2001;**8**:101–8.

46. Lens M. Sentinel lymph node biopsy in melanoma patients. *J Eur Acad Dermatol Venereol.* 2010;**24**:1005–12.

47. Morton DL, Thompson JF, Cochran AJ, et al. Sentinel-node biopsy or nodal observation in melanoma. *N Engl J Med.* 2006;**355**:1307–17.

48. Marsden JR, Newton-Bishop JA, Burrows L, et al. Revised U.K. guidelines for the management of cutaneous melanoma. *Br J Dermatol.* 2010;**163**:238–56.

49. Kirkwood JM, Manola J, Ibrahim J, et al. A pooled analysis of eastern cooperative oncology group and intergroup trials of adjuvant high-dose interferon for melanoma. *Clin Cancer Res.* 2004;**10**:1670–7.

50. Wheatley K, Ives N, Eggermont A, et al. Interferon-alpha as adjuvant therapy for melanoma: an individual patient data meta-analysis of randomized trials. [Abstract]. *J Clin Oncol.* 2007;**25**:8526.

51. Mocellin S, Pasquali S, Rossi CR, Nitti D. Interferon alpha adjuvant therapy in patients with high-risk melanoma: a systematic review and meta-analysis. *J Natl Cancer Inst.* 2010;**102**:493–501.

52. Hiratsuka M, Minakami H, Koshizuka S, Sato I. Administration of interferon-alpha during pregnancy: effects on fetus. *J Perinatal Med.* 2000;**28**:372–6.

53. Mubarak AAS, Kakil IR, Awidi A, et al. Normal outcome of pregnancy in chronic myeloid leukemia treated with interferon-alpha in 1st trimester: report of 3 cases and review of the literature. *Am J Hematol.* 2002;**69**:115–8.

54. Melillo L, Tieghi A, Candoni A, et al. Outcome of 122 pregnancies in essential thrombocythemia patients: a report from the Italian registry. *Am J Hematol.* 2009;**84**:636–40.

55. Pons JC, Lebon P, Frydman R, Delfraissy JF. Pharmacokinetics of interferon-alpha in pregnant women and fetoplacental passage. *Fetal Diagn Ther.* 1995;**10**:7–10.

56. Williams JM, Schlesinger PE, Gray AG. Successful treatment of essential thrombocythaemia and recurrent abortion with alpha interferon. *Br J Haematol.* 1994;**88**:647–8.

57. Grange JD, Abergel A, Amiot X, et al. Treatment of chronic hepatitis C with interferon alpha before pregnancy. *Gastroenterology.* 1995;**108**(suppl):A1075.

58. Hauschild A, Gogas H, Tarhini A, et al. Practical guidelines for the management of interferon-alpha-2b side effects in patients receiving adjuvant treatment for melanoma: expert opinion. *Cancer.* 2008;**112**:982–94.

59. International Federation of Gynecology and Obstetrics. Staging announcement: FIGO staging of gynecologic cancers: cervical and vulva. *Int J Gynecol Cancer.* 1995;**5**:319.

60. Wornom IL III, Smith JW, Soong SJ, Urist MM, Balch CM. Surgery as palliative treatment for distant metastases of melanoma. *Ann Surg.* 1986;**204**:181–5.

61. Overett TK, Shiu MH. Surgical treatment of distant metastatic melanoma: indications and results. *Cancer.* 1985;**56**:1222–30.

62. Gutman H, Hess KR, Kokotsakis JA, Ross MI, Guinee VF, Balch CM. Surgery for abdominal metastases of cutaneous melanoma. *Worl J Surg.* 2001;**25**:750–8.

63. Nicholson HO. Cytotoxic drugs in pregnancy: review of reported cases. *J Obstet Gynaecol Br Commonw.* 1968;**75**:307–12.

64. Doll DC, Ringenberg QS, Yarbro JW. Management of cancer during pregnancy. *Arch Intern Med.* 1988;**48**:2058–64.

65. Zemlickis D, Lishner M, Koren G. Review of fetal effects of cancer chemotherapeutic agents. In: Koren G, Lishner M, Farine D, editors. *Cancer in pregnancy.* 1st ed.

Cambridge: Press Syndicate of the University of Cambridge; 1996. p. 168.

66. Blatt J, Milvihill JJ, Ziegler JL, Young RC, Poplack DG. Pregnancy outcome following cancer chemotherapy. *Am J Med.* 1980;**39**:828–32.

67. Aviles A, Diaz-Maqueo JC, Talavera A, Guzman R, Garcia EL. Growth and development of children of mothers treated with chemotherapy during pregnancy: current status of 43 children. *Am J Hematol.* 1991;**36**:243–8.

68. Toussi T, Blais M, Langevin P, Ngassam P, Gelinas-MacKay C. Metastatic melanoma treated in a pregnant woman: pre- and postnatal implications. *Union Med Can.* 1974;**103**:1968–73.

69. Harkin KP, Drumm JE, O'Brien P, Daly A. Metastatic malignant melanoma in pregnancy. *Ir Med J.* 1990;**83**:116–7.

70. DiPaola RS, Goodin S, Ratzell M, Florczyk M, Karp G, Ravikumar TS. Chemotherapy for metastatic melanoma during pregnancy. *Gynecol Oncol.* 1997;**66**:526–30.

71. Ishida I, Yamaguchi Y, Tanemura A, et al. Stage III melanoma treated with chemotherapy after surgery during the second trimester of pregnancy. *Arch Dermatol.* 2009;**145**:346–8.

72. Gottschalk N, Jacobs VR, Hein R, et al. Advanced metastatic melanoma during pregnancy: a multidisciplinary challenge. *Onkologie.* 2009;**32**:748–51.

73. Lens MB, Rosdahl I, Ahlbom A, et al. Effect of pregnancy on survival in women with cutaneous malignant melanoma. *J Clin Oncol.* 2004;**22**:4369–75.

74. Driscoll MS, Grant-Kels JM. Hormones, nevi, and melanoma: an approach to the patient. *J Am Acad Dermatol.* 2007;**57**:919–31.

75. Adami HO, Thorn M, Bergstrom R, Lambe M. Melanoma in pregnancy. *Lancet.* 1991;**337**:1164–5.

76. Grin CM, Driscoll MS, Grant-Kels JM. Pregnancy and the prognosis of malignant melanoma. *Semin Oncol.* 1996;**23**:734–6.

77. Squatrito RC, Harlow SP. Melanoma complicating pregnancy. *Obstet Gynecol Clin North Am.* 1998;**25**:407–16.

78. Alexander A, Samlowski WE, Grossman D, et al. Metastatic melanoma in pregnancy: risk of transplacental metastases in the infant. *J Clin Oncol.* 2003;**21**:2179–86.

Chapter

10

Non-Hodgkin's lymphoma during pregnancy

David Pereg and Michael Lishner

Introduction

The coexistence of non-Hodgkin's lymphoma (NHL) and pregnancy is a rare event [1]. However, the occurrence of NHL during pregnancy might increase due to evidence suggesting a high incidence of AIDS-related NHL in younger patients in developing countries [2]. The management of the pregnant woman with NHL is a challenge to the physician because it may be associated with harmful effects on the fetus. On the other hand, the most common histological NHL subtypes during pregnancy are aggressive, albeit often curable; however, they can be rapidly progressive if not treated properly. Hence, management of the pregnant woman with NHL should be multi-disciplinary to optimize the mother's chance for cure and allow delivery of a healthy child.

Diagnosis and staging

For data regarding the diagnosis and staging of lymphoma, the reader is referred to the chapter on Hodgkin's lymphoma.

Treatment
Indolent NHL

Indolent NHL includes follicular lymphoma and chronic lymphocytic leukemia/small lymphocytic lymphoma, which are extremely rare during pregnancy. The indolent NHL subtypes are characterized by a slow clinical course, and because they are not curable with standard chemotherapy, treatment is usually delayed until the patient is symptomatic. Therefore, administration of chemotherapy during the first trimester is usually unnecessary. Most patients can be followed closely without therapy until delivery. When treatment is indicated, the CVP regimen, which is actually CHOP without doxorubicin is at least as safe and may be administered during the second and third trimesters. There are no reports regarding treatment with fludarabine during pregnancy, however, because anti-metabolites tend to be more teratogenic than other anticancer drugs, its use should be avoided if possible. The use of radiolabeled monoclonal antibodies is contraindicated due to high fetal radiation exposure.

Among the different indolent NHL, gastric MALT lymphoma is considered a separate entity due to its well-recognized association with *Helicobacter pylori* infection and the

Cancer in Pregnancy and Lactation: The Motherisk Guide ed. Gideon Koren and Michael Lishner.
Published by Cambridge University Press. © Cambridge University Press 2011.

relatively high remission rates after its eradication. The first line regimen for *H. pylori* eradication is the combination of clarithromycin, amoxicillin, and a proton pump inhibitor (PPI). As with all other indolent lymphomas, treatment during the first trimester is usually not mandatory. However, because there are abundant data regarding fetal safety of penicillins, macrolides, and PPIs, it seems that *H. pylori* eradication therapy can safely be administered during pregnancy [3,4].

Aggressive NHL

Aggressive NHL, which includes large B-cell lymphomas, mantle cell lymphoma, and mature T-cell and NK-cell neoplasms, represents the majority of NHL cases diagnosed during gestation. Because of the aggressive course of these lymphomas, most patients should be treated promptly with intensive combination chemotherapy. The CHOP regimen (cyclophosphamide, doxorubicin, vincristine, and prednisone) usually in combination with rituximab has commonly been used to treat patients with diffuse large B-cell lymphoma. According to existing data, based mainly on case reports, 41 patients were treated with CHOP for diffuse large B cell lymphoma during pregnancy. There were no reports of severe fetal malformation, even in the 4 cases in which CHOP was given in the first trimester [1,5–8]. However, further studies are needed to evaluate the safety of CHOP during the first trimester, and as with all other multi-drug regimens, therapeutic abortion should be strongly considered. The existing data suggest that CHOP treatment during the second and third trimesters is safe and not associated with adverse fetal outcomes. This relatively limited information is further supported by several reports on pregnant patients with breast cancer treated with other chemotherapy regimens that share major similarities with CHOP. These regimens were based on a combination of an alkylating agent with an anthracycline, and their administration during the second and third trimesters showed neither congenital anomalies nor growth restriction [5–8].

Rituximab is a chimeric anti-CD20 monoclonal B-cell depleting antibody indicated mainly for diffuse large B cell lymphoma (in combination with CHOP) and active refractory rheumatoid arthritis. A recent study has described 231 pregnancies associated with maternal rituximab exposure [9]. Maternal indications included lymphoma, autoimmune cytopenias, and other autoimmune diseases. Most cases were confounded by concomitant use of potentially teratogenic medications (most commonly methotrexate). Of 153 pregnancies with known outcomes, 90 resulted in live births. First-trimester miscarriages were reported in 33 (21%) cases, and 28 pregnancies were electively terminated (reasons for termination were not described). Twenty-two infants were born prematurely, with 1 neonatal death at 6 weeks. Eleven neonates had hematological abnormalities, and none of them had corresponding infections. Two congenital malformations were identified: clubfoot in 1 twin, and cardiac malformation in a singleton birth. One maternal death from pre-existing severe autoimmune thrombocytopenia occurred. Based on the available limited experience, it seems that the combination of R-CHOP may be considered safe for treating diffuse large B-cell lymphoma during the second and third trimesters.

Among patients diagnosed near the end of the first trimester, a more conservative approach may be considered. Treatment options in these patients include localized radiation therapy for limited cervical disease or close observation until the end of the first trimester followed by treatment with R-CHOP. However, this option should be limited to patients with stage 1–2 NHL with low volume disease, especially with a normal LDH level and low Ki-67 on biopsy. Patients in early stage NHL but with high burden disease are not candidates for this conservative option and should be treated with full-dose chemotherapy soon after pregnancy termination.

Very aggressive NHL

This group includes precursor (B or T) lymphoblastic leukemia/lymphoma and Burkitt's lymphoma. Due to their aggressive course and poor prognosis, treatment for aggressive lymphomas should be initiated immediately after diagnosis even during the first trimester. The pregnant patient must be informed about the high teratogenic risk, and pregnancy termination should be strongly recommended. Most chemotherapy regimens for very aggressive lymphomas include high-dose methotrexate, which among the currently used anticancer drugs, poses the greatest risk to the developing fetus when administered during the first trimester. Based on the limited data available, it seems that treatment with methotrexate during the second and third trimesters is not teratogenic but can cause severe fetal myelosuppression [1,8]. It has not been determined whether conventional chemotherapy for Burkitt's and lymphoblastic lymphomas, including high-dose methotrexate can be safely administered during the second and third trimesters. Nevertheless, the intensive anticancer regimens that are given to patients with very aggressive NHL are associated with many side effects including severe infections that may also lead to adverse pregnancy outcomes.

Prognosis and outcome

When an appropriate chemotherapy regimen is given, the survival rates of pregnant patients with NHL are similar to those of nonpregnant controls matched for grade [7]. The incidence of spontaneous abortions and prematurity does not appear to be affected by pregnancy-associated NHL [10]. However, there may be a trend toward a lower birth weight in infants born to mothers who had NHL during pregnancy [7].

Placental involvement in pregnancy-associated NHL is extremely rare, but a single case of dissemination to the fetus has been reported [11].

References

1. Pereg D, Koren G, Lishner M. The treatment of Hodgkin's and non-Hodgkin's lymphoma in pregnancy. *Haematologica*. 2007;**92**:1230–7.

2. Diamond C, Taylor TH, Aboumrad T, Anton-Culver H. Changes in acquired immunodeficiency syndrome-related non-Hodgkin lymphoma in the era of highly active antiretroviral therapy: incidence, presentation, treatment, and survival. *Cancer*. 2006;**106**:128–35.

3. Lynch CM, Sinnott JT IV, Holt DA, Herold AH. Use of antibiotics during pregnancy. *Am Fam Physician*. 1991;**43**:1365–8.

4. Gill SK, O'Brien L, Einarson TR, Koren G. The safety of proton pump inhibitors (PPIs) in pregnancy: a meta-analysis. *Am J Gastroenterol*. 2009;**104**:1541–5.

5. Azim HA, Pavlidis N, Peccatori FA. Treatment of the pregnant mother with cancer: A systematic review on the use of cytotoxic, endocrine, targeted agents and immunotherapy during pregnancy. Part 2: Hematological malignancies. *Cancer Treat Rev*. 2010;**36**:110–21.

6. Cardonick E, Iacobucci A. Use of chemotherapy during human pregnancy. *Lancet Oncol*. 2004;**5**:283–91.

7. Lishner M, Zemlickis D, Sutcliffe SB, Koren G. Non-Hodgkin's lymphoma and pregnancy. *Leuk Lymphoma*. 1994;**14**:411–3.

8. Aviles A, Neri N. Hematological malignancies and pregnancy: a final report of 84 children who received chemotherapy in utero. *Clin Lymphoma*. 2001;**2**:173–7.

9. Chakravarty EF, Murray ER, Kelman A, Farmer P. Pregnancy outcomes after maternal exposure to rituximab. *Blood.* 2011;**117**:1499–506.

10. Zuazu J, Julia A, Sierra J, et al. Pregnancy outcome in hematologic malignancies. *Cancer.* 1991;**67**:703–9.

11. Meguerian-Bedoyan Z, Lamant L, Hopfner C, Pulford K, Chittal S, Delsol G. Anaplastic large cell lymphoma of maternal origin involving the placenta: case report and literature survey. *Am J Surg Pathol.* 1997; **21**:1236–41.

Chapter

11

Ovarian tumors and pregnancy

Rinat Hackmon

Introduction

Ovarian cancer is the second most frequent gynecologic cancer complicating pregnancy [1–4]. Although the overall incidence of ovarian cancer in pregnancy is low, the increased use of ultrasound in early fetal evaluation has led to more frequent findings of adnexal mass in pregnancy. The estimated incidence of ovarian masses detected during pregnancy is approximately 1% and 2%. Approximately 2%–3% of these adnexal masses are true malignant neoplasms [2,4–10]. As child-bearing among older women increases, so likely will the incidence of the diagnosis of cancer in pregnancy. Indeed, during the past 2 decades, in the Western hemisphere, the birth rate among women older than 30 years has increased [4,6].

Diagnosis

Significant numbers of patients are asymptomatic and are found to have an adnexal mass, mostly detected during routine ultrasound and less frequently detected during routine physical examination or during cesarean delivery. Because pregnant women are more subjected to routine examination than the general population, the disease is diagnosed at earlier stages [2,11–14]. Other presenting symptoms include abdominal pain, increasing abdominal girth, obstructed labor, and emergency laparatomy due to torsion or rupture of the mass [11–14].

Adnexal masses during pregnancy are managed according to characteristics of the mass, the sonographic appearance, gestational age, and patient's symptoms.

Pelvic ultrasound (US) remains the mainstay of evaluations of the adnexae [14]. High-resolution transabdominal and transvaginal ultrasounds are usually the initial imaging tool and essential diagnostic modality [11,15]. Many of those masses undergo spontaneous resolution in the second and third trimester, thus the incidence of such adnexal masses gradually decreases with advancing gestational age [14]. Therefore, the highest incidence of adnexal masses in pregnancy is during the first trimester. The American Institute of Ultrasound in Medicine includes the evaluation of the adnexae as part of the first trimester ultrasound evaluation. Observation and repeat ultrasound at 14 to 16 weeks gestational age to document resolution is appropriate for low-risk benign-appearing tumors.

Various sonographic scoring systems of the adnexal mass may include features that have been associated with ovarian malignancies, such as bilaterality, heterogeneous solid component, papillary structure, septations, size > 7 cm, low-resistance blood flow, and ascites [14]. No single system has shown superiority in detection to become the standard approach. An experienced sonographer remains one of the best available modalities [16]. Thus it is recommended that any complex lesion should be scanned or re-scanned by a fully trained sonographer [14]. Improvement in Doppler ultrasound technology for evaluation of tumor vascularity has been used lately as a predictor of malignancy. Neovascularization of malignancies is known to cause increased blood flow and decreased vascular resistance. Identification of a centrally located vessel within a solid component or papillation can be a strong predictor of malignancy [17].

Overall, the US modality may be associated with false-positive diagnosis of ovarian masses, but it remains fairly accurate in diagnosing benign masses, therefore reassuring the patient and the clinician [14,15].

Magnetic resonance imaging (MRI) may be used as an additional diagnostic imaging tool in more complex conditions, such as displacement of the ovaries up into the abdomen when the pregnant uterus is growing, or in metastatic disease, or in other diagnostic uncertainty. Unlike the US and MRI modalities, computed tomography (CT) suggests radiation exposure to the developing fetus. The highest dosage of fetal exposure reported is during pelvic CT: 2000 millirem [5]. As such, this modality should be reserved only when absolutely necessary, such as when essential to the case management [5,14].

In nonpregnant women, the epithelial ovarian tumor marker CA125 serves as a non-specific diagnostic marker for epithelial ovarian cancer, but mainly as a method for evaluation of the response of the tumor to therapy, when initially elevated. Unfortunately, pregnancy is one of the conditions during which CA125 levels are physiologically increased; thus, this is less contributory to the diagnosis and the indication of progression of the underlying disease [4].

Staging and grading

Stages referred to in this chapter are similar to those defined by the International Federation of Gynaecology and Obstetrics (FIGO) for ovarian epithelial carcinoma. It is noteworthy, that staging during pregnancy may be technically unsatisfactory (mainly of the pelvis area) and post-delivery re-staging may be warranted. Most patients with ovarian cancer diagnosed during pregnancy have disease confined to the pelvis or abdomen. Staging is primarily surgical. To establish a diagnosis of a suspicious adnexal mass, definitive histological evidence should be obtained (low malignant vs. epithelial malignant) and grading determined: differentiation of dissemination, infiltration, and localization [13].

Pathology and biology

The vast majority of adnexal masses are benign and are diagnosed at an early stage when the disease is still confined to the ovary [14]. Recently in a large retrospective review, Leiserowitz et al. report 9,375 cases of adnexal masses associated with pregnancy. Overall, 202 of 9,375 were either borderline or malignant tumors. Of them, 87 (0.93%) were diagnosed as cancer, as opposed to low malignant potential (LMP): 50.6% of the ovarian cancers were epithelial, as were 100% of the LMP ovarian tumors. An additional 39% (34 of 87) were germ cell tumors, mostly dysgerminomas [14] and malignant teratoma [12]. Pseudomyxoma peritonei was identified in 8 patients with ovarian cancer. Dysgerminoma and malignant teratomas accounted for 76.5% of all germ cells tumors [6]. The relative frequency of tumor types reflects the young age of presentation. Depending on the series, germ cell tumors are either the most common or second only to epithelial tumors [18–20]. The epithelial tumors tend to be early stage and low grade, although advanced stage tumors have been reported [21–23]. Endodermal sinus tumors have also been reported [6,24,25]. Tumor types tend to be confined to the ovary (approximately 80%) at the time of diagnosis in pregnancy. Ten retrospective cases of serous neoplasms of low malignant potential, resected during pregnancy, were reported with clinical and microscopic features suggesting aggressive behavior. However, these features subsided significantly after delivery, and years after, all patients are still alive with no evidence of disease [26]. Sex cord–stromal tumor types that have been described include granulosa, Sertoli-Leydig, and "unclassified" [27]. The differential diagnosis of sex cord–stromal tissues includes other benign conditions that can mimic malignancy. These conditions include luteoma of pregnancy, luteinized follicular cyst, granulosa cell prolif-erations, hilus cell hyperplasia, and ectopic decidua [14,19,24]. These conditions are characterized by regression after pregnancy. There is no evidence that pregnancy alters the course or affects the prognosis of pure dysgerminoma [28,29]. However, the prognosis of non-dysgerminoma germ cell tumors associated with pregnancy may be uncertain, because 2 fatal cases of rapidly progressive disease during the second trimester were described in the literature [29].

Management

For optimal management of a suspected malignant adnexal tumor, a multidisciplinary approach must be taken. A shared decision between the patient and a surgical oncologist, an obstetrician, pathologist, and a pediatrician should be the state of art [6,13].

Acute symptoms including pain, guarding, or trauma associated with a suspicious ovarian tumor may increase the likelihood of complications (torsion, hemorrhage, or rupture). Surgery should be immediately considered, and the approach should be the same as in non-emergency context [13].

Surgery should only be considered in pregnancy for suspicious ultrasound appearances of masses, obvious tumors, or acute symptoms as mentioned above.

The surgical procedure is diagnostic but can be also part of therapy: (1) Diagnostic: providing definitive histological evidence regarding type and malignancy potential (low vs. high) and grading (localized vs. disseminative); (2) Therapeutic: initial treatment (surgery or chemotherapy) [13].

Surgical exploration using a midline incision at 16–18 weeks gestation is recommended.

For benign pathology, cystectomy is warranted. A frozen section diagnosis must be made to guide further decisions. Careful examination of both ovaries is essential as well as standard surgical exploration and staging for more advanced cancers.

Confirmed low malignant potential

Confirmed low malignant potential lesions, such as borderline tumors and non-epithelial neoplasm (germ-cell, sex-cord), are usually diagnosed in stage I. They can be treated by midline laparotomy with unilateral salpingo-oophorectomy, omentectomy, peritoneal cytology, and biopsy. In borderline tumors in selected cases, laparoscopy can be performed [12]. A super-conservative treatment (cystectomy alone) should only be indicated in a patient with 1 ovary or with bilateral borderline tumor. If this borderline tumor is revealed by the histology of a surgical specimen, it seems reasonable, considering the good prognosis, to defer surgical treatment until after delivery [13]. Surgical staging should be completed 3–6 weeks after delivery [30,31].

Invasive epithelial ovarian carcinoma

1. Low-stage low-grade: surgical staging similar to borderline.
2. Low stage intermediate grade: lymphadenectomy and adjuvant-platin based chemotherapy are mandatory.
3. Upstaged cases: paclitaxel and platinum chemotherapy during pregnancy and final surgery after delivery is needed.
4. Advanced-stage ovarian tumors: there are different approaches as follows:

    A) Before 24 weeks termination of pregnancy and primary debulking; B) Delivery; C) Expectant management; D) Surgery during pregnancy followed by postpartum chemotherapy; E) Surgery and chemotherapy during pregnancy followed by final surgery postdelivery.

There are reported cases of successful pregnancy and preservation of normal ovarian function, in cases of advanced-stage metastatic low malignant potential tumors, treated by successful tumor debulking [32,33]. For those patients with advanced disease, decisions regarding debulking procedures should take into account fetal viability, patient health, and patient desires at the time of surgery. Hysterectomy during pregnancy is rarely indicated unless it contributes significantly to tumor debulking. A retrospective study of 174 patients undergoing adnexal surgery during pregnancy showed no evidence of increasing risk of fetal loss when surgery was performed after the seventh week of gestation [34].

Chemotherapy

Paclitaxel–carboplatin chemotherapy until fetal maturity is the regimen of choice in ovarian cancer.

Cancer chemotherapeutic drugs are potentially very potent teratogens. There are no sufficient data regarding the teratogenicity of most cytotoxic drugs. Almost all cytotoxic drugs are capable of crossing the placenta [35].

Chemotherapy in the first trimester may increase the risk of spontaneous abortions, fetal death, and major malformation [5]. The risk for major malformations during this period is 10% for single-agent chemotherapy and 25% for combination therapy [36]. The second trimester is not associated with teratogenic effects but increases the risk for intrauterine growth retardation, intrauterine fetal death, and low birth weight [37].

Most germ cell tumors and invasive epithelial carcinoma require adjuvant chemotherapy with the exception of low-grade and stage IA ovarian malignancies. Given the poor prognosis of ovarian malignancy, treatment is seldom delayed in affected patients [35].

The decision to use chemotherapy while in pregnancy should be weighed against the risk of delayed maternal treatment on maternal survival.

The knowledge on pregnancy outcome following bleomycin, etoposide, and cisplatin for germ cell tumors during pregnancy is still scarce. Small cases series and case reports of this regimen for malignant germ cell tumors have been published with an overall impression of good neonatal outcome [38–41].

When chemotherapy is administered during pregnancy, timing of delivery of the infant should take into account the expected bone marrow depression and potential problems such as bleeding or infections. Self-limiting fetal hematopoietic depression has been described and the neonate should be monitored for this complication [35]. Furthermore, neonates, especially preterm babies, have limited capacities to metabolize and eliminate drugs due to liver immaturity. The delay of delivery after chemotherapy will allow fetal drug excretion by means of the placenta (65).

Long-term neurodevelopmental complications of *in utero* chemotherapy exposure have not been extensively studied. Other concerns are childhood malignancy and long-term fertility. Data regarding late effect of chemotherapy on children's neurodevelopment, malignancy, and fertility are limited and are based mainly on retrospective reports [42,43]. However, the general impression based on the available data suggests that chemotherapy does not have a major impact on these outcomes [5].

Prognosis

There is no evidence that pregnancy alters the prognosis of ovarian tumors compared to the nonpregnant population when patients are matched for tumor histology and stage. Leiserowitz *et al.* in their large series report a low maternal mortality rate of 4.7% at 2.4 years follow-up [4,6]. Thus, in general, pregnant patients with ovarian cancer have a better prognosis overall due to the age-related tumor distribution and early stage of diagnosis in a significant number of patients [4,44].

Lactation

Cytotoxic agents administered systemically may reach significant levels in breast milk and thus breastfeeding while on chemotherapy is contraindicated. A similar situation exists for the use of radioiodine.

References

1. Boulay R, Podczaski E. Ovarian cancer complicating pregnancy. *Obst Gynecol Clinic North Am.* 1998;**25**:385–99.

2. Oheler MK, Wain GV, Brand A. Gynaecological malignancies in pregnancy: a review. *Aust N Z J Obstet Gynecol.* 2003;**43**:414–20.

3. Zanotti KS, Belinson JL, Kennedy AW. Treatment of gynaecologic cancers in pregnancy. *Semin Oncol.* 2000;**27**:686–98.

4. Palmer J, Vatish M, Tidy J. Epithelial ovarian cancer in pregnancy: a review of the literature. *BJOG.* 2009;**116**:480–91.

5. Pereg D, Koren G, Lishner M. Cancer in pregnancy: Gaps, challenges and solutions. *Cancer Treat Rev.* 2008;**34**:302–12.

6. Leiserowitz GS, Xing G, Cress R, Brahmbhatt B, Darlympe JL, Smith LH. Adnexal masses in pregnancy: how often are they malignant? *Gynecol Oncol.* 2006;**101**:315–321.

7. Goff BA, Paley PJ, Koh W-J, Petersdorf SH, Douglas JG, Greer BE. Cancer in the pregnant patient. In: Hoskins WJ, Perez CA, Young RC, editors. *Principles and practice of gynecologic oncology.* 3rd ed. Philadelphia: Lipincott Williams and Wilkins; 2000 p. 501–28.

8. Whitecar MP, Turner S, Higby MK. Adnexal masses in pregnancy: a review of 130 cases undergoing surgical management. *Am J Obstet Gynecol.* 1999;**181**:19–24.

9. Agarwal N, Parul, Kriplani A, Bhatla N, Gupta A. Management and outcome of pregnancies complicated with adnexal masses. *Arch Gynecol Obstet.* 2003;**267**:148–52.

10. Machado F, Vegas C, Leon J, et al. Ovarian cancer during pregnancy: analysis of 15 cases. *Gynecol Oncol.* 2007;**105**:446–50.

11. Norton JA, Levin B, Jensen RT. Cancer of the endocrine system. In: DeVita VT, Hellman S, Rosenberg SA, editors. *Cancer: principles and practice of oncology.* 4th ed. Philadelphia: Lippincott, Williams, and Wilkins; 2001.

12. Amant F, Brepoels L, Halaska M, Gziri MM, Calsteren KV. Gynaecologic cancer complicating pregnancy: An overview. *Best Pract Res Clin Obstet Gynaecol.* 2010;**24**:61–79.

13. Marret H, Lhomme C, Lecuru F, et al. Guidelines for the management of ovarian cancer during pregnancy. *Eur J Obstet Gynecol.* 2010;**149**:18–21.

14. Schwartz N, Timor-Tristch IE, Wang E. Adnexal masses in Pregnancy. *Clin Obstet Gynecol.* 2009;**52**:570–85.

15. Bromley B, Benacerraf B. Adnexal masses during pregnancy: accuracy of sonographic diagnosis and outcome. *J Ultrasound Med.* 1997;**16**:447–52; quiz 453–4.

16. Ameye L, Valentin L, Testa AC, et al. A scoring system to differentiate malignant from benign masses in specific ultrasound-based subgroups of adnexal tumors. *Ultrasound Obstet Gynecol.* 2009;**33**:92–101.

17. Gurriero S, Alcazar JL, Coccia ME, et al. Complex pelvic mass as a target of evaluation of vessel distribution by color Doppler sonography for the diagnosis of adnexal malignancies: results of a multicenter European study. *J Ultrasound Med.* 2002;**21**:1105–11.

18. Beischer NA, Buttery BW, Fortune DW, Macafee CA. Growth and malignancy of ovarian tumors in pregnancy. *Aust N Z Obstet Gynaecol.* 1971;**11**:208–20.

19. Dgani R, Shoham Z, Atar E, Zosmer A, Lancet M. Ovarian carcinoma during pregnancy: a study of 23 cases in Israel between the years 1960 and 1984. *Gynecol Oncol.* 1989;**33**:326–31.

20. Creasman WT, Rutledge F, Smith JP. Carcinoma of the ovary associated with pregnancy. *Obstet Gynecol.* 1971;**38**:111–6.

21. Munnell EW. Primary ovarian cancer associated with pregnancy. *Clin Obstet Gynecol.* 1963;**6**:983–93.

22. Rosvoll R, Winship T. Thyroid carcinoma and pregnancy. *Surg Gynecol Obstet.* 1965;**121**:1039–42.

23. Gustafsson DC, Kottmeier HL. Carcinoma of the cervix associated with pregnancy. *Acta Obstet Gynecol Scand.* 1962;**41**:1–21.

24. El-Yahia AR, Rahman J, Rahman MS, al-Suleiman SA. Ovarian tumors in pregnancy. *Aust N Z J Obstet Gynecol.* 1991;**31**:327–30.

25. Shivvers SA, Miller DS. Preinvasive and invasive breast and cervical cancer prior to or during pregnancy. *Clin Perinatol.* 1997;**24**:369–89.

26. Mooney J, Silva E, Tornos C, Gershenson D. Unusual features of serous neoplasms of low malignant potential during pregnancy. *Gynecol Oncol.* 1997;**65**:30–5.

27. Ashkenazy M, Kessler I, Czernobilsky B, Nahshoni A, Lancet M. Ovarian tumors in pregnancy. *Int J Obstet Gynecol.* 1988;**27**:79–83.

28. Antonelli NM, Dotters DJ, Katz VL, Kuller JA. Cancer in pregnancy: a review of the literature. *Obstet Gynecol Survey.* 1996;**51**:125–34.

29. Bakri YN, Ezzat A, Akhta, Dohami, Zahrani. Malignant germ cell tumors of the ovary. Pregnancy considerations. *Eur J Obst Gynecol Reprod Biol.* 2000;**90**:87–91.

30. Yinon Y, Beiner M, Gotlieb W, Perri T, Ben-Baruch G. Clinical outcome of cystectomy compared with unilateral salpingo-oophorectomy as fertility-sparing treatment of borderline-ovarian tumors. *Fert Steril.* 2007;**88**:479–84.

31. Zanetta G, Mariani E, Lissoni A, et al. A prospective study of the role of ultrasound in the management of adnexal masses in pregnancy. *BJOG.* 2003;**110**:578–83.

32. Miller DM, Ehlen TG, Saleh EA. Successful term pregnancy following conservative debulking surgery for a stage IIIA serous low-malignant potential tumor of the

ovary: a case report. *Gynecol Oncol.* 1997;**66**:535–8.

33. Shibahara H, Wacimoto E, Mitsuo M, Ogasawara T, Takemura T, Koyana K. A case of a patient diagnosed with malignant mixed Mullerian tumor of the ovary who conceived after conservative surgery and adjuvant chemotherapy. *Gynecol Oncol.* 1997;**65**:363–5.

34. Wang PH, Chao HT, Yuan CC, Lee WL, Chao KC, Ng HT. Ovarian tumors complicating pregnancy. Emergency and elective surgery. *J Reprod Med.* 1999;**44**:279–87.

35. Ghemmaghami F, Hazanzadeh M. Good fetal outcome of pregnancies with gynecologic cancer conditions: cases and literature review *Int J Gynecol Cancer.* 2006;**16**(suppl 1):225–30.

36. Sivanesaratnam V. Management of the pregnant mother with malignant conditions. *Curr Opin Obstet Gynecol.* 2001;**13**:121–5.

37. Disaia PJ, Creasman WT *Clinical gynecology oncology.* St. Louis, MO: CV Mosby; 2002. p. 432–72.

38. Horbelt D, Delmore J, Meisel R, Cho S, Roberts D, Logan D. Mixed germ cell malignancy of the ovary concurrent with pregnancy. *Obstet Gynecol.* 1995;**84**:662–4.

39. Han JY, Nava-Ocampo AA, Kim TJ, Shim JU, Park CT. Pregnancy outcome after prenatal exposure to bleomycin, etoposide and cisplatin for malignant ovarian germ cell tumors: report of 2 cases. *Reprod Toxicol.* 2005;**19**:557–61.

40. Christman JE, Teng NNH, Lebovic GS, Sikic BL. Delivery of a normal infant following cisplatin, vinblastine, and bleomycin (PVB) chemotherapy for malignant teratoma of the ovary during pregnancy. *Gynecol Oncol.* 1990;**37**:292–5.

41. Buller RE, Darrow V, Manetta A, Porto M, DiSaia PJ. Conservative surgical management of dysgerminoma concomitant with pregnancy. *Obstet Gynecol.* 1992;**79**:887–90.

42. Aviles A, Neri N. Hematological malignancies and pregnancy: a final report of 84 children who received chemotherapy in utero. *Clin Lymphoma.* 2001;**2**:173–7.

43. Nulman I, Laslo D, Fried S, Uleryk E, Lishner M, Koren G. Neurodevelopment of children exposed in utero to treatment of maternal malignancy. *Br J Cancer.* 2001;**85**:1611–8.

44. Zemlickis D, Lishner M, Koren G. Review of fetal effects of cancer chemotherapeutic agents. In: Koren G, Lishner M, Farine D, editors. *Cancer in pregnancy.* 1st ed. New York: University of Cambridge; 1996. p. 231–2.

Thyroid cancer and pregnancy

12

Michael P. Tan

Introduction

Thyroid cancer is the most commonly diagnosed tumor of the endocrine glands and the second most frequent tumor among those diagnosed during pregnancy [1]. The differentiated thyroid cancer (DTC), subtypes papillary and follicular, often present with an indolent, asymptomatic course during pregnancy, and represent a significant proportion of all cancers in women of child-bearing age [2,3]. Approximately 10% of thyroid cancers that arose during the reproductive age are diagnosed during pregnancy or in the first year after delivery [4]. The prevalence in pregnancy ranges from 3.6 to 14 per 100,000 births. Medullary thyroid cancer (MTC) accounts for only approximately 5–10% of thyroid cancers. The clinical history of MTC is usually more aggressive than DTC [5].

Diagnosis

Thyroid gland changes that occur during pregnancy have been well described. An increase in size of the thyroid gland, up to 20–30%, may occur due to glandular hyperplasia and increased vascularity [1]. Thyroid stimulating activity has been demonstrated in the sera of normal pregnant women and has been shown to correlate with levels of human chorionic gonadotropin (hCG). The thyrotropic role of hCG is also supported by the observation that patients with trophoblastic tumors and hyperthyroidism have greatly increased hCG levels [6]. The presence of estrogen receptor alpha (ERα) in the majority of tumors diagnosed during pregnancy led to speculations that estrogen may also play a role in thyroid cancer growth by means of induction of the receptor expression and activation of intracellular signaling pathways [7]. Other changes include increased thyroxine-binding globulin (TBG), resulting in an increase in total triiodothyronine (T3) and thyroxine (T4). Free thyroid hormone levels increase slightly during the first trimester and then decrease but remains within the normal range for nonpregnant level [8].

DTC have a female predominance, approximately 2–3 times more frequent than in males. This had led some researchers to suspect that reproductive and hormonal factors play a role in increasing the risk for thyroid cancer. So far, inconsistent correlations have been found between DTC and factors such as number of parity, miscarriage during first pregnancy, artificial menopause, late age at menarche, late age at first or last birth, and oral contraceptive use [9–14]. The effect of pregnancy on the incidence of carcinoma in solitary

Cancer in Pregnancy and Lactation: The Motherisk Guide ed. Gideon Koren and Michael Lishner. Published by Cambridge University Press. © Cambridge University Press 2011.

thyroid nodules is also unclear. A few studies suggest that thyroid stimulation during both pregnancy and lactation may result in transient increase in risk of papillary thyroid cancer [7,12,15] especially among women diagnosed with thyroid cancer at a younger age [16].

Some series have reported a higher incidence of carcinoma in solitary nodules in pregnancy compared to the nonpregnant state, but this has not been substantiated in larger, well designed studies [17–19].

Kung *et al.* screened by means of real-time ultrasound pregnant women in the first trimester. Of 221 followed, only 34 (15.3%) patients had thyroid nodule. The group followed the growth of thyroid nodules by ultrasound in these women during the course of their pregnancy. The volume of the nodules was noted to increase during the study period, as well as development of new nodules. On biopsy, none were noted to be malignant nor have malignant changes occurred during the course of pregnancy [20]. The data in this study seem to suggest that pregnancy does not exacerbate the development of thyroid malignancy. Other studies showed 39–43% incidence of malignancy during pregnancy [18,19]. The later studies with high incidence recruited pregnant women with palpable neck nodules, whereas only 8 out of 54 nodules detected by ultrasound were palpable in the study by Kung *et al.*

Similar to the nonpregnant population, the presenting signs and symptoms of a well differentiated thyroid carcinoma are nonspecific. A solitary thyroid nodule is a common presentation. Other patients may report an increase in size of a pre-existing nodule, pain in the neck region, or hoarseness. The approach to thyroid nodules in pregnancy should be similar to the approach with nonpregnant patients [21].

Physical examination should be directed to the evaluation of the following characteristics of the nodule: size, consistency, mobility, and associated lymphadenopathy. Other signs such as a Horner's syndrome may be present. The thyroid function testing is usually normal in patients with cancer with the exception of medullary carcinoma where the serum calcitonin is elevated. Thyroiditis and a parathyroid lesion may be diagnosed with alterations in TSH, antithyroid antibodies, free T3,T4, and calcium levels.

Fine needle aspiration biopsy (FNAB) is recommended for thyroid nodules > 1 cm, preferably guided by ultrasound to minimize inadequate sampling [22]. It is the procedure of choice for histologic confirmation of a malignancy and has a diagnostic accuracy of 90% when diagnosing medullary or undifferentiated tumors, 80% for papillary tumors and 40% for follicular subtype [1]. For nodules detected before 20 weeks gestation, FNAB is recommended. It has been suggested that FNAB after 20 weeks gestation can be delayed until after pregnancy except for rapidly growing nodules or those that fail to suppress with thyroxine [19,24,25].

Ultrasound may be used to characterize the nodule (solid vs. cystic or mixed), detect other nodules missed on physical examination, measure nodule growth during pregnancy, and to guide the fine needle aspiration [1]. It has a low specificity for thyroid pathology. High-resolution, real-time ultrasound can be used to assess these patients [23]. Radionuclide scanning of the thyroid is rarely used in pregnancy.

Therapeutic abortion

There is no evidence that therapeutic abortion increases survival [26,27].

Staging

In this population, most patients present with well-differentiated, localized disease, and extensive staging investigations are not indicated. Due to the iodine concentrating abilities of the fetus, radioactive iodine for diagnosis is contraindicated during pregnancy. Decisions regarding the use of radiological investigations must take into account the age of the fetus and the estimated dose of radiation delivered with the respective imaging study. Magnetic resonance imaging may be preferred if benefit outweighs the risk.

Pathology and biology

Although isolated case reports exist describing rapid growth of papillary cancer during pregnancy, they appear to be the exception rather than the rule [28]. There are no data supporting altered tumor biology or more aggressive course of cancer during pregnancy [1,3].

Treatment

Surgery remains the treatment of choice for well-differentiated thyroid cancer. Due to the relatively indolent course but potential impact on long-term survival, therapy during pregnancy can be tailored to the stage of pregnancy. Thyroidectomy during pregnancy was not associated with worst maternal or neonatal outcome including preterm delivery [4]. A recent population-based study looking at outcome following thyroid and parathyroid surgery revealed an increased length of hospital stay and a 2-fold increase in complication rates (not specified) among pregnant women. However, factors contributing to the negative impact include Hispanic and black race, low surgeon volume, higher comorbidity, and government insurance [29]. For those presenting in the first trimester, surgery and general anesthesia can be delayed until the second trimester to reduce the risks associated with surgery to the fetus [1,19,21]. A few reports suggested that the risk of fetal loss related to surgery is minimal [30]. For those patients who present in the later stages of pregnancy with a well-differentiated tumor, surgery can usually be delayed safely until the postpartum period [3,22,31,32].

The use of postoperative radioiodine therapy in patients with well-differentiated thyroid cancer is controversial, although there is evidence that benefits include decreases in cancer death, tumor recurrence, and development of metastatic disease [33–35]. Radioiodine therapy is contraindicated during pregnancy as it can cross the placenta and cause fetal hypothyroidism and cretinism [36]. However, exposure before the 10 weeks of gestation is unlikely to cause fetal harm because the underdeveloped fetal thyroid is unable to take up iodine before this time [37]. It has been suggested that women receiving radioiodine should not become pregnant for at least 12 months post-therapy to ensure elimination of I-131, confirm disease remission, and allow stabilization of thyroid hormone level [22,38]. This should help avoid the higher miscarriage rate seen in the first few months after radioiodine treatment and/or surgery. The increase rate of miscarriage after treatment is thought to be due to inadequate control of thyroid hormone status after thyroidectomy/ablation [39,40]. Lin *et al.* suggested that an even shorter period does not result in demonstratable adverse effect toward subsequent pregnancies [41,42]. Other guidelines suggest avoiding pregnancy for 4–6 months after treatment is acceptable [21,22,38,43]. Several studies have shown that 1 year post-treatment of I-131(including high ablative dose), there was no evidence of increased spontaneous abortions, malformations, stillbirth, and cancer in offspring in subsequent pregnancies [40,42,44,45]. Approximately 12%–31% of women may experience changes in their menstruation post-treatment, as well as early menopause had been reported. Transient amenorrhea/oligomenorrhea may occur in 8%–27% of women but resolved within 1 year after radioiodine treatment [38].

Prior history of treatment for thyroid cancer in women of child-bearing age does not seem to cause exacerbation of this disease during pregnancy or in the pospartum period. Delivery of a healthy child after thyroidectomy and complementary treatment should be expected [46]. Postoperative treatment with exogenous thyroid hormone in suppressive doses is suggested to decrease recurrence [22,47].

Thyroxine treatment should be started immediately after surgery. Because it takes approximately 4 weeks for levothyroxine to alter the TSH level, a 4–6 weeks interval of TSH monitoring is advisable. Medication should be adjusted until the TSH stabilizes [43].

Benign or indeterminate cytology may be treated with observation or suppressive therapy using thyroxine until the pregnancy is completed. In general, malignant nodules do not suppress with exogenous thyroid hormone, although this is not absolute. Thyroxine is considered safe in pregnancy and adequate therapy should result in a suppressed but detectable TSH level [22,47]. However, the free T4 should be maintained in the upper nonpregnant normal range or trimester-specific normal pregnancy range if available, or total T4 to 1.5 times the normal nonpregnant range [22].

Treatment for undifferentiated cancer is more problematic and must be individualized to the patient and extent of disease. These aggressive cancers have a much worse prognosis and will not be discussed in this brief review. Treatment of metatastic follicular or papillary thyroid cancer is usually not curative. Palliation may occur with I-131, external beam radiation, suppressive exogenous thyroid hormone, and investigational protocols including chemotherapy.

Chemotherapy

Cancer chemotherapeutic drugs are very potent teratogens. There is very little information on the effect of cancer chemotherapy on the fetus. The risk of malformations when chemotherapy is administered in the first trimester has been estimated to be around 7.5–17% for single agent chemotherapy and 25% for combination chemotherapy [48,49]. Excluding concomitant irradiation and anti-folate medications, the risk of malformation for single agent chemotherapy exposure dropped to 6% [49]. It is generally suggested that chemotherapy be avoided during the first trimester, when cells are actively dividing. Use of these agents in the second and third trimesters has been associated with an increased risk of stillbirth, intrauterine growth retardation, and low birth weight [50,51]. When chemotherapy is administered during pregnancy, timing of delivery of the infant should take into account the potential for bone marrow depression and associated problems such as bleeding or infections. Self-limiting fetal hematopoietic depression after maternal exposure to chemotherapy has been described and the neonate should be monitored for complications of this [52]. Long-term neurodevelopmental complications of *in utero* chemotherapy exposure have not been extensively studied. Doxorubicin, bleomycin, and cisplatin have been the principal agents used for nonpregnant women with recurrent or inoperable or metastatic thyroid cancer [53]. In most cases, chemotherapy does not offer benefit to the pregnant woman to warrant the risk to the fetus [49]. Further details based on case reports can be found in Chapter 14, Chemotherapy During Pregnancy.

Prognosis

Although controversial, it appears that pregnancy does not alter the prognosis of well differentiated thyroid carcinoma. A retrospective cohort study with 61 patients with thyroid cancer diagnosed during pregnancy compared to 528 age-matched, nonpregnant controls found no statistical significant difference between the groups' cancer recurrence, distant recurrences, and cancer death [3]. Survival rates did not differ among pregnant and nonpregnant women [4,54]. In a population-based study, Yasmeen et al. compared the outcome of 595 pregnant women diagnosed with thyroid cancer (129 antepartum and 466 postpartum) to 2270 age-matched nonpregnant cohort and found similar survival rates between the groups [4]. Most studies that have examined this issue suffer from methodological problems such as limited sample size, limited length of follow-up, variable follow-up, non-standardized treatments, and inadequate control groups. Vannucchi et al. reported a poorer prognosis among pregnant women due to the negative iodine balance, several growth factors, and to the secretion of hormones with thyroid stimulatory activity such as chorionic gonadotropin and estrogen. However, the study had a small sample size, with a more advanced stage of cancer in the pregnant group and limited length of follow-up [7].

Fetal consequences

There is no evidence that fetal outcome is adversely affected by maternal thyroid cancer [4].

Lactation

Cytotoxic agents administered systemically may reach significant levels in breast milk; thus, breastfeeding while on chemotherapy is usually contraindicated.

Breastfeeding should be avoided for at least 120 days after receiving I-131 treatment [43]. However, the length of time that one should abstain from breastfeeding is dependent on the amount or dosage that the mother received and should be adjusted accordingly. Once an effective dose of <1 millisievert in breast milk has been reached, it is safe to resume breastfeeding [55].

Fertility

Fertility does not appear to be affected by thyroid cancer [38]. Current information based on follow-up studies of women having subsequent pregnancies after radioiodine treatment have failed to show statistically significant effects on chromosomal abnormalities, congenital malformation, and childhood malignancies [5].

References

1. Fanarjian N, Athavale SM, Herrero N, Fiorica J, Padhya TA. Thyroid cancer in pregnancy. *Laryngoscope.* 2007;**117**: 1777–81.

2. Parkin DM, Whelan SL, Ferlay J, et al. *Cancer incidence in five continents.* Vol VII. Lyon, IARC: IARC Sci Publ. No. 143, 1997.

3. Moosa M, Mazzaferri EL. Outcome of differentiated thyroid cancer diagnosed in pregnant women. *J Clin Endocrinol Metab.* 1997;**82**:2862–6.

4. Yasmeen S, Cress R, Romano PS, et al. Thyroid cancer in pregnancy. *Int J Gynecol Obstet.* 2005;**91**:15–20.

5. Zamperini P, Gibelli B, Gilardi D, Tradati N, Chiesa F. Pregnancy and thyroid cancer: ultrasound study of foetal thyroid. *Acta Otorhinolaryngol Ital.* 2009;**29**:339–44.

6. Yoshimura M, Hershman JM. Thyrotropic action of human chorionic gonadotropin. *Thyroid*. 1995;**5**:425–34.

7. Vannucchi G, Perrino M, Rossi S, et al. Clinical and molecular features of differentiated thyroid cancer diagnosed during pregnancy. *Eur J Endocrinol*. 2010;**162**:145–51.

8. Burrow GN, Fisher DA, Larsen PR. Mechanisms of disease: maternal and fetal thyroid function. *N Engl J Med*. 1994;**331**:1072–8.

9. Pham TM, Fujino Y, Mikami H, et al. Reproductive and menstrual factors and thyroid cancer among Japanese women: the Japan Collaborative Cohort Study. *J Womens Health (Larchmt)*. 2009;**18**:331–5.

10. Zivaljevic V, Vlajinac H, Jankovic R, et al. Case-control study of female thyroid cancer- menstrual, reproductive and hormonal factors. *Eur J Cancer Prev*. 2003;**12**:63–6.

11. Memon A, Darif M, Al-Saleh K, Suresh A. Epidemiology of reproductive and hormonal factors in thyroid cancer: evidence from a case-control study in the Middle East. *Int J Cancer*. 2002;**97**:82–9.

12. Rossing MA, Voigt LF, Wicklund KG, Daling JR. Reproductive factors and risk of papillary thyroid cancer in women. *Am J Epidemiol*. 2000;**151**:765–72.

13. Franceschi S, Fassina A, Talamini R, et al. The influence of reproductive and hormonal factors on thyroid cancer in women. *Rev Epidemiol Sante Publique*. 1990;**38**:27–34.

14. Levi F, Franceschi S, Gulie C, Negri E, La Vecchia C. Female thyroid cancer: the role of reproductive and hormonal factors in Switzerland. *Oncology*. 1993;**50**:309–15.

15. Mack WJ, Preston-Martin S, Bernstein L, Qian D, Xiang M. Reproductive and hormonal risk factors for thyroid cancer in Los Angeles County females. Cancer Epidemiol *Biomarkers Prev*. 1999;**8**:991–7.

16. Negri E, Dal Maso L, Ron E, et al. A pooled analysis of case-control studies of thyroid cancer. II. Menstrual and reproductive factors. *Cancer Causes Control*. 1999;**10**:143–55.

17. Cunningham MP, Slaughter DP. Surgical treatment of disease of the thyroid gland in pregnancy. *Surg Gynecol Obstet*. 1970;**131**:486–8.

18. Rosen IB, Walfish PG. Pregnancy as a predisposing factor in thyroid neoplasia. *Arch Surg*. 1986;**121**:1287–90.

19. Doherty C, Shindo M, Rice D, Montero M, Mestman JH. Management of thyroid nodules during pregnancy. *Laryngoscope*. 1995;**105**:251–5.

20. Kung AW, Chau MT, Lao TT, Tam SC, Low LC. The effect of pregnancy on thyroid nodule formation. *J Clin Endocrinol Metab*. 2002;**87**:1010–4.

21. Papini E, Negro R, Pinchera A, et al. Thyroid nodule and differentiated thyroid cancer management in pregnancy an Italian Association of Clinical Endocrinologists (AME) and Italian Thyroid Association (AIT) joint statement for clinical practice. *J Endocrinol Invest*. 2010;**33**:579–86.

22. Abalovich M, Amino N, Barbour LA, et al. Management of thyroid dysfunction during pregnancy and postpartum: an Endocrine Society Clinical Practice Guideline. *J Clin Endocrinol Metab*. 2007;**92**(suppl):S1–S47.

23. Solbiati L, Charboneau JW, James EM, Hay ID. The thyroid gland. In: Rumack CM, Wilson SR, Charboneau JW, editors. *Diagnostic ultrasound*. 2nd ed. St. Louis: Mosby; 1998. p. 703–29.

24. Pelsang RE. Diagnostic imaging modalities during pregnancy. *Obstet Gynecol Clin North Am*. 1998;**25**:287–300.

25. Morris PC. Thyroid cancer complicating pregnancy. *Obstet Gynecol Clin North Am*. 1998;**25**:401–5.

26. Chong KM, Tsai YL, Chuang J, Hwang JL, Chen KT. Thyroid cancer in pregnancy: a report of 3 cases. *J Reprod Med*. 2007;**52**:416–8.

27. Rosen IB, Korman M, Walfish PG. Thyroid nodular disease in pregnancy: current diagnosis and management. *Clin Obstet Gynecol*. 1997;**40**:81–9.

28. Hod M, Sharony R, Friedman S, Ovadia J. Pregnancy and thyroid carcinoma: a review

of incidence, course and prognosis. *Obstet Gynecol Surv.* 1989;**44**:774–9.

29. Kuy S, Roman SA, Desai R, Sosa JA. Outcomes following thyroid and parathyroid surgery in pregnant women. *Arch Surg.* 2009;**144**:399–406.

30. Driggers RW, Kopelman JN, Satin AJ. Delaying surgery for thyroid cancer in pregnancy. A case report. *J Reprod Med.* 1998;**43**:909–12.

31. Nam KH, Yoon JH, Chang HS, Park CS. Optimal timing of surgery in well-differentiated thyroid carcinoma detected during pregnancy. *J Surg Oncol.* 2005;**91**:199–203.

32. Vini L. Hyer S, Pratt B, Harmer C. Management of differentiated thyroid cancer diagnosed during pregnancy. *Eur J Endocrinol.* 1999;**140**:404–6.

33. Krishnamurthy GT, Blahd WH. Radioiodine I-131 therapy in the management of thyroid cancer: a prospective study. *Cancer.* 1977;**40**:195–202.

34. Samaan NA, Maheshwari YK, Nader S, et al. Impact of therapy for differentiated carcinoma of the thyroid: an analysis of 706 cases. *J Clin Endocrinol Metab.* 1983;**56**:1131–8.

35. Massin JP, Savoie JC, Garnier H, Guiraudon G, Leger FA, Bacourt F. Pulmonary metastases in differentiated thyroid carcinoma. Study of 58 cases with implication for the primary tumor treatment. *Cancer.* 1984;**53**:982–92.

36. Ringenberg QS, Droll DC. Endocrine tumors and miscellaneous cancers in pregnancy. *Semin Oncol.* 1989;**16**:445–55.

37. Shepard TH. Onset of function in the human fetal thyroid: biochemical and radioautographic studies from organ culture. *J Clin Endocrinol Metab.* 1967;**27**:945–58.

38. Sawka AM, Lakra DC, Lea J, et al. A systematic review examining the effects of therapeutic radioactive iodine on ovarian function and future pregnancy in female thyroid cancer survivors. *Clin Endocrinol.* 2008;**69**:479–90.

39. Schlumberger M, De Vathaire F, Ceccarelli C, Francese C, Pinchera A, Parmentier C. Outcome of pregnancy in women with thyroid carcinoma. *J Endocrinol Invest.* 1995;**18**:150–1.

40. Garsi JP, Schlumberger M, Rubino C, et al. Therapeutic administration of 131I for differentiated thyroid cancer: radiation dose to ovaries and outcome of pregnancies. *J Nucl Med.* 2008;**49**: 845–52.

41. Lin JD, Wang HS, Weng HF, Kao PF. Outcome of pregnancy after radioactive iodine treatment for well differentiated thyroid carcinoma. *J Endocrinol Invest.* 1998;**21**:662–7.

42. Chow SM, Yau S, Lee SH, Leung WM, Law, SC. Pregnancy outcome after diagnosis of differentiated thyroid carcinoma: no deleterious effect after radioactive iodine treatment. *Int J Radiat Oncol Biol Phys.* 2004;**59**:992–1000.

43. American College of Obstetricians and Gynecologists. ACOG Practice Bulletin. Clinical management guidelines for obstetrician-gynecologists. Number 37, August 2002. (Replaces Practice Bulletin Number 32, November 2001). Thyroid disease in pregnancy. *Obstet Gynecol.* 2002;**100**:387–96.

44. Fard-Esfahani A, Hadifar M, Fallahi B, et al. Radioiodine treatment complications to the mother and child in patients with differentiated thyroid carcinoma. *Hell J Nucl Med.* 2009;**12**:37–40.

45. Casara D, Rubelllo D, Saladini G, et al. Pregnancy after high therapeutic doses of iodine-131 in differentiated thyroid cancer: potential risks and recommendations. *Eur J Nucl Med.* 1993;**20**:192–4.

46. Pomorski L, Bartos M, Narebski J. Pregnancy following operative and complementary treatment of thyroid cancer. *Zentralbl Gynacol.* 2000;**122**:383–6.

47. O'Doherty MJ, McElhatton PR, Thomas SHL. Treating thyrotoxicosis in pregnant or potentially pregnant women: the risk to the fetus is low. *Br Med J.* 1999;**318**:5–6.

48. Nicholson H. Cytotoxic drugs in pregnancy: review of reported cases. *J Obstet Gynecol Br Commonw.* 1968;**75**:307–12.

49. Doll DC, Ringenberg S, Yarbro DW. Management of cancer during pregnancy. *Arch Intern Med*. 1988;48:2058–64.

50. Zemlickis D, Lishner M, Degendorfer P, et al. Maternal and fetal outcome after breast cancer in pregnancy. *Am J Obstet Gynecol*. 1992;166:781–7.

51. Zemlickis D, Lishner M, Degendrofer P, Panzarella T, Sutcliffe SB, Koren G. Fetal outcome after in utero exposure to cancer chemotherapy. *Arch Intern Med*. 1992;15:573–6.

52. Blatt J, Milvihill JJ, Ziegler JL, Young RC, Poplack DG. Pregnancy outcome following cancer chemotherapy. *Am J Med*. 1980;39:828–32.

53. Lessin LS. Chemotherapy of differentiated papillary or follicular thyroid carcinoma. In: Wartofsky L, Van Nostrand D, editors. *Thyroid cancer. A comprehensive guide to clinical management*. Humana Press Inc. Totowa, NJ. 2006. p. 494–5.

54. Herzon FS, Morris DM, Segal MN, Rauch G, Parnell T. Coexistent thyroid cancer and pregnancy. *Arch Otolaryngol Head Neck Surg*. 1994;120:1191–3.

55. Bennett PN, editor. *Drugs and Human Lactation: a comprehensive guide to the content and consequences of drugs, micronutrients, radiopharmaceuticals, and environmental and occupational chemicals in human milk*. 2nd ed. Amsterdam: Elsevier Science BV; 1996. p. 637–8.

Chapter

13

Pregnancy and radiation

Eyal Fenig

Introduction

The risk of embryo–fetal irradiation during pregnancy is discussed. It seems that, due to the low level of x-ray exposure to the fetus, neither diagnostic radiography nor nuclear diagnostic examination justifies termination of pregnancy. Radiotherapy for breast cancer, Hodgkin's disease, and cervical cancer in pregnant women is reviewed. Radiation therapy for breast cancer is not an absolute contraindication for pregnancy and the risk-benefit assessment should be discussed with the mother. The risk to the fetus during radiotherapy for supradiaphragmatic Hodgkin's disease appears to be minimal, provided special attention is paid to shielding the fetus and to the treatment techniques. Treatment of cervical cancer should be undertaken even during pregnancy, but the timing should be adjusted taking into consideration gestational age. Offspring of cancer patients who were treated by radiotherapy appear to be at little risk of childhood cancer or birth defects. Cancer patients should not be discouraged from having children and can expect a good outcome of pregnancy. However, in the nonpregnant woman, to further reduce any risk, it is advisable to delay pregnancy for 12 months following completion of radiation therapy.

Radiologic modes

The risks of fetal exposure to X-rays have been the subject of numerous studies over the past 50 years. The lack of clear information has given rise to unjustified panic among the public [1–3]. Indeed, fear of X-ray-induced fetal defects has led some women with unsuspected pregnancy that underwent radiography to terminate the pregnancy. In addition, many doctors tend to refrain from prescribing necessary dental, chest, or other X-rays to pregnant women.

The possible embryonic or fetal damage from radiation may be classified into two principal types. The first is teratogenic, or abnormal fetal development, which may occur on exposure to radiation in the first 12 weeks of pregnancy, when the embryo is in the stage of organogenesis [4,5]. The second type is carcinogenic, or the induction of malignancy. Gilman *et al.* suggested that the risk due to radiation is higher in the first trimester than in the second and third trimesters, but this is not fully established [6]. These effects are manifested in the first decade of life [7–12].

The available information on radiation-induced embryonic damage is derived from animal studies [13,14], follow-up of individuals exposed to atomic bomb explosions in

Cancer in Pregnancy and Lactation: The Motherisk Guide ed. Gideon Koren and Michael Lishner.
Published by Cambridge University Press. © Cambridge University Press 2011.

Japan [5,15–17], and statistical analyses [3,4]. In the laboratory studies, researchers found they had to use high levels of radiation before any effect could be noted. As long as the level remained below 15 cGy, no differences were observed between the control and the irradiated group [13,14,18]. Follow-up of Japanese women exposed to radiation levels of 10–19 cGy showed that, in Hiroshima, babies were born with relatively small head circumferences, but this was not true in Nagasaki [4,5,15,19]. These authors speculated that the significantly greater prevalence of malnutrition and multiple diseases in Hiroshima may have played an important role in this finding. Based on these studies, the report of the United States National Council on Radiation Protection [4] recommends that even radiation levels of 5–10 cGy [3] present no real danger to the embryo–fetus and the advantages gained by clinical diagnosis by far outweigh the negligible risk of embryonic damage. In conclusion, for fetal doses of less than 0.1 Gy, there is no medical justification for termination of pregnancy (ICRP 2000) [76].

The subject of the carcinogenic effects of X-ray radiation was first raised 42 years ago by a group of researchers from Oxford, United Kingdom [8]. The bulk of the data accumulated up to the 1980s was summarized by Monson and MacMahon [20]. Around the same time Harvey *et al.* [7] conducted a broad-based follow-up of 32,000 twins with 31 cases of prenatal radiation-induced cancer which indicated that radiation had no significant effect: only in cases of low birth weight did the risk of cancer increase to approximately 1:1000, as opposed to 1:2000 for the overall population. However, an editorial in the same publication [21] questioned the validity of the findings owing to the small number of cancer cases and the authors' failure to exclude all the other indications for radiography (besides twin birth). Furthermore, the lower incidence of cancer in the twin series than among singleton births in the general population, despite the greater exposure of the twin fetuses to radiation, raises the possibility that even the minuscule effects noted in the low-birth-weight twins may not have been due to radiation at all.

To gain a proper perspective of the issue, natural radiation should be considered as well. All of us are exposed to cosmic radiation, even when we are far away from X-ray institutes and hospitals. In the Rocky Mountain areas of Colorado, New Mexico, and Utah in the United States, the natural uranium content of the soil is very high and the attenuation of cosmic radiation by the atmosphere is diminished by the high altitudes. Thus, the annual level of radiation exposure per person exceeds that in other areas of the country by some 100 millirem. We might conclude that a fetus whose mother-to-be lives in, say, Colorado, will receive, during the 9 months of pregnancy, a surplus irradiation of 85 millirems. Because a routine chest X-ray of a pregnant woman exposes the fetus to 0.5 millirems [22], the fetus of a pregnant Colorado resident is exposed to a dose equal to that of 150 chest X-rays. Likewise, with regard to dental X-rays, which many pregnant women refuse, if we assume a radiation level of 0.06 millirems per X-ray (Table 1), some 1,250 dental X-rays would be required to equal the amount of surplus radiation absorbed by any fetus whose mother-to-be lives in Colorado. At the same time, while millions of people, obviously including pregnant women, reside in Colorado, the state's incidence of cancer is actually approximately 35% below the national average [2]. The same is true for some regions of India and China where background radiation is up to 2000 millirems per year, but no increase in radiation-induced morbidity has been documented [23].

Going back to the study of Harvey *et al.* [7], even if we accept its conclusions despite the reservations of the editorial, only 1 out of every 1,000 children prenatally exposed to 1 rem (1000 millirems) radiation will, by statistical probability, be damaged. Assuming that the

Table 1. Estimated average dose to fetus per radiographic examination (in millirems)*

Dental	0.06
Head	<0.5
Cervical spine	<0.5
Extremities	<0.5
Shoulder	0.5
Thoracic spine	11
Chest	0.5
Mammography	<10
Upper GI series	170
Femur (distal)	1
Lumbar spine	720
Pelvis	210
Hip and femur (proximal)	120
Intravenous pyelography	590
Cystography	1,500
Barium enema	900
Abdomen	220
Pelvimetry	1,270

* Values are taken from NCRP [4] and Monson and MacMahon [20].
* Values listed here are averages. The precise amount of fetal irradiation depends upon the device, the operator, the site, etc.

probability of damage to this 1 fetus is equal to that of damage to 2000 fetuses each irradiated with 0.5 millirems, the chest X-ray examination of 2,000,000 pregnant women will result in the birth of, at most, 1 damaged baby. By contrast, the number of spontaneously naturally damaged babies born to these 2,000,000 women, irrespective of radiation, will be at least 80,000. In short, the probability of developmental damage or childhood cancer due to embryonic–fetal irradiation of 1 cGy does not exceed 1:1,000, and may well be only 1:10,000 or even zero [1,4,16,17]. (For purposes of this discussion, 1 rad = 1 rem = 1000 millirem = 1 cGy.) These figures are negligible when compared to the overall 4–6% rate of birth defects in the general population. Furthermore, in only 1 of every 1,000 diagnostic X-ray examinations of pregnant women is the level of radiation to which the fetus is exposed equal to or greater than 1 cGy [12]. As shown in Table 1, in radiologic examinations outside the abdominal region, the dose to the embryo–fetus is almost always lower than 1 cGy (usually much lower) and the risk of damage is negligible, and in pelvic and lower-abdominal X-rays the dose to the fetus is rarely above 5 cGy, i.e., within safe limits [3,4,24,25].

   We conclude that only very rarely, if at all, will the level of embryo–fetal irradiation in diagnostic radiography justify the termination of a pregnancy. Only in women who have undergone several X-ray examinations in which the fetus is directly exposed to radiation, or when both radiographic and fluoroscopic examinations have been performed, is it necessary to calculate or measure the level of radiation; and only when that level is found to be above 5–10 cGy should abortion be considered.

Radionuclide examinations

The amount of time radioactive atoms remain in the body depends on the combination of the isotope's biological half-life or rate of its elimination by excretion, and its physical half-life. In pregnant patients undergoing radionuclide examinations, radiation may reach the embryo–fetus by means of the penetrating gamma rays and X-rays emitted by radionuclides concentrated in maternal organs or the placenta, or by radionuclides taken up by the fetus after they cross the placenta. In either case, the dose to the embryo–fetus from most nuclear diagnostic examinations will be less than 1 cGy [26,27].

When radioactive isotopes of iodine are used, and especially when a pregnant woman is administered a therapeutic dose of I-133, the irradiation of the fetal thyroid depends to a large degree on the amount of radioactive material crossing the placenta, the degree of uptake by the gland itself, and the gestational age (the normal period for onset of thyroid function is 10–12 weeks).

Detailed information regarding both x-ray exposure and radionuclide examination can be found in *Exposure of the pregnant patient to diagnostic radiation: A guide to medical management*, by L.K. Wagner, R.G. Lester, L.R. Saldana (Medical Physics Publishing, Madison, Wisconsin, 1997).

Radiotherapy

Physicians faced with a pregnant woman who requires radiation therapy for cancer may be inclined to advocate abortion for fear of possible injury to the fetus. Radiation doses used in cancer therapy are usually in the range of 4000–7000 cGy, i.e., 10^4–10^5 times the level in diagnostic radiology. The dose to the embryo–fetus will depend on several factors: (1) the teletherapy machine used and its leakage; (2) the target dose; (3) the size of the radiation fields; (4) the distance from the edges of the fields to the embryo-fetus; and (5) the use of wedges, lead blocks, compensators and other scattering objects. Lesser leakage, lower target dose, smaller radiation fields, greater distance of the edges of the radiation fields from the embryo–fetus, and avoidance of wedges and other scattering objects will all decrease the radiation dose to the embryo–fetus. A distance of over 30 cm from the field edges will yield an exposure of the embryo–fetus to only 4–20 cGy [28]. Thus, many areas (head and neck, breast, extremities) can be treated with radiation without significantly irradiating the embryo [29]. Lead shielding over the embryo–fetus can also be used to reduce the dose. A qualified medical physicist should be consulted, and the dose levels to the embryo–fetus should be determined for every case.

Types of cancer requiring radiotherapy

The following sections discuss specific cancers complicating pregnancy that may require radiation therapy. These cancers are usually divided into extrapelvic and pelvic. We will discuss the most common types: breast cancer, Hodgkin's disease (extrapelvic), and cervical cancer (pelvic).

Breast cancer

The growing interest in pregnancy-associated breast cancer has been prompted by the rising incidence of breast cancer in young women, combined with the modern trend to delay child-bearing. Diagnosed breast cancers occur in 1:10,000 to 1:3000 pregnancies [30–32]. In a review of 32 series reported in the past few decades, Wallack et al. [33] noted an incidence of 0.2–3.8%.

Breast or chest wall irradiation should generally be avoided in pregnant women because of fetal risk [34–37]. Indeed, the Steering Committee on Clinical Practice Guidelines for the Care and Treatment of Breast Cancer states that pregnancy is an absolute contraindication for breast irradiation [38]. Therefore, when breast or chest wall irradiation is necessary for tumor control, a risk assessment must be performed by an experienced medical physicist and a radiation oncologist. As mentioned earlier, embryos in the first 8 weeks of organogenesis are the most susceptible to the teratogenic effects of radiation. Nevertheless, because the internal scatter depends mostly on the distance of the fetus from the central beam, if the embryo is in the true pelvis, maternal breast or chest wall irradiation will expose it to only 0.1%–0.3% of the total dose, or 5–15 cGy for a typical breast treatment course of 5000 cGy. Toward the end of pregnancy, the now larger fetus lies closer to the radiation field and could receive more than 200 cGy for the same treatment course, but radiation-induced congenital defects at this gestational age are extremely rare [39]. However, the life-time risk of radiation-induced cancer is higher than normal and should not be ignored. According to NRPB (1993) [40] the risk of radiation-induced cancer is approximately 9.3% for a typical breast treatment.

Successful breast cancer radiation therapy during pregnancy has been reported in the literature. Ngu et al. [41] treated a patient in the third trimester with 6 Mv photons with tangential wedged fields using a 9-mm lead shielding over the abdomen and a lead block inferior to the breast. The estimated fetal dose was 14–18 cGy for a total dose of 5000 cGy to the breast. Antypas et al. [29] treated a patient in the first trimester with a 6 Mv photon beam with opposing tangential unwedged fields. In vivo and phantom measurements showed the fetal dose to be 0.05% of the tumor dose, corresponding to a cumulative fetal dose of 3.9 cGy for a total dose of 4600 cGy to the breast. In 1997, Van der Giessen [42] published a data set to estimate the fetal dose as a function of stage of pregnancy. This methodology is considered sufficiently accurate for risk assessment.

Another issue of concern is the effect of breast lumpectomy and irradiation on lactation. A national survey of 2582 members of the American Society of Therapeutic Radiology and Oncology revealed that approximately 1 in 4 women can achieve successful bilateral lactation after conservative surgery and radiation therapy [43].

In conclusion, we believe that radiation therapy to the breast or chest wall is not an absolute contraindication for pregnancy. The risk–benefit assessment should be presented to the patient, and the final decision should depend on the strength of the indication for treatment and the woman's desire to continue the pregnancy. The use of wedges and/or lead blocks should be avoided to decrease external scatter to the fetus. In the third trimester, when adjuvant chemotherapy can be safely administered, radiation therapy should be postponed until after delivery.

Hodgkin's disease

The incidence of Hodgkin's disease peaks during the reproductive years, and its rate of association with pregnancy is 1:1,000 to 1:6,000 [44]. Hodgkin's disease most commonly presents with supradiaphragmatic lymphadenopathy, so radiation therapy is feasible. Its use during pregnancy has been extensively investigated [45–57]. In 1992 Woo *et al* [56]. described 16 pregnant patients (estimated gestational age 6 to 32 weeks) presenting with supradiaphragmatic nodal disease who underwent definitive radiation therapy, typically with "mantle" fields. Lead was used to shield the uterus. The estimated dose to the mid-fetus ranged from 1.4 to 5.5 cGy for treatment with 6 MV photons, and from 10 to 13.6 cGy for cobalt 60. In all 16 patients, the babies were born at term, without congenital anomalies, growth retardation, or subsequent childhood malignancies. The same year, Lishner *et al.* [44] compared 48 pregnant women with Hodgkin's disease with matched controls and found no between-group differences in 20-year survival. Although 21 women of this group received radiation therapy during pregnancy (16 definitive radiotherapy, 5 with chemotherapy), there was no significant difference in fetal or maternal outcome.

Although definitive radiation therapy (4000 cGy) is still considered the standard for early stages of Hodgkin's disease, some authors have recently recommended a combination of chemotherapy with low-dose, low-volume radiation fields [58]. This approach in pregnant women can reduce the fetal dose.

In conclusion, radiotherapy is an appropriate treatment for supradiaphragmatic presentation of Hodgkin's disease during pregnancy, provided special attention is paid to shielding and treatment techniques. The outcome of treatment for women with early-stage disease is not adversely affected by pregnancy, and the risk to the fetus appears to be minimal.

Cervical cancer

The incidence of pregnancy-associated cervical cancer [59–61] is difficult to interpret because (1) the major studies have been conducted at referral centers; (2) different definitions are used for the postpartum period (2–18 months); and (3) cervical intraepithelial neoplasia is often reported together with invasive malignancy. It is generally estimated that 1:2,000 pregnancies is associated with cervical cancer, and pregnancy is a complication in approximately 3% of patients with cervical carcinoma [62].

The treatment of carcinoma of the cervix should be stage-related regardless of the presence of a pregnancy. Surgery and radiotherapy (for advanced disease) should be used in the same manner as in nonpregnant patients [63]. However, the timing of treatment may be adjusted according to the gestational age. Late second- or early third-trimester pregnancies should be allowed to continue to 35 weeks, unless there is evidence of a rapidly growing tumor [64]. Vaginal delivery should be avoided because of the risk of tumor implantation in the episiotomy site [65,66]. Patients in whom cervical cancer is diagnosed in the first or second trimester are not good candidates for delay of treatment and should be given external radiotherapy immediately, with the fetus *in situ*. Usually, spontaneous abortion will occur after a few days and intracavitary radiation can be added. In case no spontaneous abortion occurs, curettage of the fetus should be performed.

The majority of reports indicate that survival is not altered by pregnancy [63,64,67,68].

Hereditary effects of radiation

The gonads are one of the most radiosensitive organs in the human body. The threshold radiation dose for permanent sterility in men is 350–600 cGy, and for women 250–600 cGy [69]. In a retrospective cohort study of survivors of cancer, it was found that radiation therapy directed below the diaphragm depressed fertility in both sexes by approximately 25% [70].

Even if fertility is preserved, there is concern regarding the induction of genetic abnormalities (germ-line mutation, chromosomal aberrations) that could potentially produce birth defects and cancer in the offspring. However, a 40-year follow-up of survivors of the nuclear blasts in Japan showed no significant increase in genetically linked disorders in children born thereafter compared to matched controls of the general population [71]. Based on animal experiments, the estimated dose of gonadal radiation required to produce a mutation rate equal to the baseline spontaneous rate in humans (mutation doubling dose) is between 100 and 150 cGy, with an approximate risk of 100 per 10,000 live-born infants per 100 cGy exposure [69]. Some publications suggest lower doses of around 50 cGy and a threshold of approximately 10 cGy. Yet, recent studies of children of cancer treatment survivors [28] have found no more birth defects than expected for healthy parents [72–74], although an increase in low-birth-weight infants or spontaneous abortions was noted, particularly if conception occurred less than 1 year after cessation of radiation.

Radiation exposure has been shown to increase the risk of cancers in both adult and children. It is likely that late stage of fetogenesis is the period of highest radiosensitivity with respect to cancer induction. The fetus is assumed to be susceptible to the carcinogenic effects of radiation as a young child (ICRP 2003). The relative risk may be up to 1.4 (40% of normal incidence) following a fetal dose of 10 mGy, but the individual risk remains small due to the low incidence of childhood cancer. For 0- to 15-year-olds, this equates to 1 excess cancer death per 1,700 children exposed to 10 mGy *in utero* (ICRP2000) [75].

In conclusion, offspring of survivors of cancer who were treated by radiotherapy appear to be at little risk of childhood cancer or birth defects [76]. Thus, in most instances, survivors of cancer should not be discouraged from having children and can expect a good outcome of pregnancy. To reduce the likelihood of an adverse fetal outcome, it is advisable to delay pregnancy for 12 months following completion of radiation therapy.

References

1. Mole RH. Radiation effects on prenatal development and their radiological significance – review article. *Br J Radiol*. 1979;**52**:89–101.

2. Cohen LB. *Before it's too late*. New York: Plenum Press; 1983. p. 157–68.

3. Baker ML, Vandergrift A, Dalrymple GV. Fetal exposure in diagnostic radiology. *Health Phys*. 1979;**37**:237–9.

4. NCRP. (National Council of Radiation Protection). *Medical radiation exposure of pregnant and potentially pregnant women*. NCRP Report No. 54, Washington, DC, 1977, 7–13.

5. Miller RW, Mulvihill JJ. Small head size after atomic irradiation. *Teratology*. 1976;**14**:355–7.

6. Gilman EA, Kneale GW, Knox EG, Steward AM. Pregnancy, x-rays and childhood cancers: effect of exposure, age and radiation dose. *J Radiol Prot*. 1988;**8**:3–8.

7. Harvey EB, Boice JD Jr, Huneyman M, Flannery JT. Prenatal X-ray exposure and childhood cancer in twins. *N Engl J Med*. 1985;**312**:541–5.

8. Stewart A, Webb J. Malignant disease in childhood and diagnostic irradiation in utero. *Lancet*. 1956;**2**:447–50.

9. Gaulden ME. *Genetic effects of radiation. Medical Radiation Biology*. Philadelphia: WB Saunders; 1973.

10. Bross ID, Natarajan N. Genetic damages from diagnostic radiation. *JAMA*. 1977;**237**:2399–401.

11. Mole RH. Antenatal radiography and the ten day rule. *Lancet*. 1976;**1**:378–9.

12. BRH. (Bureau of Radiological Health). *Population exposure to X-rays. DHEW Publication (FDA) 73–8047*. Washington, DC: US Government Printing Office; 1973.

13. Rugh R. X-ray induced teratogenesis in the mouse and its possible significance to man. *Radiology*. 1971;**99**:433–43.

14. Hicks SP, D'Amato CJ. Effects of ionizing radiation on mammalian development. *Adv Teratol*. 1966;**1**:195–9.

15. Jablon S, Kato H. Childhood cancer in relation to prenatal exposure to atomic bomb radiation. *Lancet*. 1970;2:1000–3.

16. ICRP. (International Commission on Radiological Protection). *ICRP Publication* **60**. Oxford: Pergamon Press; 1990.

17. UNSCEAR (United Nations Scientific Committee on the Effects of Atomic Radiation). *Genetic and somatic effects of ionizing radiation*. United Nations, NY; 1986, 16–18, 332–4.

18. Russel LB, Badgett SK. Comparison of the effects of acute, continuous and fractionated irradiation during embryonic development. *Int J Radiat Biol Suppl*. 1960.

19. Shigematsu I, Katoo H. *Late health effects among Hiroshima and Nagasaki atomic bomb survivors. Radiation-Risk-Protection Compacts*, Volume 1, 6th Congress, International Association, Berlin; 1984, 2:89–95.

20. Monson RR, MacMahon B. Prenatal X-ray exposure and cancer in children. In: Boice JDJr, Fraumeni JF Jr, editors. *Radiation carcinogenesis: epidemiology and biological significance*. New York: Raven Press; 1984.

21. MacMahon B. Prenatal x-ray exposure and twins. *N Engl J Med*. 1985;**312**:576–7.

22. Donagi A, Leser Y. *National evaluation of trends in X-ray exposure of medical patients in Israel. Proceedings of the 4th Congress of the International Radiation Protection Association (IRPA)*, Paris, April 23–30, 1977, I:10–27.

23. Feige Y, Kahan RS. *Practical implications of new approaches in evaluating risks from ionizing radiation*. Transactions of the Nuclear Societies of Israel, December 1976, 71–103.

24. NCRP. (National Council of Radiation Protection). *Review of NCRP radiation dose limit for embryo and fetus in occupationally exposed women*. NCRP Report No. 53, Washington, DC; 1977, 25–53.

25. Hamer-Jacobsen E. Therapeutic abortion on account of X-ray. *Denver Med Bull*. 1959;**6**:113–7.

26. Brent RI. Radiation and other medical agents. In: Wilson LG, Fraser FC, editors. *Handbook of teratology*, Volume **1**, Chapter 5. New York: Plenum Press; 1977. p. 60–83.

27. Steenvoorde P, Pauwels EK, Harding LK, Bourguignon M, Mariere B, Broerse JJ. Diagnostic nuclear medicine and risk to the fetus. *Eur J Nucl Med*. 1998;**25**:193–9.

28. Stovall M, Blackwell RC, Cundiff J, et al. Fetal dose from radiotherapy with photon beams: report of AAPM Radiation Therapy Committee Task Group No. 36. *Med Phys*. 1995;**22**:63–82.

29. Antypas C, Sandilos P, Kauvaris J, et al. Fetal dose evaluation during breast cancer radiotherapy. *Int J Radiat Oncol Biol Phys*. 1998;**40**:995–9.

30. White TT. Carcinoma of the breast and pregnancy. *Ann Surg*. 1954;**139**:9–18.

31. Peete CH Jr, Honeycutt HC Jr, Cherny WB. Cancer of the breast in pregnancy. *N C Med J*. 1966;**27**:514–20.

32. Anderson JM. Mammary cancers and pregnancy. *Br Med J*. 1979;**1**:1124–7.

33. Wallack MK, Wolf JA Jr, Bedwinek J, Denes AE, Glasgow G, Kumar B. Gestational carcinoma of the female breast. *Curr Probl Cancer*. 1983;7:1–58.

34. Petrek JA. Breast cancer during pregnancy. *Cancer*. 1994;**84**(suppl):518–27.

35. Espie M, Cuvier C. Treatment of breast cancer during pregnancy. *Contracept Fertil Sex*. 1996;**24**:805–10.

36. Isaacs JH. Cancer of the breast in pregnancy. *Surg Clin North Am*. 1995;**75**:47–51.

37. van der Vange N, van Dongen JA. Breast cancer and pregnancy. *Eur J Surg Oncol*. 1991;**17**:1–8.

38. The Steering Committee on Clinical Practice Guidelines for the Care and Treatment of Breast Cancer. Mastectomy or lumpectomy? The choice of operation

for clinical stages I and II breast cancer. *CMAJ*. 1998;**158**(suppl 3):S15–S21.

39. Orr JW, Shingleton HM. Cancer in pregnancy. *Curr Probl Cancer*. 1983;**8**:1–50.

40. Muirhead CR, Cox R, Stather JW, MacGibbon BH, Edwards AA, Laylock RGE. Estimates of late radiation risks to the UK population. *NRPB*. 1998;**4**:15–157.

41. Ngu SL, Duval P, Collins C. Foetal radiation dose in radiotherapy for breast cancer. *Austral Radiol*. 1992;**36**:321–2.

42. Van der Giessen PH. Measurement of the peripheral dose for the tangential breast treatment technique with Co-60 gamma radiation and high energy X-rays. *Radiother Oncol*. 1997;**42**:257–64.

43. Tralins AH. Lactation after conservative breast surgery combined with radiation therapy. *Am J Clin Oncol*. 1995;**18**:40–3.

44. Lishner M, Zemlickis D, Degendorfer P, et al. Maternal and foetal outcome following Hodgkin's disease in pregnancy. *Br J Cancer*. 1992;**65**:114–7.

45. Becker MH. Hodgkin's disease and pregnancy. *Radiol Clin North Am*. 1968;**6**:111–4.

46. Becker MH, Hyman GA. Management of Hodgkin's disease coexistent with pregnancy. *Radiology*. 1965;**85**:725–8.

47. Conley JG, Jacobson A. Modified radiation therapy regimen for Hodgkin's disease in the third trimester of pregnancy. *AJR Am J Roentgenol*. 1977;**128**:666–7.

48. Covington EE, Baker AS. Dosimetry of scattered radiation to the fetus. *JAMA*. 1969;**209**:414–5.

49. Jacobs C, Donaldson SS, Rosenberg SA, Kaplan HS. Management of the pregnant patient with Hodgkin's disease. *Ann Intern Med*. 1981;**95**:669–75.

50. Nisce LZ, Tome MA, He S, Lee BJ, Kutcher GJ. Management of coexisting Hodgkin's disease and pregnancy. *Am J Clin Oncol*. 1986;**9**:146–51.

51. Sharma SC, Williamson JF, Khan FM, Lee CK. Measurement and calculation of ovary and fetus dose in extended field radiotherapy for 10 MV x-rays. *Int J Radiat Oncol Biol Phys*. 1981;**7**:843–6.

52. Spitzer M, Citron M, Ilardi CF, Saxe B. Non-Hodgkin's lymphoma during pregnancy. *Gynecol Oncol*. 1991;**45**:309–12.

53. Tawil E, Mercier JP, Dandavino A. Hodgkin's disease complicating pregnancy. *J Can Assoc Radiol*. 1983;**36**:133–7.

54. Thomas PR, Biochem D, Peckham MJ. The investigation and management of Hodgkin's disease in the pregnant patient. *Cancer*. 1976;**38**:1443–51.

55. Wong PS, Rosemark PJ, Wexler MC, Greenberg SH, Thompson RW. Doses to organs at risk from mantle field radiation therapy using 10 MV x-rays. *Mt Sinai J Med*. 1985;**52**:216–20.

56. Woo SY, Fuller LM, Cundiff JH, et al. Radiotherapy during pregnancy for clinical stages IA–IIA Hodgkin's disease. *Int J Radiat Oncol Biol Phys*. 1992;**23**:407–12.

57. Zacali R, Marchesini R, De Palo G. Abdominal dosimetry for supradiaphragmatic irradiation of Hodgkin's disease in pregnancy. Experimental data and clinical considerations. *Tumori*. 1981;**67**:203–8.

58. Hoppe RT. *Treatment of early-stage Hodgkin's disease: consideration in the use of radiation therapy*. Alexandria, VA: American Society of Clinical Oncology Educational Book;1998. p. 188–200.

59. Waldrop GM, Palmer JP. Carcinoma of the cervix associated with pregnancy. *Am J Obstet Gynecol*. 1963;**86**:202–12.

60. Stander RW, Lein JN. Carcinoma of the cervix and pregnancy. *Am J Obstet Gynecol*. 1960;**79**:164–7.

61. Gustafsson DC, Kottmeier HL. Carcinoma of the cervix associated with pregnancy. *Acta Obstet Gynecol Scand*. 1962;**41**:1–12.

62. Hacker NF, Berek JS, Lagasse LD, Charles EH, Savage EW, Moore JG. Carcinoma of the cervix associated with pregnancy. *Obstet Gynecol*. 1982;**59**:735–46.

63. Nevin J, Soeters R, Dehaeck K, Bloch B, Van Wyk L. Cervical carcinoma associated with pregnancy. *Obstet Gynecol Surv*. 1995;**50**:228–39.

64. Greer BE, Easterling TR, McLennan DA, et al. Fetal and maternal considerations in

the management of stage IB cervical cancer during pregnancy. *Gynecol Oncol.* 1989;**34**:61–5.

65. Gordon AN, Jensen R, Jones HW III. Squamous carcinoma of the cervix complicating pregnancy: recurrence in episiotomy after vaginal delivery. *Obstet Gynecol.* 1989;**73**:850–2.

66. Copeland LJ, Saul PB, Sneige N. Cervical adenocarcinoma: tumor implantation in the episiotomy sites of two patients. *Gynecol Oncol.* 1987;**28**:230–5.

67. Sood AK, Sorosky JI, Mayr N, et al. Radiotherapeutic management of cervical carcinoma that complicates pregnancy. *Cancer.* 1997;**80**:1073–8.

68. Zemlickis D, Lishner M, Degendorfer P, Panzarella T, Sutcliffe SB, Koren G. Maternal and fetal outcome after invasive cervical cancer in pregnancy. *J Clin Oncol.* 1991;**9**:1956–61.

69. Hall EJ. Hereditary effects of radiation. In: Hall EJ, editor. *Radiobiology for the radiologist.* 4th ed. Philadelphia: JB Lippincott; 1994. p. 351–67.

70. Byrne J, Mulvihill JJ, Myers MH, et al. Effects of treatment on fertility in long-term survivors of childhood or adolescent cancer. *N Engl J Med.* 1987;**317**:1315–21.

71. Schull WL, Otake M, Neal JV. Genetic effects of the atomic bomb: a reappraisal. *Science.* 1981;**213**:1220–7.

72. Aisner J, Wiernik RH, Pearl P. Pregnancy outcome in patients treated for Hodgkin's disease. *J Clin Oncol.* 1993;**11**:507–12.

73. Hawkins MM. Is there evidence of a therapy-related increase in germ cell mutation among childhood cancer survivors? *J Natl Cancer Inst.* 1991;**83**:1643–50.

74. Mulvihill JJ, McKeen EA, Rosner F, Zarrabi MH. Pregnancy outcome in cancer patients: experience in a large cooperative group. *Cancer.* 1987;**60**:1143–50.

75. Cousins C. Medical radiation and pregnancy. *Health Phys.* 2008;**95**:551–3.

76. Kal HB, Stunkman H. Radiotherapy during pregnancy: fact and fiction. *Lancet Oncol.* 2005;**6**:328–33.

Chapter

14

Chemotherapy during pregnancy

Israel Mazin, David Pereg, and Michael Lishner

Introduction

The diagnosis of pregnancy-associated cancer is a dramatic event that poses difficult dilemmas for the pregnant patient, her family, and the medical team. The main challenge is to treat the patient with the optimal anticancer regimen without harming the developing fetus. This issue is further complicated; because of the lack of large prospective studies, the available experience regarding the treatment of pregnancy-associated cancer is based mainly on small, retrospective studies and case reports. Almost all chemotherapeutic agents are teratogenic in animals and for some drugs, only experimental data exist [1]. Furthermore, because cytotoxic drugs are usually not administered as a single drug, most human reports arise from exposure to multi-drug regimens, making it difficult to estimate the direct effect of each drug [2].

Decisions about the management of pregnancy-associated cancer should be made individually for each patient after careful consideration of possible treatment alternatives as well as maternal and fetal risks. However, when there is a clear risk to the pregnant patient, her safety may supersede fetal risk.

In this chapter, we critically review the current information and controversies regarding different aspects of the administration of chemotherapy during pregnancy. We also review the available experience with the most common anticancer regimens as well as each chemotherapeutic agent.

Pharmacology

Due to their relatively low molecular weight, most cytotoxic agents can cross the placenta and reach the fetus [1,3]. The pharmacology of the various anticancer drugs may be altered by the normal physiological changes that occur during pregnancy such as increased plasma volume, enhanced renal and hepatic elimination, and decreased albumin concentration. These changes may decrease active drug concentrations. Dosing similar to that of nonpregnant women of the same weight may lead to undertreatment of patients with pregnancy-associated cancer [3]. However, it is still not clear whether pregnant women should be treated with different doses of chemotherapy.

Cancer in Pregnancy and Lactation: The Motherisk Guide ed. Gideon Koren and Michael Lishner.
Published by Cambridge University Press. © Cambridge University Press 2011.

Effects of chemotherapy during pregnancy [4–9]

Chemotherapy during the first trimester may increase the risk of spontaneous abortions, fetal death, and major congenital malformations. The teratogenic effects depend on the dosage, time of administration, and cumulative exposure to the chemotherapeutic agent. Fetal malformations reflect the gestational age at exposure and the most vulnerable period is during weeks 2–8 when organogenesis occurs. The eyes, ears, teeth-palate, genitalia, hematopoietic system, and the central nervous system remain vulnerable to chemotherapy even after organogenesis [1].

Overall, the risk of teratogenesis in humans following cancer treatment appears to be lower than that commonly estimated from animal data. First-trimester exposure to chemotherapy has been associated with 10–20% risk of major malformations. Furthermore, it has been suggested that this risk may decline to approximately 6% when folate antagonists (which are considered the most teratogenic anticancer drugs) are excluded [1,10].

The administration of chemotherapy during the second and third trimesters is not associated with major congenital malformations but may increase the risk for intrauterine growth restriction (IUGR) and low birth weight. A review of 376 cases of fetuses exposed to chemotherapy *in utero*, most after organogenesis, demonstrated 5% fetal death rate and 1% neonatal death rate, respectively. Other complications included premature delivery (5%), IUGR (7%), and transient myelosuppression (4%) [1].

A recent American registry [11] of 152 women exposed to chemotherapy mostly after the first trimester, demonstrated a single case of intrauterine fetal death and another case of neonatal death. The malformation rate was 3.8%, with a 7.6% risk for IUGR. Only 2 of the 159 live-born infants suffered transient myelosuppression. A European [12] study compared the rates of adverse pregnancy outcomes of patients exposed to chemotherapy (117 pregnancies) during the second and third trimesters and healthy controlled patients (58 pregnancies). The incidences of major and minor malformations have not increased compared to previous reports. The rate of low birth weight was higher in the chemotherapy group 17.9% compared to 8.6% in the control group. Most of the infants with low birth weight were born to mothers treated for hematological malignancies.

Treatment strategy

Patients with a slowly growing cancer diagnosed during the first trimester may be followed at short intervals for signs of disease progression without treatment until the second trimester. However, for women with aggressive, advanced, or progressive disease, which is diagnosed in the first trimester, a delay in therapy may adversely affect maternal survival [4–9,13]. Therefore, treatment with appropriate, often combination chemotherapy, should be given promptly. However, this should be accompanied by a recommendation for therapeutic abortion due to the potential teratogenic effects of chemotherapy in the first trimester. In specific cases, the treatment with single agent chemotherapy (preferably a vinca alkaloid or an anthracycline) during the first trimester followed by conventional multi-agent therapy at the beginning of the second trimester may be considered. Such therapeutic approaches appear to be safe; however, data regarding their efficacy are lacking. Most multi-drug protocols may be administered during the second and third trimester without an apparent increase in the risk for severe malformations. Among the different regimens, those based on a combination of cyclophosphamide and an anthracycline administered to women with breast cancer or lymphomas have been most commonly used during pregnancy and their administration after the end of the first trimester was found to be safe.

Delivery should be postponed for 2–3 weeks following anticancer treatment to allow for bone marrow recovery [8,9]. Furthermore, neonates, especially preterm infants, have limited capacity to metabolize and eliminate drugs due to liver and renal immaturity. The delay of delivery after chemotherapy will allow fetal drug excretion by the placenta.

Recently, the choice of treatment for the pregnant patient with cancer has become even more complicated due to the increasing use of targeted anticancer therapies. The benefit of the targeted agents has been well demonstrated for different malignancies; however, their safety during pregnancy has not been established. Currently, significant experience with exposure during pregnancy is available only for the tyrosine kinase inhibitor imatinib and the monoclonal antibody rituximab.

The largest report regarding exposure to imatinib during pregnancy has included 180 pregnant women with chronic myeloid leukemia; of them outcome data were available for 125 patients [14]. There were 12 infants in whom congenital abnormalities were identified, 3 of which had strikingly similar complex malformations (a combination of exomphalus with severe renal and skeletal malformations) that are clearly a cause for concern. All congenital malformations were associated with first-trimester exposure to imatinib. It appears that, although most pregnancies exposed to imatinib are likely to have a successful outcome, this exposure may result in serious fetal malformations. These concerns suggest that imatinib should be avoided during the first trimester [14,15].

Rituximab is an anti-CD20 monoclonal B-cell antibody indicated mainly for diffuse large B cell and follicular non-Hodgkin's lymphomas (in combination with CHOP). Recently it has also been administered to patients with different autoimmune diseases. A recent report has described 231 pregnancies associated with maternal rituximab exposure [16]. Most cases were confounded by the concomitant use of potentially teratogenic medications (most commonly methotrexate). Of the 153 pregnancies with outcome data, 90 resulted in live births. First-trimester miscarriages were reported in 33 (21%) cases and 28 pregnancies were electively terminated (reasons for termination were not specified). Twenty-two infants were born prematurely; with one case of neonatal death. Eleven neonates had hematological abnormalities without corresponding infections. Two congenital malformations were identified: one case of clubfoot, and another case of cardiac malformation (a combination of VSD, PFO, and PDA). According to the limited available experience, it seems that the administration of rituximab may be considered safe during the second and third trimesters.

Breastfeeding and chemotherapy

There is little information regarding breastfeeding while receiving chemotherapy. Durodola [17] concluded that the administration of cyclophosphamide while breast-feeding is not recommended. He reported that an infant that had received cyclophosphmide became neutropenic from breastfeeding. He concluded that chemotherapeutic agents could reach high concentrations in the mammary glands, thus affecting the newborn. Other reports [18–20] measured the concentration of imatinib in breast milk of mothers treated for CML. They found that concentrations of the drug and active metabolite corresponded to 10% of the therapeutic dose. The authors advised against breastfeeding while receiving therapy.

Leslie [2] summarized the use of various chemotherapeutic agents during pregnancy and breastfeeding. No drug has been proven safe for breastfeeding. Although some drugs have valid subtherapeutic concentrations in breast milk, the author advised to withhold breastfeeding.

We support the common recommendation to avoid breastfeeding during chemotherapy [6].

Long-term outcomes

While treating pregnant mothers during the second and third trimesters, one should remember that the central nervous system is still developing. Thus, long-term side effects of the child's development can occur. Long-term follow-up data on children born to mothers treated for leukemia during pregnancy have been published [21]. The children's psychological, physical, and neurological developments were reported as normal. In that report the grandchildren of exposed pregnant mothers, were followed up. Even those children had normal neurological and psychological development. No congenital malformations were reported. One review [22]. included 111 children born to mothers treated during pregnancy, who were followed for up to 19 years. All the children had normal neurological development.

Another concern is the possibility of secondary malignancies in exposed children. Avilés and Neri [21] followed 84 children up to a median age of 18 years; no secondary malignancies were reported; no fertility issues were reported.

To date, there is no other large-scale follow-up. A recent registry [11] reported on well-being of infants born to treated mothers, but the follow-up period is only a few years. Ongoing observation is underway to provide a full and detailed report in the coming years.

Tables

In the following tables, we summarized important reports concerning different cytotoxic agents. We present each medication according to its pharmacological group and time of publication. A brief description of the study and the pregnancy outcome are provided (see below).

Summary

We have provided an overview of data regarding administration of common chemotherapy agents during pregnancy. Information about the new-targeted agents is naturally less available; most of the data are observational or based on case reports.

Most cytotoxic agents should be avoided during the first trimester. We have shown that most of the cytotoxic agents can be used for the treatment of pregnant women during the second and third trimesters. These infants may be born earlier than expected and small for gestational age. The timing of delivery should be planned to avoid cytopenia; however, no long-term developmental sequelae have been reported. Similarly, there was no increased risk of malignancies or fertility issues in these children.

Alkylating agents	Description of study	Pregnancy outcome	References
Cyclophosphamide	61 patients with different malignancies treated during 2nd and 3rd trimesters	1 hip subluxation (treated together with doxorubicin) 1 rectal atresia (treated with FEC protocol and epiribicin alone)	[78]
	110 patients with different malignancies exposed during 2nd and 3rd trimesters (different treatment protocols)	1 intrauterine death with normal autopsy; 1 neonatal death due to autoimmune disorder; 1 infant with IgA deficiency; 1 with pyloric stenosis; 1 with holoprosencephaly	[33]
	57 patients diagnosed with breast cancer, exposed during 2nd and 3rd trimesters (part of FAC regimen)	1 child with Down syndrome; 1 with ureteral reflux; 1 with clubfoot	[46]
	28 patients treated for breast cancer with different regimens during 2nd and 3rd trimesters	No congenital malformations	[69]
	24 mothers treated for breast cancer during 2nd and 3rd trimesters (part of FAC regiment)	Normal deliveries; no congenital malformations	[30]
	21 patients treated with different regimens; 11 during the 1st trimester	No congenital malformations	[26]
	5 case reports of treatment during 1st trimester with various regimens	Absent big toes bilateral, single left coronary artery, imperforated anus, umbilical hernia, cleft palate, multiple eye defects, esophageal atresia	[44,52,76,80,82]
Dacarbazine (DTIC)	19 patients treated for lymphoma with ABVD protocol	1 infant with plagiocephaly 1 infant with 4th and 5th syndactyly that was surgically repaired	[33]

Alkylating agents	Description of study	Pregnancy outcome	References
Ifosfamide	2 case reports, treated together with doxorubicin for Ewing sarcoma during 2nd trimester	No congenital malformations	[59,63]
Mechlorethamine	1 patient treated with MOPP/ABV during 2nd trimester	Bilateral partial syndactyly digits II-III	[78]
	12 patients treated for HD with MOPP, MOPP/ABVD or MOPP/ABD protocols (some during 1st trimester)	No congenital malformations	[27]
	1 patient treated with MOPP during 1st trimester	Hydrocephaly and death	[56]
Procarbazine	1 patient treated with MOPP/ABV during 2nd trimester	Bilateral partial syndactyly digits II-III	[78]
	12 patients treated for HD with MOPP, MOPP/ ABVD and MOPP/ABD (some during 1st trimester)	No congenital malformations	[27]
	1 patient treated with MOPP during 1st trimester	Hydrocephaly and death	[56]

Platinum compounds	Description of study	Pregnancy outcome	References
Carboplatin	3 patients treated for ovarian cancer during 2nd and 3rd trimesters 1 patient treated for CNS malignancy during 2nd trimester	No congenital malformations Spontaneous abortion of a fetus with gastroschisis	[33]
	1 patient treated for ovarian cancer from 18th week of gestation	No congenital malformations	[74]
Cisplatin	7 patients treated for various malignancies with different drug regimens	1 infant with genetic hearing loss – both parents were carriers (disease unspecified)	[33]

Platinum compounds	Description of study	Pregnancy outcome	References
	during 2nd and 3rd trimesters		
	1 patient with small cell lung carcinoma at 26 weeks gestation, treated also with etoposide	No congenital malformations	[81]
	1 patient treated with cisplatin from week 17 of gestation	No congenital malformations	[40]
	1 patient treated for teratoma during 3rd trimester (together with bleomycin and etoposide)	Normal delivery, no congenital malformations	[50]
	4 case reports of cervical cancer during pregnancy all treated from 2nd trimester	No congenital malformations	[29,32,41,66]

Antibiotics	Description of study	Pregnancy outcome	References
Bleomycin	23 patients with varying malignancies and regimens (20 lymphoma, 3 ovarian) treated during 2nd and 3rd trimesters	1 infant with plagiocephaly; 1infant with 4th and 5th finger syndactyly 1 infant with genetic hearing loss – both parents were carriers	[33]
	1 patient treated for teratoma during 3rd trimester (together with etoposide and cisplatin)	Normal delivery, no congenital malformations	[50]

Topoisomerase inhibitors	Description of study	Pregnancy outcome	References
Doxorubicin and Daunorubicin	36 patients with various malignancies treated with doxorubicin during 2nd and 3rd trimesters	1 hip subluxation (treated together with cyclophosphamide) 1 infant born with doubled cartilage ring in both ears (FAC regimen)	[78]

Topoisomerase inhibitors	Description of study	Pregnancy outcome	References
	25 patients treated with various regimens during 2nd and 3rd trimesters; (treated with daunorubicin)	1 infant born with bilateral partial syndactyly digits II-III 1 infant born with rectal atresia	[78]
	118 patients treated for breast cancer (98) and lymphoma (20) with various regimens; all treated during 2nd or 3rd trimester	1 infant with IgA deficiency, 1 neonatal death due to autoimmune disorder, 1 infant with pyloric stenosis, 1 infant born with holoprosencephaly,1 intrauterine death with normal autopsy	[33]
	11 patients treated together with cyclophosphamide during 2nd and 3rd trimesters	No congenital malformations	[69]
	1 patient treated for AML and ATRA; started at second trimester	No congenital malformations Transient dilated cardiomyopathy.	[72]
Epirubicin	5 patients treated together with cyclophosphamide during 2nd and 3rd trimesters	No congenital malformations	[69]
Etoposide (VP16–213)	4 patients treated during 2nd and 3rd trimesters for various malignancies	1 infant born with genetic hearing loss – both parents were carriers	[33]
	1 patient with small cell lung cancer at 26 weeks gestation; treated together with cisplatin	No congenital malformations	[81]
	1 patient treated for teratoma during 3rd trimester (together with bleomycin and cisplatin)	Normal delivery, no congenital malformations	[50]
Idarubicin	1 patient treated for AML during 1st	No congenital malformations	[77]

Topoisomerase inhibitors	Description of study	Pregnancy outcome	References
	trimester together with ATRA		
	9 cases of patients treated for various malignancies during 2nd and 3rd trimesters	1 infant with transient dilated cardiomyopathy 2 cases of permanent dilated cardiomyopathy 1 infant born with short limbs, digits and macrognathia	[23,36,58,65,72]
Mitoxantrone	1 patient treated for teratoma during 3rd trimester (together with bleomycin and cisplatin)	Normal delivery, no congenital malformations	[50]

Antimetabolites	Description of study	Pregnancy outcome	References
5-Fluorouracil	18 patients treated for breast and colorectal cancer during 2nd and 3rd trimesters	No congenital malformations	[33]
	35 patients treated with the FAC protocol during 2nd and 3rd trimesters	1 infant with Down syndrome; 1 with clubfoot; 1 with congenital bilateral ureteral reflux	[46]
	12 patients treated together with cyclophosphamide and methotrexate during 2nd and 3rd trimesters	No congenital malformations	[69]
	53 patients, 5 treated during 1st trimester	6 cases of IUGR; 1 case of spontaneous neonatal death – miscarriage	[34]
Capecitabine	1 patient treated for colorectal cancer with oxaloplatin during 1st trimester	No congenital malformations	[33]
Cytosine arabinoside	1 patient treated for NHL during 3rd trimester	No congenital malformations	[33]

Antimetabolites	Description of study	Pregnancy outcome	References
	1 patient treated for ALL during 2nd and 3rd trimesters		
	9 patients treated for leukemia, 5 during 1st trimester with varying regimens	No congenital malformations	[26]
Gemcitabine	1 patient treated for pancreatic tumor during 2nd and 3rd trimesters	No congenital malformations	[33]
	1 patient treated for NSCLC during 3rd trimester	No congenital malformations; delivered at 28 weeks gestation	[45]
Methotrexate	12 patients treated together with cyclophosphamide and 5-FU during 2nd and 3rd trimesters	No congenital malformations	[69]
	20 cases treated during 1st trimester	7 cases developed a pattern very similar to the aminopterin syndrome (cranial dysotosis with delayed ossification, hypertelorism, wide nasal bridge, micrognathia, and ear abnormalities); 1 case of skeletal abnormalities and ambiguous genitalia 5 cases of spontaneous abortion	[24,28,31,37,38,39, 53,60,67]

Antimitotic agents	Description of study	Pregnancy outcome	References
Docetaxel	19 patients, two treated during 1st trimester; 3 with paclitaxel. All treated with different regimens	2 infants with ventriculomegaly, noted not related to docetaxel; 1 infant with holoprosencephaly; 1 infant with pyloric stenosis (treated with paclitaxel)	[61]

Antimitotic agents	Description of study	Pregnancy outcome	References
Paclitaxel	16 patients treated for varying malignancies during 2nd and 3rd trimesters	1 infant with pyloric stenosis; 1 intrauterine fetal death with normal autopsy	[33]
	24 patients treated for cancer, 3 with docetaxel. All treated with different chemotherapy regimens	1 infant had pyloric stenosis (treated with docetaxel)	[61]
	1 patient treated weekly from 20 weeks gestation	No congenital malformations	[43]
Vincristine	11 patients treated for various cancers during 2nd and 3rd trimesters	1 infant died at 30 weeks gestation, normal autopsy	[33]
Vinblastine	20 patients treated for HD and NHL during 2nd and 3rd trimesters	1 infant with plagiocephaly 1 infant with syndactyly 4th and 5th digits	[33]

Molecularly targeted agents	Description of study	Pregnancy outcome	References
Imatinib	180 patients, 103 exposed during 1st trimester; Outcome data were available for 125 cases	18 spontaneous abortions; 35 cases of elective pregnancy termination (unspecified reasons) 12 cases of congenital malformations, Including 3 cases with similar malformations (a combination of exomphalus with severe renal and skeletal malformations). Other malformations included hypospadias, cerebellar hypoplasia, ASD, pyloric stenosis, hypoplastic lung	[68] (Pharmaceutical company data report)
Lapatinib	Patient conceived during treatment; treatment stopped at 14 weeks of gestation	No congenital malformations	[51]

Molecularly targeted agents	Description of study	Pregnancy outcome	References
Rituximab	2 patients treated for NHL	1 case of intrauterine fetal death at week 30, normal autopsy	[33]
	231 patients treated for NHL and auto-immune diseases. Outcome data were available for 153 patients Most cases were confounded by the concomitant use of other medications- most commonly methotrexate	33 spontaneous abortions. 28 cases of elective pregnancy termination (unspecified reasons) 1 maternal death from severe underlying thrombocytopenia (ITP). 2 cases of congenital malformations. One infant born with clubfoot, and another one with cardiac malformations (VSD+PFO+PDA).	[35] (Pharmaceutical company data base report)
Tretinoin (ATRA)	1 patient treated for AML during 1st trimester together with idarubicin	No congenital malformations	[77]
	1 patient treated for AML together with idarubicin, starting at the 2nd trimester.	Transient dilated cardiomyopathy; no congenital malformations	[72]
	1 patient treated for APL; 13 patients previously reported at this chapter. 3 were treated during 1st trimester	No congenital malformations No congenital malformations	[42,47,48,49,54,55,57, 62,64,70,71,73,75,79]

References

1. Cardonick E, Iacobucci A. Use of chemotherapy during human pregnancy. *Lancet Oncol.* 2004;5:283–91.

2. Leslie KK. Chemotherapy and pregnancy. *Clin Obstet Gynecol.* 2002;45:153–64.

3. Van Calsteren K, Verbesselt R, Ottevanger N, et al. Pharmacokinetics of chemotherapeutic agents in pregnancy: a preclinical and clinical study. *Acta Obst Gynecol.* 2010;89:1338–45.

4. Pentheroudakis G. Cancer and pregnancy. *Ann Oncol.* 2008;19(suppl 5):v38–9.

5. Pentheroudakis G, Orecchia R, Hoekstra HJ, Pavlildis N, EMSO Guidelines Working Group. Cancer, fertility and pregnancy: ESMO Clinical Practice Guidelines for diagnosis, treatment and follow-up. *Ann Oncol.* 2010;21(suppl 5):v266–73.

6. Lishner M. Cancer in pregnancy. *Ann Oncol.* 2003;14(suppl 3):iii31–iii36.

7. Pereg D, Koren G, Lishner M. The treatment of Hodgkin and non-Hodgkin's

lymphoma in pregnancy. *Haematologica.* 2007;**92**:1230–7.

8. Shapira T, Pereg D, Lishner M. How I treat acute and chronic leukemia in pregnancy. *Blood Rev.* 2008;**22**:247–59.

9. Pereg D, Koren G, Lishner M. Cancer in pregnancy: gaps, challenges and solutions. *Cancer Treat Rev.* 2008;**34**:302–12.

10. Doll DC, Ringenberg QS, Yarbro JW. Antineoplastic agents and pregnancy. *Semin Oncol.* 1989;**16**:337–46.

11. Cardonick E, Usmaniv A, Ghaffar S. Perinatal outcome of a pregnancy complicated by cancer, including neonatal follow-up after in utero exposure to chemotherapy. *Am J Clin Oncol.* 2010;**33**:221–8.

12. Van Calsteren K, Heyns L, De Smet F, et al. Cancer during pregnancy: an analysis of 215 patients emphasizing the obstetrical and the neonatal outcomes. *J Clin Oncol.* 2010;**28**:683–9.

13. Azim HA Jr, Paclidis N, Peccatori FA. Treatment of the pregnant mother with cancer: a systemic review on the use of cytotoxic, endocrine, targeted agents and immunotherapy during pregnancy. Part I and II. *Cancer Treat Rev.* 2010;**36**:101–21.

14. Pye SM, Cortes J, Ault P, et al. The effects of imatinib on pregnancy outcome. *Blood.* 2008;**111**:5505–8.

15. Cole S, Kantarjian H, Ault P, Cortés JE. Successful completion of pregnancy in patient with CML without active intervention: a case report and review of the literature. *Clin Lymphoma Myeloma.* 2009;**9**:324–7.

16. Chakravarty EF, Murray ER, Kelman A, Farmer P. Pregnancy outcomes following maternal exposure to rituximab. *Blood.* 2011;**117**:1499–506.

17. Durodola JI. Administration of cyclophosphamide during late pregnancy and early lactation: a case report. *J Natl Med Assoc.* 1979;**71**:165–6.

18. Ali R, Ozkalemkes F, Kimya Y, et al. Imatinib use during pregnancy and breast feeding: a case report and review of the literature. *Arch Gynecol Obstet.* 2009;**280**:169–75.

19. Gambacorti-Passerini CB, Tornaghi L, Marangon E, et al. Imatinib concentrations in human milk. *Blood.* 2007;**109**:1790.

20. Russell MA, Carpenter MW, Akhtar MS, Lagattuta TF, Egorin MJ. Imatinib mesylate and metabolite concentrations in maternal blood, umbilical cord blood, placenta and breast milk. *J Perinatol.* 2007;**27**:241–3.

21. Avilés A, Neri N. Hematological malignancies and pregnancy: a final report of 84 children who received chemotherapy in utero. *Clinical Lymphoma.* 2001;**2**:173–7.

22. Nulman I, Laslo D, Fried S, Uleryke E, Lishner M, Koren G. Neurodevelopment of children exposed in utero to treatment of maternal malignancy. *Br J Cancer.* 2001;**85**:1611–8.

23. Achtari C, Hohlfeld P. Cardiotoxic transplacental effect of idarubicin administered during the second trimester of pregnancy. *Am J Obstet Gynecol.* 2000;**183**:511–2.

24. Addar MH. Methotrexate embryopathy in a surviving intrauterine fetus after presumed diagnosis of ectopic pregnancy: case report. *J Obstet Gynaecol Can.* 2004;**26**:1001–3.

25. Ali R, Ozkalemkes F, Kimya Y, et al. Imatinib use during pregnancy and breast feeding: a case report and review of the literature. *Arch Gynecol Obstet.* 2009;**280**:169–75.

26. Avilés A, Díaz-Maqueo JC, Talavera A, Guzmán R, García EL. Growth and development of children of mothers treated with chemotherapy during pregnancy: current status of 43 children. *Am J Hematol.* 1991;**36**:243–8.

27. Avilés A, Neri N. Hematological malignancies and pregnancy: a final report of 84 children who received chemotherapy in utero. *Clin Lymphoma.* 2001;**2**:173–7.

28. Bawle EV, Conard JV, Weiss L. Adult and two children with fetal methotrexate syndrome. *Teratology.* 1998;**7**;51–5.

29. Benhaim X, Pautier P, Bensaid C, Lhomme C, Haie-Meder C, Morice P. Neoadjuvant

chemotherapy for advanced stage cervical cancer in a pregnant patient: report of one case with rapid tumor progression. *Eur J Obstet Gynecol Reprod Biol.* 2008;**136**:267–8.

30. Berry DL, Theriault RL, Holes FA, et al. Management of breast cancer during pregnancy using a standardized protocol. *J Clin Oncol.* 1999;**17**:855–61.

31. Buckley LM, Bullboy CA, Leichtman L, Marquez M. Multiple congenital anomalies associated with weekly low dose methotrexate treatment of the mother. *Arthritis Rheum.* 1997;**40**:971–3.

32. Caluwaerts S, Van Calsteren K, Mertens L, et al. Neoadjuvant chemotherapy followed by radical hysterectomy for invasive cervical cancer diagnosed during pregnancy: report of a case and review of the literature. *Int J Gynecol Cancer.* 2006;**16**:905–8.

33. Cardonick E, Usmani A, Ghaffar S. Perinatal outcome of a pregnancy complicated by cancer, including neonatal follow-up after in utero exposure to chemotherapy. *Am J Clin Oncol.* 2010;**33**:221–8.

34. Cardonick E, Iacobucci A. Use of chemotherapy during human pregnancy. *Lancet Oncol.* 2004;**5**:283–91.

35. Chakravarty EF, Murray EF, Kelman A, Farmer P. Pregnancy outcomes after maternal exposure to rituximab. *Blood.* 2010;**117**:1499–506.

36. Claahsen HL, Semmekrot BA, van Dongen PW, Mattijssen V. Successful outcome after exposure to idarubicin and cytosine-arabinoside during second trimester of pregnancy-a case report. *Am J Perinatol.* 1998;**15**:295–7.

37. Dara P. Slater LM. Armentrout SA. Successful pregnancy during chemotherapy for acute leukemia. *Cancer.* 1981;**47**:845–6.

38. Diniz EM, Corradini HB, Ramos JL, Brock R. Effect of the fetus of methotrexate (amethopterin) administered to the mother. Presentation of a case. *Rev Hosp Clin Fac Med Sao Paulo.* 1978;**33**:286–90.

39. Feliu J, Juarez S, Ordonez A, Garcia-Paredes ML, Gonzalez-Baron M, Montero JM. Acute leukemia and pregnancy. *Cancer.* 1988;**61**:580–4.

40. Ferrandina G, Distefano M, Testa A, De Vincenzo R, Scambia G. Management of an advanced ovarian cancer at 15 weeks of gestation: case report and literature review. *Gynecol Oncol.* 2005;**97**:693–6.

41. Giacalone PL, Laffargue F, Benos P, Rousseau O, Hedon B. Cisplatinum neoadjuvant chemotherapy in a pregnant woman with invasive carcinoma of the uterine cervix. *Br J Obstet Gynaecol.* 1996;**103**:932–4.

42. Giagounidis AA, Beckmann MW, Giagounidis AS, et al. Acute promyelocytic leukemia and Pregnancy. *Eur J Haematol.* 2000;**64**:267–71.

43. Gonzalez-Angulo AM, Walters RS, Carpenter RJ Jr, et al. Paclitaxel chemotherapy in pregnant patient with bilateral breast cancer. *Clin Breast Cancer.* 2004;**4**:317–9.

44. Greenberg LH, Tanaka KR. Congenital anomalies probably induced by cyclophosphamide. *JAMA* 1964;**188**:423–6.

45. Gurumurthy M, Koh P, Singh R, et al. Metastatic non-small-cell lung cancer and the use of gemcitabine during pregnancy. *J Perinatol.* 2009;**29**:63–5.

46. Hahn K, Johnson P, Gordon N, et al. Treatment of pregnant breast cancer patients and outcomes of children exposed to chemotherapy in utero. *Cancer.* 2006;**107**:1219–26.

47. Harrison P, Chipping P, Fothergill GA. Successful use of all-trans-retinoic acid in acute promyelocytic leukaemia presenting during the second trimester of pregnancy. *Br J Haematol.* 1994;**86**:681–2.

48. Heistinger M, Schume J, Isak E, et al. Acute promyelocytic leukemia (APL) in late pregnancy: successful treatment with all-trans-retinoic acid (ATRA) – a case report. *Onkologie.* 1995;**18**:137.

49. Incerpi MH, Miller DA, Posen R, Byrne. All-transretinoic acid for the treatment of acute promyelocytic leukemia in pregnancy. *Obstet Gynecol.* 1997;**89**:826–8.

50. Karimi Zarchi M, Behtash N, Modares Gilani M. Good pregnancy outcome after

prenatal exposure to bleomycin, etoposide and cisplatin for ovarian immature teratoma: a case report and literature review. *Arch Gynecol Obstet.* 2008; **277**:75–8.

51. Kelly H, Graham M, Humes E, et al. Delivery of a healthy baby after first trimester maternal exposure to lapatinib. *Clin Breast Cancer.* 2006;**7**:339–41.

52. Kirshon B, Wasserstrum N, Willis R, Herman GE, McCabe ER. Teratogenic effects of first-trimester cyclophosphamide therapy. *Obstet Gynecol.* 1988;**72**:462–4.

53. Kozlowski RD, Steinbrunner JV, Mackenzie AH, Clough JD, Wilke WS, Segal AM. Outcome of first trimester exposure to low dose methotrexate in eight patients with rheumatic disease. *Am J Med.* 1990;**88**:589–92.

54. Lin CP, Huang MJ, Liu HJ, Chang IY, Tsai CH. Successful treatment of acute promyelocytic leukemia in a pregnant Jehovah's witness with all-trans-retinoic acid, rhG-CSF, and erythropoietin. *Am J Hematol.* 1996;**51**:251.

55. Lipovsky MM, Biesma DH, Christiaens GC, Petersen EJ. Successful treatment of acute promyelocytic leukaemia with all-trans-retinoic-acid during late pregnancy. *Br J Haematol.* 1996;**97**:699–701.

56. Lishner M, Zemlickis D, Degendorfer P, Panzarella T, Sutcliffe SB, Koren G. Maternal and foetal outcome following Hodgkin's disease in pregnancy. *Br J Cancer.* 1992;**65**:114–7.

57. Maeda M, Tyugu H, Okubo T, Yamamoto M, Nakamura K, Dan K. Neonate born to a mother with acute promyelocytic leukemia treated by all-trans-retinoic acid. *Rinsho Ketsueki.* 1997;**38**:770–5.

58. Matsuo K, Shimoya K, Ueda S, Wada K, Doyama M, Murata Y. Idarubicin administered during pregnancy: its effect on the fetus. *Gynecol Obstet Invest.* 2004;**58**:186–8.

59. Merimsky O, Le Chevalier T, Missenard G, et al. Management of cancer in pregnancy: a case of Ewing's sarcoma of the pelvis in the third trimester. *Ann Oncol.* 1999;**10**:345–50.

60. Milunsky A, Greaf JW, Gaynor MF Jr. Methotrexate induced congenital malformations. *J Pediatr.* 1968;**72**:790–5.

61. Mir O, Berveilleret P, Ropert S, Goffinet F, Goldwasser F. Use of platinum derivatives during pregnancy. *Cancer.* 2008;113,**11**:3069–74.

62. Morton J, Taylor K, Wright S. Successful maternal outcome following the use of ATRA for the induction of APML late in the first trimester. *Blood.* 1995;**86**:772a.

63. Nakajima W, Ishida A, Takahashi M, et al. Good outcome for infant of mother treated with chemotherapy for Ewing sarcoma at 25 to 30 weeks' gestation. *J Pediatr Hematol Oncol.* 2004;**26**:308–11.

64. Nakamura K, Dan K, Kwakiri R, Gomi S, Nomura T. Successful treatment of acute promyelocytic leukemia in pregnancy with all-trans retinoic acid. *Ann Hematol.* 1995;**71**:263–4.

65. Niedermeier DM, Frei-Lahr DA, Hall PD. Treatment of acute myeloid leukemia during the second and third trimesters of pregnancy. *Pharmacotherapy.* 2005;**25**:1134–40.

66. Palaia I, Pernice M, Graziano M, Bellati F, Panici PB. Neoadjuvant chemotherapy plus radical surgery in locally advanced cervical cancer during pregnancy: a case report. *Am J Obstet Gynecol.* 2007;**197**:e5–6.

67. Powell HR, Ekert H. Methotrexate induced congenital malformations. *Med J Aust.* 1971;**2**:1076–7.

68. Pye SM, Cortes J, Ault P, et al. The effects of imatinib on pregnancy outcome. *Blood.* 2008;**111**:5505–8.

69. Ring AE, Smith IE, Jones A, Shannon C, Galani E, Ellis PA. Chemotherapy for breast cancer during pregnancy: an 18-year experience from five London teaching hospitals. *J Clin Oncol.* 2005;**23**:4192–7.

70. Sham RL. All-trans-retinoic acid-induced labor in a pregnant patient with acute promyelocytic leukemia. *Am J Hematol.* 1996;**53**:145.

71. Simone MD, Stasi R, Venditti A. All-trans-retinoic acid (ATRA) administration

during pregnancy in relapsed acute Promyelocytic leukemia [letter]. *Leukemia.* 1995;**9**:1412–3.

72. Siu BL, Alonzo MR, Varga TA, Ferich AL. Transient dilated cardiomyopathy in a newborn exposed to idarubicin and all-trans-retinoic acid (ATRA) early in the second trimester of pregnancy. *Int J Gynecol Cancer.* 2002;**12**:399–402.

73. Stentoft J, Nielsen JL, Hvidman LE. All-trans retinoic acid in acute promyelocytic leukemia in late pregnancy. *Leukemia.* 1994;**8**:1585–8.

74. Tabata T, Nishiura K, Tanida K, Kondo E, Okugawa T, Sagawa N. Carboplatin chemotherapy in a pregnant patient with undifferentiated ovarian carcinoma: case report and review of the literature. *Int J Gynecol Cancer.* 2008;**18**:181–4.

75. Terada Y, Shindo T, Endoh A, Watanabe M, Fukaya T, Yajima A. Fetal arrhythmia during treatment of pregnancy associated acute promyelocytic leukemia with all-transretinoic acid and favorable outcome. *Leukemia.* 1997;**11**:454–5.

76. Toledo TM, Harper RC, Moser RH. Fetal effects during cyclophosphamide and irradiation therapy. *Ann Intern Med.* 1971;**74**:87–91.

77. Valappil S, Kurkar M, Howell R. Outcome of pregnancy in women treated with all-trans retinoic acid: a case report and review of literature. *Hematology.* 2007;**12**:415–8.

78. Van Calsteren K, Heyns L, De Smet F, et al. Cancer during pregnancy: an analysis of 215 patients emphasizing the obstetrical and the neonatal outcomes. *J Clin Oncol.* 2010;**28**:683–9.

79. Watanabe R, Okamoto S, Moriki T, Kizaki M, Kawai Y, Ikeda Y. Treatment of acute promylocytic leukemia with all-transretinoic acid during the third trimester of pregnancy. *Am J Hematol.* 1995;**48**:210–1.

80. Zemlickis D, Lishner M, Erlich R, Koren G. Teratogenicity and carcinogenicity in a twin exposed in utero to cyclophosphamide. *Teratog Carcinog Mutagen.* 1993;**13**:139–43.

81. Kluetz PG, Edelman MJ. Successful treatment of small cell lung cancer during pregnancy. *Lung Cancer.* 2008;**61**:129–30.

82. Murry CL, Reichery JA, Anderson J, Twiggs LB. Multimodal cancer therapy for breast cancer in the first trimester of pregnancy. A case report. *JAMA.* 1984;**252**:2607–8.

Chapter

15

Nonobstetrical surgical interventions during pregnancy

Bi Lan Wo, Angela Mallozzi, and Alon Shrim

Introduction

It is estimated that 8,000 to 50,000 nonobstetrical surgical procedures are performed on pregnant women every year in the United States [1,2]. and between 5,700 to 76,000 in Europe [3]. The incidence of nonobstetrical general surgery procedures during pregnancy is reported at 0.75% to 2% of all pregnancies [4–6]. The largest cohort of nonobstetrical procedures during pregnancy was reported by Mazze and Kallen (1989) who analyzed the reproductive outcomes in 5,405 nonobstetrical surgeries in 720,000 pregnant women from the Swedish healthcare registries between 1973 and 1981. The greatest proportion of procedures, 41.6%, occurred in the first trimester, followed by the second and third trimesters at 34.8% and 23.5%, respectively [6]. Improved diagnostic and imaging techniques with minimal radiation exposure, including computed tomography scan, magnetic resonance imaging, and ultrasound, has generated a shift away from diagnostic laparoscopy over the past 20 years. In the 1990s, laparoscopic surgery, including appendectomy and cholecystectomy, was in its infancy with most cases being done through a traditional open approach or laparotomy compared to the preponderance of the laparoscopic approach used currently. Based on most recent data, with the decrease of diagnostic laparotomy, the most common nonobstetrical intervention during pregnancy is appendectomy, including both open and laparoscopic [7].

Additional conditions requiring surgery during pregnancy include ovarian cysts, masses or torsions, cholecystitis, symptomatic cholelithiasis, adrenal tumors, complicated inflammatory bowel diseases, and abdominal pain of unknown etiology [8,9].

Recommendations regarding timing of surgery have been based on experience with open surgical procedures. Historically, general guidelines emphasized delay of surgery until the second trimester to minimize the possibility of first-trimester miscarriage following surgery and teratogenicity from exposure of the developing fetus to anesthetic agents [6]. This experience has not been reproduced in the most recent literature reporting laparoscopic cases. Several recent studies have shown that pregnant patients may undergo laparoscopic surgery safely at any time without any appreciated increased risk to the mother or the fetus [10–16].

This present chapter summarizes current data on the maternal and fetal effects of nonobstetrical surgeries during pregnancy, including anesthesia, diagnostic and therapeutic management, laparoscopy, and the common general surgical pathologies found in the pregnant patient. We have only included publications that reported a series of at least 10 patients.

Cancer in Pregnancy and Lactation: The Motherisk Guide ed. Gideon Koren and Michael Lishner. Published by Cambridge University Press. © Cambridge University Press 2011.

Anesthesia during pregnancy

Six reviews have been published on anesthesia in pregnant women for nonobstetrical surgery [3,17–21]. Changes in maternal physiology during pregnancy due to gestational hormones and mechanical effects of the increasingly gravid uterus have an impact on anesthesia during nonobstetrical surgery.

The safety of nonobstetrical surgery and anesthesia has been well established for nearly every operative procedure [4,6,8,20,22–27]. No differences in congenital abnormalities have been described in groups of women undergoing nonobstetrical surgery during pregnancy compared with women who did not have surgery [6,28,29]. Two studies showed a small increase in preterm birth (PTB)[6] and higher rate of miscarriage [29]. Many outcome studies show that women who have surgery during pregnancy deliver earlier and have smaller babies. However, the majority of studies suggests that it is probably the primary disease or the site of surgery that has the greater impact on the rates of PTB or miscarriages [30].

A recent meta-analysis reviewed 12452 pregnant women who underwent nonobstetrical surgeries in 54 publications. It was concluded that maternal mortality is a rare event, with only 1 case out of their entire study population being reported. There was no increase in risk of major birth defects, or miscarriages, and fetal loss was only increased with appendicitis complicated by peritonitis [30].

The American College for Obstetrics and Gynecology (ACOG) concluded that although there are no data to support specific recommendations for nonobstetrical surgery and anesthesia in pregnancy, it is important for physicians to obtain obstetric consultation before surgery. The decision to use intraoperative fetal monitoring should be individualized, and each case warrants a team approach for the optimal safety of the woman and her baby [31].

Only 1 recent publication examined the long-term consequences of exposure to anesthetic agents *in utero* and reported that it was associated with learning disabilities in children who received multiple anesthetic agents; however, no effects were shown when a single-agent anesthetic was used [32].

Appendectomy

We identified 37 studies that focused on the treatment of appendicitis during pregnancy (Table 1), with the last review published in 2007 [33].

Incidence

Appendectomy is the most common nonobstetrical surgical intervention during pregnancy [5,34]. However, it is less common in pregnant than nonpregnant women. The third trimester appears to be particularly protective, with an odds ratio (OR) reported at 0.33, 95% confidence interval (CI): 0.28–0.39 for nonperforated appendicitis and OR = 0.49, 95% CI: 0.30–0.79 for perforated appendicitis [35] The incidence ranging from 1 in 614 pregnancies [36] to 1 in 5,529 pregnancies [37].

The diagnosis of appendicitis can still be challenging during pregnancy. First, the presenting complaints may be less specific (e.g., nausea, vomiting, vague abdominal discomfort). Second, an enlarging uterus gradually displaces the appendix out of the pelvis into the right upper quadrant. Third, diagnostic imaging like ultrasound may not be able to

Table 1. Children exposed in utero to glucocorticoids

Author	Year of publication	Procedure	Study design	N [trimesters: 1,2,3]	Pregnancy outcome			Fetal outcome			Maternal mortality	Addressing confounders
					SA	TA	Surgery-induced delivery	Death	Prematurity	MM		
Finch[105]	1974	Appendectomy	Retro. Series	56[16,25,15]	0	0	0	4	2	0	0	No
Mohammed[106]	1975	Appendectomy	Retro. Series	20[12,6,2]	2	0	0	1	2	0	0	No
Cunningham[34]	1975	Appendectomy	Retro. Series	34[10,16,8]	2	0	NA	1	3	0	0	No
Townsend[107]	1976	Appendectomy	Retro. Series	29[8,14,7]	1	1	1	2	2	0	0	No
Gomez[42]	1979	Appendectomy	Retro. Series	35[9,17,9]	NA	NA	1	0	3	0	0	No
Punnonen[108]	1979	Appendectomy	Retro. Series	24[2,14,8]	0	0	2	1	1	0	0	No
Frisenda[41]	1979	Appendectomy	Retro. Series	37[10,16,11]	1	0	0	0	1	0	0	No
Farquharson[109]	1980	Appendectomy	Retro. Series	25[9,13,3]	NA	NA	1	1	4	0	0	No
McComb[110]	1980	Appendectomy	Retro. Series	19[3,9,7]	1	NA	NA	1	3	0	0	No
Horowitz[37]	1985[†]	Appendectomy	Retro. Series	10[1,9,0]	1	0	1	3	1	0	0	No
Doberneck[111]	1985	Appendectomy	Retro. Series	29[9,14,6]	0	2	3	0	3	0	0	No

Table 1. (cont.)

Author	Year of publication	Procedure	Study design	N [trimesters: 1,2,3]	Pregnancy outcome			Fetal outcome			Maternal mortality	Addressing confounders
					SA	TA	Surgery-induced delivery	Death	Prematurity	MM	MM	
Bailey[112]	1986	Appendectomy	Retro. Series	41[NA]	1	NA	NA	1	0	1	0	No
Liang[113]	1989	Appendectomy	Retro. Series	24[6,12,6]	0	0	3	0	5	0	0	No
Tamir[114]	1990‡	Appendectomy	Retro. Series	77[27,37,13]	2	7	4	0	23	0	0	No
Mazze[23]	1991	Appendectomy	Retro. Registry	778[272,400,106]	NA	NA	39	14	57	18	NA	No
Halvorsen[53]	1992 ††	Appendectomy	Retro. Series	12[0,6,6]	0	0	0	1	2	0	0	No
To[115]	1995‡‡	Appendectomy	Retro. Series	34[13,13,8]	5	0	4	0	5	0	0	No
Al-Mulhim[36]	1996	Appendectomy	Retro. Series	49[10,31,8]	3	0	7	7	3	0	0	No
Andersen[116]	1999	Appendectomy	Retro. Series	56[12,28,16]	4	0	2	1	4	0	0	No
Hee[117]	1999‡‡†	Appendectomy	Retro. Series	117[28,67,22]	4	2	0	NA	2	NA	0	No
Nunnelee[118]	1999	Appendectomy	Retro. Series	42[NA]	0	1	0	0	0	0	0	No
Mourad[51]	2000	Appendectomy	Retro. Series	67[17,27,23]	0	0	1	0	3	0	0	No

Study	Year	Procedure	Study type									
Tracey[119]	2000	Appendectomy	Retro. Series	22[5,6,11]	0	0	1	0	5	0	0	No
Sakhri[120]	2001	Appendectomy	Retro. Series	23[2,6,15]	0	0	0	1	3	0	0	No
Hsu[121]	2001	Appendectomy	Retro. Series	35[11,19,5]	0	3	3	1	0	0	0	No
Ghazanfar[122]	2001	Appendectomy	Retro. Series	50[19,26,5]	0	0	0	7	0	0	0	No
Duqoum[123]	2001	Appendectomy	Retro. Series	10[5,4,1]	2	0	1	0	1	0	0	No
Ueberrueck[57]	2004	Appendectomy	Retro. Series	94[23,48,23]	3	3	0	3	3	0	0	No
Carver[124]	2005	Appendectomy	Retro. Series	28[9,19,0]	2	0	0	0	0	0	0	No
Wu[49]	2005	Appendectomy	Retro. Series	11[5,5,1]	0	2	1	1	0	0	0	No
McGory[52]	2007	Appendectomy	Retro. Series	3133[NA]	NA	NA	NA	119	217	NA	0	Yes
Kazim[48]	2009	Appendectomy	Retro. Series	37[11,14,12]	1	0	3	0	5	0	0	No
Kirshtein[125]	2009	Appendectomy	Retro. Series	42[23,19,0]	0	0	NA	2	0	NA	0	No
Lemieux[126]	2009	Appendectomy	Retro. Series	45[15,22,8]	0	8	0	0	7	0	0	No
Machado[127]	2009	Appendectomy	Retro. Series	20[8,9,3]	1	0	0	0	0	0	0	No
Zhang[55]	2009	Appendectomy	Retro. Series	78[24,46,8]	NA	NA	NA	4	5	0	0	No

Table 1. (cont.)

Author	Year of publication	Procedure	Study design	N [trimesters: 1,2,3]	Pregnancy outcome			Fetal outcome		MM	Maternal mortality	Addressing confounders
					SA	TA	Surgery-induced delivery	Death	Prematurity			
Sadot[128]	2010	Appendectomy	Retro. Series	65[14,44,7]	0	0	0	1	15	0	0	No
Greene[29]	1963	Cholecystect.	Retro. Series	17[10,5,2]	0	0	0	3	1	0	0	No
Hill[71]	1975	Cholecystect.	Retro. Series	20[NA]	1	1	0	1	0	0	0	No
Dixon[30]	1987	Cholecystect.	Retro. Series	18[3,14,1]	0	2	0	0	1	0	0	No
Swisher[131]	1994	Cholecystect.	Retro. Series	16[5,11,0]	0	0	0	0	2	0	0	No
Davis[132]	1995	Cholecystect.	Retro. Series	19[4,10,5]	0	0	0	0	5	0	0	No
Steinbrook[133]	1996	Cholecystect.	Retro. Series	10[NA]	0	0	0	0	0	0	0	No
Barone[11]	1999	Cholecystect.	Retro. Series	46[NA]	0	0	1	2	1	1	1	No
Cosenza[134]	1999	Cholecystect.	Retro. Series	32[8,22,2]	1	2	0	1	1	0	0	No
Daradkeh[135]	1999	Cholecystect.	Retro. Series	16[2,10,4]	0	0	0	0	0	0	0	No
Muench[136]	2001	Cholecystect.	Retro. Series	14[NA]	0	0	0	0	1	0	0	No

Study	Year	Procedure	Study type	N [...]								
Patel[137]	2002	Cholecystect.	Retro. Series	10[3,6,1]	1	0	0	0	0	0	0	No
Lu[138]	2004	Cholecystect.	Retro. Series	10[0,8,2]	0	0	0	0	0	0	0	No
Bani Hani[77]	2007	Cholecystect.	Retro. Series	10[5,3,2]	0	0	0	0	0	0	0	No
Curet[64]	1996	Laparoscopy	Case control	34[15,19,0]	0	0	0	0	0	0	0	No
Amos[139]	1996	Laparoscopy	Retro. Series	12[NA]	2	0	0	4	0	0	0	No
Andreoli[140]	1996	Laparoscopy	Retro. Series	18[4,11,3]	0	0	0	0	1	0	0	No
Reedy[15]	1997	Laparoscopy	Retro. Registry	3,704[NA]	NA	NA	NA	30	NA	173	NA	Yes
Conron[141]	1998	Laparoscopy	Retro. Series	21[12,0,9]	1	0	0	1	1	0	0	No
Akira[142]	1999	Laparoscopy	Retro. Series	35[NA]	1	0	NA	1	0	0	0	No
Affleck[10]	1999	Laparoscopy	Retro. Series	98[NA]	0	0	NA	0	11	0	0	No
Lyass[143]	2001	Laparoscopy	Pros. Cohort	22[7,8,7]	0	0	0	0	0	0	0	No
Rojansky[144]	2002	Laparoscopy	Retro. Series	37[NA]	2	1	0	0	3	2	0	No
Oelsner[13]	2003	Laparoscopy	Retro. Series	389[204,156,29]	0	22	NA	0	11	7	0	No
Rizzo[68]	2003	Laparoscopy	Retro. Series	11[0,11,0]	0	NA	NA	0	0	0	0	No

Table 1. (cont.)

Author	Year of publication	Procedure	Study design	N [trimesters: 1,2,3]	Pregnancy outcome			Fetal outcome			Maternal mortality	Addressing confounders
					SA	TA	Surgery-induced delivery	Death	Prematurity	MM		
Rollins[16]	2004	Laparoscopy	Retro. Series	59[9,32,18]	0	0	0	1	4	0	0	No
Halkic[22]	2006	Laparoscopy	Retro. Series	16[0,13,3]	0	0	0	0	0	0	0	No
Palanivelu[145]	2007	Laparoscopy	Retro. Series	19[0,19,0]	NA	NA	NA	0	NA	NA	0	No
Buser[i] [146]	2009	Laparoscopy	Retro. Series	36[8,22,7]	NA	NA	NA	0	1	0	0	No
Corneille[ii] [147]	2010	Laparoscopy	Retro. Series	54[NA]	3	NA	0	1	8	0	0	No
Hess[148]	1988	Adnexal	Retro. Series	54[9,41,4]	5	1	0	0	3	0	0	Yes
Platek[149]	1995	Adnexal	Retro. Series	19[NA]	1	0	0	0	0	0	0	No
Soriano[150]	1999	Adnexal	Retro. Series	93[64,29,0]	7	NA	0	0	8	3	0	No
Moore[86]	1999	Adnexal	Retro. Series	14[0,9,0]	0	0	0	1	3	0	0	No
Whitecar[151]	1999	Adnexal	Retro. Series	129[15,65,49]	0	0	1	2	12	0	0	No

Study	Year	Type	Design	N[...]								Outcome
Usui[152]	2000	Adnexal	Retro. Series	60[NA]	2	0	0	3	7	2	0	No
Mathevet[84]	2003	Adnexal	Retro. Series	48[17,27,4]	0	0	0	1	3	0	0	No
Sherard[79]	2003	Adnexal	Retro. Series	51[NA]	2	1	0	0	10	0	0	No
Steppl[153]	2003	Adnexal	Retro. Series	11[0,11,0]	0	0	0	0	0	0	0	No
Carter[154]	2004	Adnexal	Retro. Series	16[NA]	1	0	0	0	4	NA	0	No
Yuen[155]	2004	Adnexal	Retro. Series	67[0,67,0]	0	0	0	1	4	0	0	No
Oguri[156]	2005	Adnexal	Retro. Series	13[9,4,0]	0	0	0	0	0	0	0	No
Schmeler[157]	2005	Adnexal	Case control	17[NA]	0	0	0	0	2	0	0	No
Hong[158]	2006	Adnexal	Retro. Series	235[109,122,4]	12	2	0	2	18	3	0	No
Ribic[85]	2007	Adnexal	Retro. Series	51[28,21,2]	2	0	0	0	2	1	0	No
Ko[159]	2009	Adnexal	Retro. Series	11[11,0,0]	0	0	0	0	0	0	0	No
Turkcuoglu[160]	2009	Adnexal	Retro. Series	35[7,7,21]	0	3	0	0	10	0	0	No
Hamilton[98]	1968	Thyroidectomy	Retro. Series	24[5,18,1]	0	0	0	0	1	0	0	No

Table 1. (cont.)

Author	Year of publication	Procedure	Study design	N [trimesters: 1,2,3]	Pregnancy outcome			Fetal outcome			Maternal mortality	Addressing confounders
					SA	TA	Surgery-induced delivery	Death	Prematurity	MM		
Duncan[29]	1986	Various	Retro. Registry	2,565[NA]	181	NA	NA	NA	NA	82	NA	No
Mazze[6]	1989	Various	Retro. Registry	5,405 [2252,1881,1272]	NA	NA	NA	99	423	102	NA	No
Kort[5]	1993	Various	Retro. Series	78[0,36,42]	NA	0	NA	3	17	0	0	No

SA, spontaneous abortion; TA, therapeutic abortion; MM, major malformation; NA, not available (information missing or not clear); Pros, prospective; Retro, retrospective.

[†]Horowitz et al. reports on 12 patients. However, two patients were operated on at the puerperium.

[‡]The study by Tamir reported on 84 patients; however, only 77 were eligible for the pregnancy outcome analysis, 7 were diagnosed at puerperium.

[††]Halvorsen et al. reported on a group of 16 patients; however, the report considers only those who were diagnosed with acute appendicitis.

[‡‡]To et al. reported on a group of 38 patients, however, four patients were treated in the postpartum period, therefore only 34 were considered for analysis.

[†††]Missing data on several patients, information on preterm termination is not available for five patients out of eleven.

[i]One patient had 2 surgeries in same pregnancy.

[ii]Corneille reported 94 patients but data available for only 54 patients.

Updated version of previous edition: Koren G. *The Motherisk Guide to Cancer in Pregnancy and Lactation*. 2nd ed: Toronto: Motherisk, Hospital for Sick Children, 2005.

visualize the appendix with a gravid uterus [33]. A delay in diagnosis increases the risk of fetal and maternal mortality [34,38,39]. The major predictor of fetal mortality is perforation of the appendix. The risk of perforation increases with gestational age [40] and the rate of accurate diagnosis of appendicitis ranges from 54% [41] to close to 100% in different reports [42].

Medical management

In addition to broad spectrum antibiotic coverage, in the presence of acute appendicitis, the treatment is immediate surgical intervention within the first 24 hours in a pregnant woman to avoid perforation and possible severe complications [43].

Maternal morbidity and mortality

Maternal mortality rates for acute appendicitis in pregnancy have declined from 40% in 1908 [44]. to 0.5% in 1977 [38]. In our review of the literature, there was no maternal death except for 1 case describing a patient who developed peritonitis following perforation of the appendix and subsequent appendectomy [37]. The decrease in maternal death can be explained by prompt surgery and improved antimicrobial coverage. It has been stated over 100 years ago by Balber that "the mortality of appendicitis complicating pregnancy is the mortality of delay" [44]. This has been confirmed by numerous studies [34,38,45,46]. When associated with perforation and peritonitis, there is considerable maternal morbidity and morta-lity [34,38,45,46] with the most common complication being wound infection [37,47–49].

Fetal morbidity and loss

The rate of PTB with appendicitis ranges from 8% [48] to 15% [5,50,51], significantly higher when compared to other medical conditions during pregnancy [30]. McGory and associates conducted a retrospective study of 3133 pregnant women who underwent appendectomy. As expected they reported a higher rate of negative appendectomies in pregnant women (23% vs. 18%, $P < 0.05$). They also reported considerably higher rates of fetal loss and early delivery in cases of complicated appendicitis (6% and 11%, respectively; $P < 0.05$) when compared with negative (4% and 10%) and simple append-ectomy (2% and 4%) [52].

The role of tocolytics to prevent PTB in the context of appendectomy is not well defined in the literature [48,53]. However, their use should be limited to obstetrical indications and not administered prophylactically [27,54].

The fetal loss rate is significantly greater for pregnant patients undergoing appendec-tomy when compared to other surgical procedures during pregnancy ($P < 0.001$) [30]. It ranges from 3% to 5% with early appendicitis [33] to 25% when complicated by perforation/peritonitis [33,55] and tends to increase during the week following the appendectomy if performed before 24 weeks gestation [23].

Most publications on appendectomy in pregnancy conclude that delaying diagnosis and surgery increases the risk of appendiceal perforation and peritonitis, therefore worsens maternal and fetal outcomes [48,55,56]. The greatest risk of perforation appears to be highest in the third trimester of pregnancy [57], therefore, early surgical intervention is essential [48,55,56].

Laparoscopic surgery during pregnancy

Numerous reviews were published in the English medical literature on this subject [58–62]. We identified 16 studies on laparoscopic appendectomy and cholecystectomy (Table 1). Historically, it was safer to postpone laparoscopic surgery to the second trimester. All the 16 studies concluded that laparoscopic surgery did not increase the maternal/fetal morbidity and mortality. In 2007, the Society of American Gastrointestinal and Endoscopic Surgeons (SAGES) published guidelines for diagnostic, treatment and use of laparoscopy for surgical problems during pregnancy [27].

In the second trimester, open laparoscopy is recommended [63]. The advantages of laparoscopy versus laparotomy in pregnancy is early ambulation, early return of bowel function, short hospital stay, rapid return to normal activity, low rate of wound infection and hernia, less pain, and less fetal depression due to reduced narcotic use in post-operative period [64]. CO_2 insufflation of 10–15 mmHg can be safely used for laparoscopy in the pregnant patient [65,66]. Laparoscopy is safe at any time in pregnancy, even in late third trimester [10,16,67]. Although, laparoscopy can be performed safely in pregnancy with good maternal/fetal outcomes, the long-term effects on children have not been well studied. In a recent study with follow-up from 1 to 8 years, the offspring of 11 patients who underwent laparoscopy while pregnant (in their 16th to 28th week of pregnancy), showed no evidence of developmental or physical abnormalities [68].

Cholecystectomy

We identified 13 articles on the treatment of cholecystitis in pregnancy that fit our inclusion criteria (Table 1). They used both open and laparoscopic cholecystectomy. The last review of the literature pertaining to management of gravid women with biliary tract disease was published in 2008 by Date and associates [69].

Incidence

Acute cholecystitis may affect between 10% and 15% of the general population [70]. The physiologic changes of pregnancy can predispose women to gallstones and sludge formation. Gallstones in pregnancy has been reported in 1–3% of patients [70]. Acute cholecystitis only affects 0.1% of pregnant women despite predilection toward biliary sludge and stone formation [7]. Cholecystectomy is the second most common nonobstetrical surgical procedure in pregnancy. It is performed in 1 to 8 out of every 10,000 pregnancies [71].

Diagnosis

Gallbladder disease can present a diagnostic challenge to the obstetrician as many healthy pregnant women report upper digestive complaints that mimic biliary symptoms [43]. Most authors report no major differences in symptoms and in classic sonographic findings (an increased gallbladder wall thickness more than 3–5 mm, pericholecystic fluid, calculi, and a sonographic Murphy's sign) between pregnant and nonpregnant patients [12,43].

Medical management

The majority of the patient population in the 13 studies identified was medically managed with surgery being performed when medical management failed. Initially, conservative treatment may be an option in an attempt to avoid surgery during pregnancy. Patients with cholecystitis and biliary colic should be admitted to the hospital for intravenous hydration, opioid analgesia, and bowel rest. Broad spectrum antibiotic use is recommended for systemic symptoms and for the patient in whom there is no improvement in 12–24 hours [43].

Several experts advocate an earlier surgical intervention to avoid complications and relapses (40%–70% of cases) [72,73]. An alternative to surgical intervention includes successful percutaneous cholecystostomy [74] and endoscopic retrograde cholangiopancreatography (ERCP). The theoretical risk of radiation exposure to the fetus from ERCP (approximately 180 to 310 mrad) is not a concern when conducted after the first trimester [75,76]. Due to a lack of data these two approaches cannot be recommended routinely.

Maternal morbidity and mortality

In 238 cases, 1 maternal death was reported [11]. It was a 27-year-old patient who died from postsurgical hemorrhage after undergoing laparoscopic cholecystectomy in the 20th week of pregnancy. Very few other maternal complications were reported with either open or laparoscopic cholecystectomy [72].

Fetal morbidity and loss

Fetal loss occurred in 2.5% of cholecystectomies and PTB in 5% of cases. Prophylactic use of tocolytics in laparoscopic cholecystectomy is controversial; there is no dispute that, if uterine contractions are detected during surgery, tocolytic therapy should be initiated [77]. Overall, there are fewer fetal complications compared to appendectomy.

Adnexal masses

This topic was last reviewed by Leiserowitz in 2006 [78]. The 17 retrospective case series that matched our criteria, including 924 patients, are included in Table 1.

Incidence

The frequency of ovarian tumors is approximately 1 in 632 [79] to 1 in 1,000 pregnancies [80]. Ovarian tumor in pregnancy requiring surgical intervention has an incidence ranging from 0.13% to 0.36% [79,81].

Diagnosis

With the availability of routine ultrasound examination during the first trimester of pregnancy, the diagnosis of ovarian cysts is relatively common. Most are benign with 30% being corpus luteum cysts and 24% to 40% dermoid cysts [5,82]. Ovarian cancer in pregnancy is rare and is usually histologically borderline. Frankly malignant epithelial lesions are found in approximately 1 of 15,000–32,000 pregnancies [83]. It has been suggested that the diagnosis of adnexal masses during pregnancy should be deferred until the second trimester because most of the cysts are functional undergoing spontaneous resolution during the second trimester [84]. Surgical treatment for a persistent mass in the second trimester is justified because of the high risk of torsion, rupture, and malignancy [85].

Laparoscopic management of adnexal masses in pregnancy is a safe and effective procedure compared to traditional surgery [84,86].

Maternal morbidity and mortality

There were no maternal deaths reported and there appeared to be a minimum of maternal complications from the procedure.

Fetal morbidity and loss

Fetal loss occurred in 10 cases out of the 924 cases (1.1%) and PTB occurred in 86 cases (9.3%). Given the retrospective nature from which these data are derived, no specific conclusions can be drawn regarding any variables that may contribute to fetal morbidity in relation to maternal adnexal masses.

Miscellaneous
Pheochromocytoma

This topic was last reviewed in 1983 by Geelhoed [87] Pheochromocytoma is a rare endocrine tumor accounting for 0.1%–1% of all cases of hypertension, with fewer than 250 cases reported during pregnancy [88]. Schenker has published 2 case series of pregnant women with pheochromocytoma spanning from 1955 to 1979. The 2 case series included a total of 48 patients. Before 1969, there were 4 deaths in 22 cases diagnosed during pregnancy (18%) and an overall maternal death rate of 43% (pregnancy and postpartum), including tumor resections at cesarean section [89]. Between 1969 and 1979, 1 maternal death was reported in 26 cases of pheochromocytoma diagnosed during pregnancy (4%). An additional 24 patients undergoing cesarean section and abdominal exploration were reported, 12 of whom died for an overall maternal death rate of 40% [90]. Before 1969, the fetal loss rate was 61%; between 1969 and 1979, there was a slight decrease to 47%. Since the advent of laparoscopic adrenelectomy in 1992, there have been only 6 cases reported in pregnancy with good maternal and fetal outcomes [91–95]. However, we should keep in mind that pheochromocytoma in pregnancy is a serious condition that can have significant, adverse maternal/fetal outcomes.

Thyroidectomy

Six articles on thyroid surgery in pregnancy [96–101] were reviewed. Due to the low number of cases, it was not possible to establish an incidence rate of the disease. No maternal deaths were reported. Specific fetal outcomes were not available.

Carpal tunnel decompression

The last review on this topic was by Massey in 1978 [102]. Carpal tunnel syndrome occurs in 1.2–10% of pregnant women. Stahl in 1996 described 50 pregnant patients who required surgery after failed conservative approach. No maternal or fetal adverse outcomes were reported [103].

Rectal neoplasm surgery

In 1967, O'Leary published 17 cases of rectal carcinoma during pregnancy [104]. Between 1917 and 1966, there were 3 maternal deaths: 1 due to sepsis, 2 due to advanced cancer; and 2 fetal deaths: 1 secondary to maternal death and the other due to prematurity. There have not been any recent publications from which to draw any meaningful conclusions on this subject.

Conclusion

1. Maternal morbidity and mortality are low except in the cases of appendicitis complicated by peritonitis.
2. The rate of spontaneous abortion appears to be in the range of the general population.
3. Surgery and general anesthesia do not appear to be major risk factors for miscarriages.
4. The risk of major birth defects was not increased.
5. In acute appendicitis, increased fetal loss can be related to delay in surgery; therefore, surgery should be performed as soon as possible.
6. The majority of studies do not address possible confounders. Results in this review highlight that we need better data that take into account underlying maternal conditions, its management, smoking, alcohol consumption, socioeconomic status, etc.

References

1. Jenkins TM, Mackey SF, Benzoni EM, Tolosa JE, Sciscione AC. Non-obstetric surgery during gestation: risk factors for lower birthweight. *Aust N Z J Obstet Gynaecol.* 2003;**43**:27–31.

2. Pedersen H, Finster M. Anesthetic risk in the pregnant surgical patient. *Anesthesiology.* 1979;**51**:439–51.

3. Van De Velde M, De Buck F. Anesthesia for non-obstetric surgery in the pregnant patient. *Minerva Anestesiol.* 2007;**73**: 235–40.

4. Brodsky JB, Cohen EN, Brown BW Jr, Wu ML, Whitcher C. Surgery during pregnancy and fetal outcome. *Am J Obstet Gynecol.* 1980;**138**:1165–7.

5. Kort B, Katz VL, Watson WJ. The effect of nonobstetric operation during pregnancy. *Surg Gynecol Obstet.* 1993;**177**:371–6.

6. Mazze RI, Kallen B. Reproductive outcome after anesthesia and operation during pregnancy: a registry study of 5405 cases. *Am J Obstet Gynecol.* 1989;**161**:1178–85.

7. Dietrich CS III, Hill CC, Hueman M. Surgical diseases presenting in pregnancy. *Surg Clin North Am.* 2008;**88**:403–19, vii–viii.

8. Chestnut DH. *Obstetric anesthesia: principles and practice.* St. Louis: Mosby; 2004.

9. Kammerer WS. Nonobstetric surgery during pregnancy. *Med Clin North Am.* 1979;**63**:1157–64.

10. Affleck DG, Handrahan DL, Egger MJ, Price RR. The laparoscopic management of appendicitis and cholelithiasis during pregnancy. *Am J Surg.* 1999;**178**:523–9.

11. Barone JE, Bears S, Chen S, Tsai J, Russell JC. Outcome study of cholecystectomy during pregnancy. *Am J Surg.* 1999;**177**:232–6.

12. Glasgow RE, Visser BC, Harris HW, Patti MG, Kilpatrick SJ, Mulvihill SJ. Changing management of gallstone disease during pregnancy. *Surg Endosc.* 1998;**12**:241–6.

13. Oelsner G, Stockheim D, Soriano D, et al. Pregnancy outcome after laparoscopy or laparotomy in pregnancy. *J Am Assoc Gynecol Laparosc.* 2003;**10**:200–4.

14. Reedy MB, Galan HL, Richards WE, Preece CK, Wetter PA, Kuehl TJ. Laparoscopy during pregnancy. A survey of laparoendoscopic surgeons. *J Reprod Med.* 1997;**42**:33–8.

15. Reedy MB, Kallen B, Kuehl TJ. Laparoscopy during pregnancy: a study of

five fetal outcome parameters with use of the Swedish Health Registry. *Am J Obstet Gynecol.* 1997;**177**:673–9.

16. Rollins MD, Chan KJ, Price RR. Laparoscopy for appendicitis and cholelithiasis during pregnancy: a new standard of care. *Surg Endosc.* 2004; **18**:237–41.

17. Anderson EF. Anesthesia and surgery during pregnancy. *S D J Med.* 1985; **38**:19–23.

18. Barron WM. Medical evaluation of the pregnant patient requiring nonobstetric surgery. *Clin Perinatol.* 1985;**12**:481–96.

19. Cheek TG, Baird E. Anesthesia for nonobstetric surgery: maternal and fetal considerations. *Clin Obstet Gynecol.* 2009;**52**:535–45.

20. Ni Mhuireachtaigh R, O'Gorman DA. Anesthesia in pregnant patients for nonobstetric surgery. *J Clin Anesth.* 2006;**18**:60–6.

21. James FM III. Anesthesia for nonobstetric surgery during pregnancy. *Clin Obstet Gynecol.* 1987;**30**:621–8.

22. Halkic N, Tempia-Caliera AA, Ksontini R, Suter M, Delaloye J-F, Vuilleumier H. Laparoscopic management of appendicitis and symptomatic cholelithiasis during pregnancy. *Langenbecks Arch Surg.* 2006;**391**:467–71.

23. Mazze RI, Kallen B. Appendectomy during pregnancy: a Swedish registry study of 778 cases. *Obstet Gynecol.* 1991;**77**:835–40.

24. Kuczkowski KM. Nonobstetric surgery during pregnancy: what are the risks of anesthesia? *Obstet Gynecol Surv.* 2004;**59**:52–6.

25. Kuczkowski KM. The safety of anaesthetics in pregnant women. *Expert Opin Drug Saf.* 2006;**5**:251–64.

26. Kuczkowski KM. Nonobstetric surgery in the parturient: anesthetic considerations. *J Clin Anesth.* 2006;**18**:5–7.

27. Yumi H. Guidelines for diagnosis, treatment, and use of laparoscopy for surgical problems during pregnancy: this statement was reviewed and approved by the Board of Governors of the Society of American Gastrointestinal and Endoscopic Surgeons (SAGES),tember 2007. It was prepared by the SAGES Guidelines Committee. *Surg Endosc.* 2008;**22**: 849–61.

28. Czeizel AE, Pataki T, Rockenbauer M. Reproductive outcome after exposure to surgery under anesthesia during pregnancy. *Arch Gynecol Obstet.* 1998;**261**:193–9.

29. Duncan PG, Pope WD, Cohen MM, Greer N. Fetal risk of anesthesia and surgery during pregnancy. *Anesthesiology.* 1986;**64**:790–4.

30. Cohen-Kerem R, Railton C, Oren D, Lishner M, Koren G. Pregnancy outcome following non-obstetric surgical intervention. *Am J Surg.* 2005;**190**:467–73.

31. ACOG Committee Opinion Number 284, August 2003: Nonobstetric surgery in pregnancy. *Obstet Gynecol.* 2003;**102**:431.

32. Wilder RT, Flick RP, Sprung J, et al. Early exposure to anesthesia and learning disabilities in a population-based birth cohort. *Anesthesiology.* 2009;**110**:796–804.

33. Borst AR. Acute appendicitis: pregnancy complicates this diagnosis. *JAAPA.* 2007;**20**:36–8, 41.

34. Cunningham FG, McCubbin JH. Appendicitis complicating pregnancy. *Obstet Gynecol.* 1975;**45**:415–20.

35. Andersson RE, Lambe M. Incidence of appendicitis during pregnancy. *Int J Epidemiol.* 2001;**30**:1281–5.

36. Al-Mulhim AA. Acute appendicitis in pregnancy. A review of 52 cases. *Int Surg.* 1996;**81**:295–7.

37. Horowitz MD, Gomez GA, Santiesteban R, Burkett G. Acute appendicitis during pregnancy. Diagnosis and management. *Arch Surg.* 1985;**120**:1362–7.

38. Babaknia A, Parsa H, Woodruff JD. Appendicitis during pregnancy. *Obstet Gynecol.* 1977;**50**:40–4.

39. Brant HA. Acute appendicitis in pregnancy. *Obstet Gynecol.* 1967;**29**:130–8.

40. Malangoni MA. Gastrointestinal surgery and pregnancy. *Gastroenterol Clin North Am.* 2003;**32**:181–200.

41. Frisenda R, Roty AR Jr, Kilway JB, Brown AL Jr, Peelen M. Acute appendicitis during pregnancy. *Am Surg.* 1979;**45**:503–6.

42. Gomez A, Wood M. Acute appendicitis during pregnancy. *Am J Surg.* 1979;**137**:180–3.

43. Gilo NB, Amini D, Landy HJ. Appendicitis and cholecystitis in pregnancy. *Clin Obstet Gynecol.* 2009;**52**:586–96.

44. Balber EA. Perforative appendicitis complicating pregnancy with a report of a successful case. *JAMA.* 1908;**51**:1310–4.

45. Black WP. Acute appendicitis in pregnancy. *Br Med J.* 1960;**1**:1938–41.

46. Lee RA, Johnson CE, Symmonds RE. Appendicitis during pregnancy. *JAMA.* 1965;**193**:966–8.

47. Hoshino T, Ihara Y, Suzuki T. Appendicitis during pregnancy. *Int J Gynaecol Obstet.* 2000;**69**:271–3.

48. Kazim SF, Pal KM. Appendicitis in pregnancy: experience of thirty-eight patients diagnosed and managed at a tertiary care hospital in Karachi. *Int J Surg.* 2009;**7**:365–7.

49. Wu JM, Chen KH, Lin HF, Tseng LM, Tseng SH, Huang SH. Laparoscopic appendectomy in pregnancy. *J Laparoendosc Adv Surg Tech A.* 2005;**15**:447–50.

50. Allen JR, Helling TS, Langenfeld M. Intraabdominal surgery during pregnancy. *Am J Surg.* 1989;**158**:567–9.

51. Mourad J, Elliott JP, Erickson L, Lisboa L. Appendicitis in pregnancy: new information that contradicts long-held clinical beliefs. *Am J Obstet Gynecol.* 2000;**182**:1027–9.

52. McGory ML, Zingmond DS, Tillou A, Hiatt JR, Ko CY, Cryer HM. Negative appendectomy in pregnant women is associated with a substantial risk of fetal loss. *J Am Coll Surg.* 2007;**205**: 534–40.

53. Halvorsen AC, Brandt B, Andreasen JJ. Acute appendicitis in pregnancy: complications and subsequent management. *Eur J Surg.* 1992-Dec; **158**:603–6.

54. Moreno-Sanz C, Pascual-Pedreno A, Picazo-Yeste JS, Seoane-Gonzalez JB. Laparoscopic appendectomy during pregnancy: between personal experiences and scientific evidence. *J Am Coll Surg.* 2007;**205**:37–42.

55. Zhang Y, Zhao YY, Qiao J, Ye RH. Diagnosis of appendicitis during pregnancy and perinatal outcome in the late pregnancy. *Chin Med J (Engl).* 2009;**122**:521–4.

56. Guttman R, Goldman RD, Koren G. Appendicitis during pregnancy. *Can Fam Physician.* 2004;**50**:355–7.

57. Ueberrueck T, Koch A, Meyer L, Hinkel M, Gastinger I. Ninety-four appendectomies for suspected acute appendicitis during pregnancy. *World J Surg.* 2004;**28**:508–11.

58. Chohan L, Kilpatrick CC. Laparoscopy in pregnancy: a literature review. *Clin Obstet Gynecol.* 2009;**52**:557–69.

59. Fatum M, Rojansky N. Laparoscopic surgery during pregnancy. *Obstet Gynecol Surv.* 2001;**56**:50–9.

60. Lachman E, Schienfeld A, Voss E, et al. Pregnancy and laparoscopic surgery. *J Am Assoc Gynecol Laparosc.* 1999;**6**:347–51.

61. O'Rourke N, Kodali BS. Laparoscopic surgery during pregnancy. *Curr Opin Anaesthesiol.* 2006;**19**:254–9.

62. Shay DC, Bhavani-Shankar K, Datta S. Laparoscopic surgery during pregnancy. *Anesthesiol Clin North America.* 2001;**19**:57–67.

63. Al-Fozan H, Tulandi T. Safety and risks of laparoscopy in pregnancy. *Curr Opin Obstet Gynecol.* 2002;**14**:375–9.

64. Curet MJ, Allen D, Josloff RK, et al. Laparoscopy during pregnancy. *Arch Surg.* 1996;**131**:546–50; discussion 50–1.

65. Curet MJ, Vogt DA, Schob O, Qualls C, Izquierdo LA, Zucker KA. Effects of CO_2 pneumoperitoneum in pregnant ewes. *J Surg Res.* 1996;**63**:339–44.

66. Reedy MB, Galan HL, Bean-Lijewski JD, Carnes A, Knight AB, Kuehl TJ. Maternal and fetal effects of laparoscopic insufflation in the gravid baboon. *J Am Assoc Gynecol Laparosc.* 1995;**2**:399–406.

67. Geisler JP, Rose SL, Mernitz CS, Warner JL, Hiett AK. Non-gynecologic laparoscopy in second and third trimester pregnancy: obstetric implications. *JSLS*. 1998;**2**:235–8.

68. Rizzo AG. Laparoscopic surgery in pregnancy: long-term follow-up. *J Laparoendosc Adv Surg Tech A*. 2003;**13**:11–5.

69. Date RS, Kaushal M, Ramesh A. A review of the management of gallstone disease and its complications in pregnancy. *Am J Surg*. 2008;**196**:599–608.

70. Ramin KD, Ramsey PS. Disease of the gallbladder and pancreas in pregnancy. *Obstet Gynecol Clin North Am*. 2001;**28**:571–80.

71. Hill LM, Johnson CE, Lee RA. Cholecystectomy in pregnancy. *Obstet Gynecol*. 1975;**46**:291–3.

72. Dhupar R, Smaldone GM, Hamad GG. Is there a benefit to delaying cholecystectomy for symptomatic gallbladder disease during pregnancy? *Surg Endosc*. 2010;**24**:108–12.

73. Swisher SG, Schmit PJ, Hunt KK, et al. Biliary disease during pregnancy. *Am J Surg*. 1994;**168**:576–9; discussion 80–1.

74. Allmendinger N, Hallisey MJ, Ohki SK, Straub JJ. Percutaneous cholecystostomy treatment of acute cholecystitis in pregnancy. *Obstet Gynecol*. 1995;**86** (4 Pt 2):653–4.

75. Kahaleh M, Hartwell GD, Arseneau KO, et al. Safety and efficacy of ERCP in pregnancy. *Gastrointest Endosc*. 2004;**60**:287–92.

76. Tham TC, Vandervoort J, Wong RC, et al. Safety of ERCP during pregnancy. *Am J Gastroenterol*. 2003;**98**:308–11.

77. Bani Hani MN. Laparoscopic surgery for symptomatic cholelithiasis during pregnancy. *Surg Laparosc Endosc Percutan Tech*. 2007;**17**:482–6.

78. Leiserowitz GS. Managing ovarian masses during pregnancy. *Obstet Gynecol Surv*. 2006;**61**:463–70.

79. Sherard GB III, Hodson CA, Williams HJ, Semer DA, Hadi HA, Tait DL. Adnexal masses and pregnancy: a 12-year experience. *Am J Obstet Gynecol*. 2003;**189**:358–62; discussion 62–3.

80. Hermans RH, Fischer DC, van der Putten HW, et al. Adnexal masses in pregnancy. *Onkologie*. 2003;**26**:167–72.

81. Wang PH, Chao HT, Yuan CC, Lee WL, Chao KC, Ng HT. Ovarian tumors complicating pregnancy. Emergency and elective surgery. *J Reprod Med*. 1999;**44**:279–87.

82. Peterson WF, Prevost EC, Edmunds FT, Hundley JM Jr, Morris FK. Benign cystic teratomas of the ovary; a clinico-statistical study of 1,007 cases with a review of the literature. *Am J Obstet Gynecol*. 1955;**70**:368–82.

83. Goffinet F. [Ovarian cysts and pregnancy]. *J Gynecol Obstet Biol Reprod (Paris)*. 2001;**30**(1 suppl):S100–8.

84. Mathevet P, Nessah K, Dargent D, Mellier G. Laparoscopic management of adnexal masses in pregnancy: a case series. *Eur J Obstet Gynecol Reprod Biol*. 2003;**108**:217–22.

85. Ribic-Pucelj M, Kobal B, Peternelj-Marinsek S. Surgical treatment of adnexal masses in pregnancy: indications, surgical approach and pregnancy outcome. *J Reprod Med*. 2007;**52**:273–9.

86. Moore RD, Smith WG. Laparoscopic management of adnexal masses in pregnant women. *J Reprod Med*. 1999;**44**:97–100.

87. Geelhoed GW. Surgery of the endocrine glands in pregnancy. *Clin Obstet Gynecol*. 1983;**26**:865–89.

88. Junglee N, Harries SE, Davies N, Scott-Coombes D, Scanlon MF, Rees DA. Pheochromocytoma in pregnancy: when is operative intervention indicated? *J Womens Health (Larchmt)*. 2007;**16**:1362–5.

89. Schenker JG, Chowers I. Pheochromocytoma and pregnancy. Review of 89 cases. *Obstet Gynecol Surv*. 1971;**26**:739–47.

90. Schenker JG, Granat M. Phaeochromocytoma and pregnancy – an updated appraisal. *Aust N Z J Obstet Gynaecol*. 1982;**22**:1–10.

91. Demeure MJ, Carlsen B, Traul D, et al. Laparoscopic removal of a right adrenal pheochromocytoma in a pregnant woman. *J Laparoendosc Adv Surg Tech A.* 1998;**8**:315–9.

92. Kim PT, Kreisman SH, Vaughn R, Panton ON. Laparoscopic adrenalectomy for pheochromocytoma in pregnancy. *Can J Surg.* 2006;**49**:62–3.

93. tinez Brocca MA, Acosta Delgado D, Quijada D, Navarro Gonzalez E, Soto Moreno A, Gonzales Duarte D, et al. Pheochromocytoma in a pregnant woman with multiple endocrine neoplasia type 2a. *Gynecol Endocrinol.* 2001;**15**:439–42.

94. Pace DE, Chiasson PM, Schlachta CM, Mamazza J, Cadeddu MO, Poulin EC. Minimally invasive adrenalectomy for pheochromocytoma during pregnancy. *Surg Laparosc Endosc Percutan Tech.* 2002;**12**:122–5.

95. Wolf A, Goretzki PE, Rohrborn A, et al. Pheochromocytoma during pregnancy: laparoscopic and conventional surgical treatment of two cases. *Exp Clin Endocrinol Diabetes.* 2004;**112**:98–101.

96. Cunningham MP, Slaughter DP. Surgical treatment of disease of the thyroid gland in pregnancy. *Surg Gynecol Obstet.* 1970;**131**:486–8.

97. Doherty CM, Shindo ML, Rice DH, Montero M, Mestman JH. Management of thyroid nodules during pregnancy. *Laryngoscope.* 1995;**105**(3 Pt 1):251–5.

98. Hamilton NT, Paterson PJ, Breidahl HD. Thyroidectomy during pregnancy. *Med J Aust.* 1968;**1**:431–3.

99. Nam KH, Yoon JH, Chang HS, Park CS. Optimal timing of surgery in well-differentiated thyroid carcinoma detected during pregnancy. *J Surg Oncol.* 2005;**91**:199–203.

100. Rosen IB, Walfish PG, Nikore V. Pregnancy and surgical thyroid disease. *Surgery.* 1985;**98**:1135–40.

101. Tan GH, Gharib H, Goellner JR, van Heerden JA, Bahn RS. Management of thyroid nodules in pregnancy. *Arch Intern Med.* 1996;**156**:2317–20.

102. Massey EW. Carpal tunnel syndrome in pregnancy. *Obstet Gynecol Surv.* 1978;**33**:145–8.

103. Stahl S, Blumenfeld Z, Yarnitsky D. Carpal tunnel syndrome in pregnancy: indications for early surgery. *J Neurol Sci.* 1996;**136**(1–2):182–4.

104. O'Leary JA, Pratt JH, Symmonds RE. Rectal carcinoma and pregnancy: a review of 17 cases. *Obstet Gynecol.* 1967;**30**:862–8.

105. Finch DR, Lee E. Acute appendicitis complicating pregnancy in the Oxford region. *Br J Surg.* 1974;**61**:129–32.

106. Mohammed JA, Oxorn H. Appendicitis in pregnancy. *Can Med Assoc J.* 1975;**112**:1187–8.

107. Townsend JM, Greiss FC. Appendicitis in pregnancy. *South Med J.* 1976;**69**:1161–3.

108. Punnonen R, Aho AJ, Gronroos M, Liukko P. Appendicectomy during pregnancy. *Acta Chir Scand.* 1979;**145**:555–8.

109. Farquharson RG. Acute appendicitis in pregnancy. *Scott Med J.* 1980;**25**:36–8.

110. McComb P, Laimon H. Appendicitis complicating pregnancy. *Can J Surg.* 1980;**23**:92–4.

111. Doberneck RC. Appendectomy during pregnancy. *Am Surg.* 1985;**51**:265–8.

112. Bailey LE, Finley RK Jr, Miller SF, Jones LM. Acute appendicitis during pregnancy. *Am Surg.* 1986;**52**:218–21.

113. Liang CC, Hsieh TT, Chang SD. Appendicitis during pregnancy. *Changgeng Yi Xue Za Zhi.* 1989;**12**:208–14.

114. Tamir IL, Bongard FS, Klein SR. Acute appendicitis in the pregnant patient. *Am J Surg.* 1990;**160**:571–5; discussion 5–6.

115. To WW, Ngai CS, Ma HK. Pregnancies complicated by acute appendicitis. *Aust N Z J Surg.* 1995;**65**:799–803.

116. Andersen B, Nielsen TF. Appendicitis in pregnancy: diagnosis, management and complications. *Acta Obstet Gynecol Scand.* 1999;**78**:758–62.

117. Hee P, Viktrup L. The diagnosis of appendicitis during pregnancy and maternal and fetal outcome after

appendectomy. *Int J Gynaecol Obstet.* 1999;**65**:129–35.

118. Nunnelee JD, Musselman R, Spaner SD. Appendectomy in pregnancy and postpartum: analysis of data from a large private hospital. *Clin Excell Nurse Pract.* 1999;**3**:298–301.

119. Tracey M, Fletcher HS. Appendicitis in pregnancy. *Am Surg.* 2000;**66**:555–9; discussion 9–60.

120. Sakhri J, Youssef S, Ben Letaifa D, Sridi K, Essaidi H, Khairi H. Acute appendicitis during pregnancy. *Tunis Med.* 2001;**79**:521–5.

121. Hsu YP, Chen RJ, Fang JF, Lin BC. Acute appendicitis during pregnancy: a clinical assessment. *Chang Gung Med J.* 2001;**24**:245–50.

122. Ghazanfar A, Nasir SM, Choudary ZA, Ahmad W. Acute appendicitis complicating pregnancy; experience with the management of 50 patients. *J Ayub Med Coll Abbottabad.* 2002;**14**:19–21.

123. Duqoum W. Appendicitis in pregnancy. *East Mediterr Health J.* 2001;**7**(4–5):642–5.

124. Carver TW, Antevil J, Egan JC, Brown CV. Appendectomy during early pregnancy: what is the preferred surgical approach? *Am Surg.* 2005;**71**:809–12.

125. Kirshtein B, Perry ZH, Avinoach E, Mizrahi S, Lantsberg L. Safety of laparoscopic appendectomy during pregnancy. *World J Surg.* 2009; **33**:475–80.

126. Lemieux P, Rheaume P, Levesque I, Bujold E, Brochu G. Laparoscopic appendectomy in pregnant patients: a review of 45 cases. *Surg Endosc.* 2009;**23**:1701–5.

127. Machado NO, Grant CS. Laparoscopic appendicectomy in all trimesters of pregnancy. *J Soc Laparoendosc Surg.* 2009;**13**:384–90.

128. Sadot E, Telem DA, Arora M, Butala P, Nguyen SQ, Divino CM. Laparoscopy: a safe approach to appendicitis during pregnancy. *Surg Endosc.* 2010;**24**:383–9.

129. Greene J, Rogers A, Rubin L. Fetal loss after cholecystectomy during pregnancy. *Can Med Assoc J.* 1963;**88**:576–7.

130. Dixon NP, Faddis DM, Silberman H. Aggressive management of cholecystitis during pregnancy. *Am J Surg.* 1987;**154**:292–4.

131. Swisher SG, Hunt KK, Schmit PJ, Hiyama DT, Bennion RS, Thompson JE. Management of pancreatitis complicating pregnancy. *Am Surg.* 1994;**60**:759–62.

132. Davis A, Katz VL, Cox R. Gallbladder disease in pregnancy. *J Reprod Med.* 1995;**40**:759–62.

133. Steinbrook RA, Brooks DC, Datta S. Laparoscopic cholecystectomy during pregnancy. Review of anesthetic management, surgical considerations. *Surg Endosc.* 1996;**10**:511–5.

134. Cosenza CA, Saffari B, Jabbour N, Stain SC, Garry D, Parekh D, et al. Surgical management of biliary gallstone disease during pregnancy. *Am J Surg.* 1999;**178**:545–8.

135. Daradkeh S, Sumrein I, Daoud F, Zaidin K, Abu-Khalaf M. Management of gallbladder stones during pregnancy: conservative treatment or laparoscopic cholecystectomy? *Hepatogastroenterology.* 1999;**46**:3074–6.

136. Muench J, Albrink M, Serafini F, Rosemurgy A, Carey L, Murr MM. Delay in treatment of biliary disease during pregnancy increases morbidity and can be avoided with safe laparoscopic cholecystectomy. *Am Surg.* 2001;**67**:539–42; discussion 42–3.

137. Patel SG, Veverka TJ. Laparoscopic cholecystectomy in pregnancy. *Curr Surg.* 2002;**59**:74–8.

138. Lu EJ, Curet MJ, El-Sayed YY, Kirkwood KS. Medical versus surgical management of biliary tract disease in pregnancy. *Am J Surg.* 2004;**188**:755–9.

139. Amos JD, Schorr SJ, Norman PF, et al. Laparoscopic surgery during pregnancy. *Am J Surg.* 1996;**171**:435–7.

140. Andreoli M, Servakov M, Meyers P, Mann WJ Jr. Laparoscopic surgery during pregnancy. *J Am Assoc Gynecol Laparosc.* 1999;**6**:229–33.

141. Conron RW Jr, Abbruzzi K, Cochrane SO, Sarno AJ, Cochrane PJ. Laparoscopic

procedures in pregnancy. *Am Surg.* 1999;**65**:259–63.

142. Akira S, Yamanaka A, Ishihara T, Takeshita T, Araki T. Gasless laparoscopic ovarian cystectomy during pregnancy: comparison with laparotomy. *Am J Obstet Gynecol.* 1999;**180**(3 Pt 1):554–7.

143. Lyass S, Pikarsky A, Eisenberg VH, Elchalal U, Schenker JG, Reissman P. Is laparoscopic appendectomy safe in pregnant women? *Surg Endosc.* 2001;**15**:377–9.

144. Rojansky N, Shushan A, Fatum M. Laparoscopy versus laparotomy in pregnancy: a comparative study. *J Am Assoc Gynecol Laparosc.* 2002;**9**:108–10.

145. Palanivelu C, Rangarajan M, Senthilkumaran S, Parthasarathi R. Safety and efficacy of laparoscopic surgery in pregnancy: experience of a single institution. *J Laparoendosc Adv Surg Tech A.* 2007;**17**:186–90.

146. Buser KB. Laparoscopic surgery in the pregnant patient: results and recommendations. *J Soc Laparoendosc Surg.* 2009;**13**:32–5.

147. Corneille MG, Gallup TM, Bening T, et al. The use of laparoscopic surgery in pregnancy: evaluation of safety and efficacy. *Am J Surg.* 2010;**200**:363–7.

148. Hess LW, Peaceman A, O'Brien WF, Winkel CA, Cruikshank DP, Morrison JC. Adnexal mass occurring with intrauterine pregnancy: report of fifty-four patients requiring laparotomy for definitive management. *Am J Obstet Gynecol.* 1988;**158**:1029–34.

149. Platek DN, Henderson CE, Goldberg GL. The management of a persistent adnexal mass in pregnancy. *Am J Obstet Gynecol.* 1995;**173**:1236–40.

150. Soriano D, Yefet Y, Seidman DS, Goldenberg M, Mashiach S, Oelsner G. Laparoscopy versus laparotomy in the management of adnexal masses during pregnancy. *Fertil Steril.* 1999;**71**:955–60.

151. Whitecar MP, Turner S, Higby MK. Adnexal masses in pregnancy: a review of 130 cases undergoing surgical management. *Am J Obstet Gynecol.* 1999;**181**:19–24.

152. Usui R, Minakami H, Kosuge S, Iwasaki R, Ohwada M, Sato I. A retrospective survey of clinical, pathologic, and prognostic features of adnexal masses operated on during pregnancy. *J Obstet Gynaecol Res.* 2000;**26**:89–93.

153. Stepp KJ, Tulikangas PK, Goldberg JM, Attaran M, Falcone T. Laparoscopy for adnexal masses in the second trimester of pregnancy. *J Am Assoc Gynecol Laparosc.* 2003;**10**:55–9.

154. Carter JF, Soper DE. Operative laparoscopy in pregnancy. *J Soc Laparoendosc Surg.* 2004;**8**:57–60.

155. Yuen PM, Ng PS, Leung PL, Rogers MS. Outcome in laparoscopic management of persistent adnexal mass during the second trimester of pregnancy. *Surg Endosc.* 2004;**18**:1354–7.

156. Oguri H, Taniguchi K, Fukaya T. Gasless laparoscopic management of ovarian cysts during pregnancy. *Int J Gynaecol Obstet.* 2005;**91**:258–9.

157. Schmeler KM, Mayo-Smith WW, Peipert JF, Weitzen S, Manuel MD, Gordinier ME. Adnexal masses in pregnancy: surgery compared with observation. *Obstet Gynecol.* 2005;**105**(5 Pt 1):1098–103.

158. Hong JY. Adnexal mass surgery and anesthesia during pregnancy: a 10-year retrospective review. *Int J Obstet Anesth.* 2006;**15**:212–6.

159. Ko ML, Lai TH, Chen SC. Laparoscopic management of complicated adnexal masses in the first trimester of pregnancy. *Fertil Steril.* 2009;**92**:283–7.

160. Turkcuoglu I, Meydanli MM, Engin-Ustun Y, Ustun Y, Kafkasli A. Evaluation of histopathological features and pregnancy outcomes of pregnancy associated adnexal masses. *J Obstet Gynaecol.* 2009;**29**:107–9.

Chapter 16

Management of complications associated with cancer or antineoplastic treatment during pregnancy

Michael P. Tan

Introduction

Cancer is the second leading cause of death in women during the reproductive years. The incidence ranges between 0.07% and 0.1% in pregnant women [1]. The diagnosis of cancer during pregnancy prompts major therapeutic decisions: optimal maternal treatment must be balanced against the risks to the fetus. The malignant disease and its treatment have specific complications that may have special importance during pregnancy. These include, among others, bone marrow depression with neutropenia and infections, anemia, and thrombocytopenic bleeding. Both pregnancy and cancer are associated with hypercoagulability and thromboembolism. Skeletal manifestations of cancer, such as osteoporosis, bone pain, pathological fractures, and hypercalcemia, may also require specific treatment during pregnancy. Thus, these complications of cancer or its treatment may expose the pregnant woman to additional medications including anticoagulants, antibiotics, analgesics, and new treatment modalities such as hematopoietic growth factors and bisphosphonates. This is a general overview of the use of these therapeutic measures during pregnancy.

Heparin

Unfractionated heparin

Unfractionated heparin (UFH) does not cross the placenta and has not been shown to increase the risk of congenital defects. In a review of the literature of fetal outcome following anticoagulant therapy during pregnancy, 186 publications reporting fetal outcome in 1,325 pregnancies were collected. Heparin compared with a coumarin was shown to be safe during pregnancy for either the prevention or treatment of thromboembolic disease [2]. Heparin is preferred as initial therapy for unstable patients with pulmonary embolism plus hypoxia, extreme venous congestion, extensive iliofemoral venous thromboembolism (VTE), or renal impairment. In pregnancy, particularly in the third trimester, an increase in heparin-binding proteins combined with elevated factor VIII levels can significantly attenuate the activated partial thromboplastin time (APTT) response leading to "heparin resistance." A plasma heparin level may be useful to guide treatment if there is difficulty achieving a therapeutic APTT range. Women with high risk of bleeding may do better with UFH as its anticoagulant effects can be rapidly reversed by protamine compared to low molecular weight heparin (LMWH) [3].

With heparin, the mother is at risk of heparin-induced thrombocytopenia (HIT) and osteoporosis. Women taking heparin for more than 6 weeks should be warned that there is a 2% risk of symptomatic vertebral collapse [4].

Low molecular weight heparins

LMWHs are formed by enzymatic depolymerization of heparin. Their molecular mass is between 4,000 and 6,000 Dalton [5]. Due to their different structure, the major difference between LMWH and UFH lies in their relative inhibitory activity against factor Xa and thrombin. The main advantages of LMWH over UFH are their predictable anticoagulant activity, no laboratory monitoring necessary, higher bioavailability, long half-life, once daily dosing, decreased bleeding incidence, decreased risk for osteoporosis, and less risk to induced thrombocytopenia associated with paradoxical thrombosis [3,6]. Several animal and human studies compared anti-Xa and anti-IIa activities in the mothers and their fetuses and demonstrated no transfer of LMWH through the placenta [7–9]. Clinical experience with LMWH (predominantly dalteparin and enoxaparin) as treatment or prophylaxis for thromboembolic phenomena in pregnancy was addressed in several studies and review [5,10–13], no teratogenic effect, no thromboembolic complications occurred, with very low bleeding risks. The LMWH has likewise been shown to be just as effective or may be even superior over a coumarin for long-term therapy as secondary prevention of VTE among cancer patients[14,15]. In the nonpregnant population, LMWH is superior to UFH for the prevention of VTE and equivalent to heparin for treatment [16]. For these reasons, LMWH is the preferred choice for initial anticoagulant therapy for clinically stable pregnant patients and for use as prophylaxis in both cancer and pregnant patients [3,14,15,17].

The need for dose adjustment in pregnancy is controversial. Some studies suggest that increasing the dose is required to maintain anti-Xa levels in the expected therapeutic range. Other experts believe this is unnecessary due to the relatively wide therapeutic window unless excessive weight changes occur, in which case, dose adjustment would either be guided based on weight or antifactor Xa level (measured 4 hours post-dose) [3,18,19]. There are also theoretical concerns with regard to the efficacy of once daily dosing versus twice daily dosing for treatment of VTE in pregnancy. There are no control data to address this issue [3].

To avoid the anticoagulant effect at delivery, experts recommend that LMWH be discontinued 24–36 hours before elective induction of labor or cesarean section. In case of no planned induction, LMWH therapy should be withheld at the onset of regular contractions [3]. Anti-Xa level may be checked and protamine administered if high or bleeding occurs. Anticoagulant therapy should be restarted 12–24 hours postdelivery as long as there are no bleeding concerns. Optimal duration of anticoagulation for women diagnosed with VTE during pregnancy remains unknown. Data are extrapolated from nonpregnant population. Experts recommend a minimum of 3–6 months with treatment continued until at least 6 weeks postpartum in all cases [19]. Further approaches to management of VTE in pregnancy for different scenarios have been extensively covered in the literature [3,17,20].

In summary, the administration of heparin and LMWH during pregnancy is safe for both the mother and the fetus. The absence of teratogenic effects, predictable anticoagulation, easy administration, and lack of need for laboratory monitoring makes LMWH preferable for thromboembolism during pregnancy. They can be administered to pregnant women with cancer for both prevention and treatment.

Apart from the anticoagulant role of heparins, its anticancer effect is currently being investigated. These agents were observed to influence multiple pathways: inhibition of tumor angiogenesis, tumor adhesion, and invasion [21].

Oral anticoagulants
Coumarin

Oral anticoagulants cross the placenta and can enter the fetal circulation. Since 1966 [22], characteristics of fetal warfarin syndrome associated with first-trimester exposure to a coumarin have been described: nasal hypoplasia due to maldevelopment of the nasal septum, depression of the nasal bridge with a flattened upturned appearance, and stippled epiphyses. Eye defects, seizures, deafness, congenital heart disease, and hypoplasia of the extremities have all been reported [23]. Exposure to warfarin during any trimester resulted in central nervous system abnormalities. Two main patterns were reported: (1) dorsal midline dysplasia with agenesis of the corpus callosum, Dandy-Walker malformations and midline cerebellar atrophy; (2) ventral midline dysplasia characterized by optic atrophy [24].

The overall risk of embryopathy is believed to be approximately 3–6% regardless of maternal dosage [25,26]. The risk to the fetus is thought to be dose dependent with less than 5 mg per day carrying a minimal risk [25]. The critical period for malformation appears to be between 6 and 12 weeks of gestation as substitution with heparin during this time appears to eliminate the risk of embryopathy [18,24,25].

A population-based cohort study of children exposed during the second and third trimester of pregnancy suggests that, when exposure during the first trimester is avoided, warfarin therapy during pregnancy has little, if any, risk to a child's skeletal development, average IQ, or educational achievements [27]. On the other hand, a study on the same population showed a marginally increased risk for minor neurological dysfunction such as decreased performance in writing and spelling for exposed boys, and for having an IQ below 80 [28,29]. The clinical significance of these impairments appears to be minimal.

The risk of delivering an anticoagulated infant can be reduced by substituting UFH or LMWH for vitamin K antagonists approximately 3 weeks before planned delivery and discontinuing these medications shortly before delivery. Others have advocated the use of planned cesarean section at 38 weeks with only a brief 2- to 3-day interruption of anticoagulant therapy with good maternal and fetal outcomes (only 30 babies) [17].

In summary, the use of oral anticoagulants during the first trimester is associated with an increased rate of fetal wastage and congenital malformations. The use of warfarin in any trimester carries an increased risk of central nervous system defects. In our view, coumarin should not be used during pregnancy for VTE unless heparin or LMWH are strongly contraindicated due to a serious adverse effect in the mother (severe thrombocytopenia, paradoxical thrombosis).

Other anticoagulant therapy

In pregnant women with HIT or allergic skin reactions to UFH or LMWH, use of danaparoid or fondaparinux may be used. This is based on limited data but reassuring [6].

In cases where thrombolysis were required, recombinant tissue plasminogen activator (rtPA), which does not cross the placenta and streptokinase, which minimally crosses the placenta, did not show significant adverse effects to the fetus nor has congenital malformation been reported, although evidence is based on very few case reports [3,30–33]. Low-dose aspirin is safe during pregnancy [20,34].

Granulocyte colony-stimulating factor (G-CSF) and Granulocyte-macrophage colony stimulating factor (GM-CSF)

These growth factors are used in a variety of situations in which rapid neutrophil recovery is needed. As they have been shown to decrease the periods of hospitalization, duration of infection, or antibiotic administration and the period of neutropenia, their use has been approved by the Food and Drug Administration for the treatment of patients with pre-specified indications after chemotherapy for hematological malignancies. They are also employed today for other conditions like bone marrow transplantation or various causes of bone marrow depression, and for preventing recurrent miscarriages.

Clinical experience with GM-CSF and G-CSF during pregnancy is very limited. No teratogenicity and negative effect on fertility were reported in animal studies for G-CSF [35] and GM-CSF [36]. One report suggested transplacental transfer of filgrastrim, despite its high molecular mass of 18.800 daltons. Whether this is due to cell receptor signaling pathway, through direct metabolite or drug effect is not clear [37]. The information in human pregnancy is limited to case reports and registry, mostly on Filgrastim. There are at least 12 case reports with exposure in pregnancy for treatment of neutropenia (including some with first-trimester exposures) with normal neonatal outcome [38–44]. The Severe Chronic Neutropenia International Registry reported 20 pregnancies in women who were on Filgrastim (median dose of 2.7 µg/kg/day daily or alternate day schedule) for a median of 2 trimesters, including the first trimester in some cases. There were 13 normal healthy live births, 3 spontaneous abortions, and 4 elective terminations (3 nonmedical and 1 severe thrombocytopenia) [45]. Scarpellini and Sbracia reported 29 of 35 women with history of recurrent miscarriages treated with Filgrastim (1 mcg/kg/day from day 6 after ovulation until the ninth week of gestation) who gave birth to 29 normal healthy babies [46].

In summary, possible transplacental transfer of G-CSF has been documented in humans at the second and third trimester. No teratogenicity was observed in animal models. The information in humans is limited to Filgrastim, but so far no teratogenic effect has been reported.

Erythropoietin

Therapy with recombinant human erythropoietin was first shown to correct the anemia caused by end-stage renal failure in dialysis patients [47]. Obviously, cancer during pregnancy by itself or due to different treatment modalities can result in anemia. Physiologic erythropoietin levels increase gradually and peak during the third trimester. With a molecular weight of 30,400 daltons, erythropoietin is not expected to cross the placenta. This is supported by the lack of association between fetal and maternal erythropoietin levels during pregnancy and at birth [48]. In animal studies, no teratogenic effects were noticed at doses used in humans, although the administration of high doses (500 U/kg) was shown to cause birth defects [49]. Blood transfusions carry both immediate and long term complications and hazards. In contrast, the complications of erythropoietin are mild and include flu like syndrome which is usually self-limited, conjunctival inflammation, and, in small percentage, seizures. Developing or worsening hypertension, which was reported during erythropoietin treatment in patients with renal failure, was not reported in pregnant women. Treatment of pregnant women with erythropoietin may obviate the need for multiple blood transfusions. There is little information in the literature on the use of erythropoietin during pregnancy. No large controlled studies exist; most of the information is reported as case reports or case series with no association with teratogenicity [50].

In summary, erythropoietin administration during pregnancy is considered to be safe. It does not seem to cross the placenta and no teratogenic effects were found among the small number of women treated during organogenesis.

Bisphosphonates

Pregnant women with cancer may have hypercalcemia. Hematological malignancies (multiple myeloma, lymphoma) as well as solid tumors (breast, kidney, lung) can be associated with hypercalcemia, which is a medical emergency. Also, painful bone metastasis or severe osteoporosis may occur during the course of neoplastic disease [51].

Bisphosphonates are a group of compounds with high affinity for bone and are concentrated in areas of high bone turnover. Their mechanism of action is thought to be inhibition of osteoclast activity. The experience with bisphosphonates during pregnancy is very limited. There are no large controlled studies in pregnant women. Both animal and human studies have shown that bisphosphonates cross the placenta [52]. Animal studies showed skeletal abnormalities when given a high dose of the drug [53]. The main adverse effect found in animal reports was their ability to decrease maternal calcium, which caused protracted parturition due to uterine contraction, a calcium-dependent process which leads to fetal demise. Intravenous calcium supplementation prevented the above-described adverse effects. Thus, in animals, the bisphosphonate-induced hypocalcemia is the main cause of maternal toxicity, rather than a direct effect on the pups [54].

Bisphosphonates can persist in mineralized bone for many years (more than 10 years for alendronate) [55]. Even if use of these drugs is stopped before conception, the fetus might still be exposed to bisphosphonates, released from the maternal skeleton [52]. There are 2 case series and several case reports involving approximately 55 pregnant women who either stopped the drug within 6 months preconception or were exposed during pregnancy, mostly first trimester, which have not shown teratogenic concerns [55,56]. Lower birth weight, earlier gestational age at delivery, and increased spontaneous abortion were noted, which may be due to maternal illness and multidrug therapy [57]. Although the information regarding the safety of bisphosphonates use during pregnancy is limited, inadvertent exposure during preconception and first trimester may not pose significant fetal risks. If the drug is used, careful monitoring of calcium levels in the mother and the neonate is advised.

Antibiotics

As the pregnant woman with malignancy might be treated with a single or combination of antibiotics, their effects on either the mother or the child should be known. Penicillins (including piperacillin-tazobactam), cephalosporins (including Cefepime, Ceftazidime), and erythromycin are considered safe [51]. Aminoglycosides and metronidazole are not contraindicated during pregnancy and can be used when indicated [50,58,59]. Quinolones were blamed for causing arthropathy when used by pediatric age group but prospective data for *in utero* exposure did not show increased risk for birth defect nor cartilage disorder. Short-term use of quinolones during pregnancy is considered safe [58–61]. The tetracyclines are not teratogenic but exposure after 4–5 months of gestation may lead to discoloration (staining) of deciduous teeth and deposition in bones [62]. Trimethoprim, a folic acid antagonist, had been associated with increased risk for birth defect including neural tube defect if used in the first trimester [63,64]. Sulfonamides and nitrofurantoin are avoided near term due to the risk of hyperbilirubinemia in the newborn due to displacement of bilirubin from albumin and hemolysis of immature erythrocytes with higher risk among neonates with glucose-6-phosphate dehydrogenase (G6PD) deficiency [65,66].

Among the broad spectrum antibiotics, imipenem-cilastatin, and meropenem are closely similar to penicillin. Animal studies revealed no teratogenic effect. No first-trimester exposures have been reported, but not expected to increase risk for birth defect. No adverse neonatal effect noted for imipenem-cilastatin when used in late trimester [67]. Reports on vancomycin used in pregnancy are limited to second and third trimester, with no neonatal adverse effects noted. Animal model revealed no teratogenic effect [50].

Antifungal

Fluconazole is a triazole antifungal agent used for treatment of vaginal candidiasis and other fungal infections. Case reports suggest risk of birth defect with continuous high-dose fluconazole ($\geq$ 400 mg/day) exposure in the first trimester [68,69], whereas a single fluconazole dose of 150–200 mg, usually prescribed for vaginal candidiasis, appears to be safe at any point during gestation [70].

Itraconazole is indicated for the treatment of various fungal infections in both immunocompetent and immunocompromised patients. It has a long half-life of 64 hours. Animal studies had shown to produce embryotoxicity and teratogenic effect in both rats and mice [71]. The use of itraconazole during pregnancy (specifically first trimester) involving approximately 400 pregnant women in 2 prospective cohort studies did not show an increased risk of major malformations [72,73]. It should be used in pregnant patients with cancer only if benefit outweighs the risk.

Amphotericin B has been shown to cross the human placenta. No teratogenic effects were noted in animal studies. Based on numerous case reports and series spanning over 50 years, no evidence of adverse effects or teratogenicity have been reported in the literature [50].

Antiviral

Acyclovir is a synthetic acyclic purine nucleoside analog used as an antiviral agent against herpes viruses. Valacyclovir is a prodrug of acyclovir. It is rapidly converted to acyclovir by the liver after absorption in the gut. The drug has been shown to cross the human placenta at term [74]. Based on manufacturer's pregnancy registry and the nationwide registries in Denmark (approximately 2,300 pregnant women exposed to acyclovir and 250 women exposed to valacyclovir in the first trimester), no increased risk for birth defect was noted [75,76]. Acyclovir and valacyclovir are considered safe to use during pregnancy.

Oseltamivir is a viral neuraminidase inhibitor for the treatment of influenza A and B reducing both the duration and severity of flu symptoms. *Ex vivo* human placenta model demonstrated it is extensively metabolized by the placenta with incomplete transplacental transfer of the metabolite, with minimal accumulation on the fetal side. The manufacturer has reported 61 pregnancy exposures with unknown timing during pregnancy, 4 of which had miscarriages. One newborn had trisomy 21, and another had anencephaly, which is not likely due to the treatment. The majority of pregnancies resulted in the birth of normal babies. The Japanese teratogen information services prospectively followed 90 pregnancies with exposure in the first trimester with 1 malformation observed [77]. Patients should only use oseltamivir when the potential benefits to the mother outweigh potential risk to the fetus.

Analgesics

Acetaminophen is the drug of choice during pregnancy. Nonsteroidal anti-inflammatory drugs (NSAIDs) such as high-dose aspirin, ibuprofen, and naproxen use in the first trimester have been associated with increased risk for spontaneous abortion if used around the time of conception and small risk for septal heart defect, gastroschisis, and oral cleft [50,78]. These observations remain inconclusive due to methodological flows, small sample size in the study group (less than 15) or due to confounders such as maternal viral illness or medical conditions. If there is a risk in the first trimester, it is most likely small. NSAIDs are avoided at and beyond 32 weeks of gestation due to potential risk of premature closure of ductus arteriosus, which may lead to fetal pulmonary hypertension [50].

Opioid analgesics are not considered teratogenic in humans. Maternal addiction, with subsequent signs of neonatal withdrawal, is expected in chronic users. Respiratory depression and decreased oxygen consumption in the newborn were all observed in children born to mothers who received morphine during labor or used the drug chronically [50].

References

1. Doll DC, Ringenberg QS, Yarbro JW. Management of cancer during pregnancy. *Arch Intern Med.* 1988;**48**:2058–64.

2. Ginsberg JS, Hirsh J, Turner DC, Levine MN, Burrows R. Risks to the fetus of anticoagulation therapy during pregnancy. *Thromb Haemost.* 1989;**61**:197–203.

3. Chunilal SD, Bates SM. Venous thromboembolism in pregnancy: diagnosis, management and prevention. *Thromb Haemost.* 2009;**101**:428–38.

4. Girling JC, De Swiet M. thromboembolism in pregnancy: an overview. *Curr Opin Obstet Gynecol.* 1996;**8**:458–63.

5. Laurent P, Dussarat GV, Bonal J, et al. Low molecular weight heparins. A Guide to their optimum use in pregnancy. *Drugs.* 2002;**62**:463–77.

6. Kher A, Bauersachs R, Nielsen JD. The management of thrombosis in pregnancy: role of low-molecular-weight heparin. *Thromb Haemost.* 2007;**97**:505–13.

7. Forestier F, Dallos F, Capella-Pavlovsky M. Low molecular weight heparin (PK 10169) does not cross the placenta during the second trimester of pregnancy study by direct fetal blood sampling under ultrasound. *Thromb Res.* 1984;**34**:557–60.

8. Doutremepuich C, Fantauzzi B, Masse A, et al. Passage of commercial heparin and LMW fragment of heparin, CY 222, across the placenta of pregnant rabbits. *Pathol Biol.* 1985;**33**:677–9.

9. Forestier F, Daffos F, Rainaut M, Toulemonde F. Low molecular weight heparin (CY216) does not cross the placenta during the third trimester of pregnancy. *Thromb Haemost.* 1987;**57**:234.

10. Nelson-Piercy C, Letsky EA, de Swiet M. Low molecular-weight heparin for obstetric thromboprophylaxis: experience of sixty-nine pregnancies in sixty-one women at high risk. *Am J Obstet Gynecol.* 1997;**176**:1062–8.

11. Blomback M, Bremme K, Hellgren M, Siegbahn A, Lindberg H. Thromboprophylaxis with low molecular mass heparin 'Fragmin' (dalteparin), during pregnancy: a longitudinal safety study. *Blood Coagul Fibrinolysis.* 1998;**9**:1–9.

12. Ellison J, Walker ID, Greer IA. Antenatal use of enoxaparin for prevention and treatment of thromboembolism in pregnancy. *BJOG.* 2000;**107**:1116–21.

13. Lepercq J, Conrad J, Borel-Derlon A, et al. Venous thromboembolism during pregnancy: a retrospective study of enoxaparin safety in 624 pregnancies. *BJOG.* 2001;**108**:1134–40.

14. Lee AY, Levine MN, Baker RI, et al. Low-molecular-weight heparin versus a coumarin for the prevention of recurrent venous thromboembolism in patients with cancer. *N Eng J Med.* 2003;**349**:146–53.

15. Louzada ML, Majeed H, Wells P. Efficacy of low-molecular weight- heparin versus Vitamin K antagonists for long term treatment of cancer-associated venous thromboembolism in adults: a systematic review of randomized controlled trials. *Thromb Res.* 2009;**123**:837–44.

16. Van Dongen CJ, van den Belt AG, Prins MH, Lensing AW. Fixed dose subcutaneous low molecular weight heparins versus adjusted dose unfractionated heparin for venous thromboembolism. *Cochrane Database Syst Rev.* 2004(4);CD001100.

17. Bates SM, Greer IA, Pabinger I, et al. Venous thromboembolism, thrombophilia, antithrombotic therapy, and pregnancy: American college of chest physicians evidence- based clinical practice guidelines (8th Edition). *Chest.* 2008;**133**(suppl):844S–86S.

18. Greer IA. Venous thromboembolism and anticoagulant therapy in pregnancy. *Gender Med.* 2005;**2**:S10–7.

19. Lim W. Using low molecular weight heparin in special patient populations. *J Thromb Thrombolysis.* 2010;**29**:233–40.

20. Bauersachs RM. Treatment of venous thromboembolism during pregnancy. *Thromb Res.* 2009;**123**:S45–S50.

21. Lee AY. The roles of anticoagulants in patients with cancer. *Thromb Res.* 2010;**125**:S8–11.

22. DiSaia PJ. Pregnancy and delivery of a patient with a Starr-Edwards mitral valve prosthesis: report of a case. *Obstet Gynecol.* 1966;**28**:469.

23. Pauli RM, Haun J. Intrauterine effects of coumarin derivatives. *Dev Brain Dysfunc.* 1993;**6**:229–47.

24. Hall JG, Pauli RM, Wilson KM. Maternal and fetal sequelae of anticoagulation during pregnancy. *Am J Med.* 1980;**68**:122–40.

25. Oakley CM. Anticoagulation and pregnancy. *Eur Heart J.* 1995;**16**:1317–9.

26. Chan WS, Anand S, Ginsberg JS. Anticoagulation of pregnant women with mechanical heart valves: a systematic review of the literature. *Arch Intern Med.* 2000;**160**:191–6.

27. Van Driel D, Wesseling J, Sauer PJ, van Der Veer E, Touwen BC, Smrkovsky M. In utero exposure to coumarins and cognition at 8 to 14 years old. *Pediatrics.* 2001;**107**:123–9.

28. Wesseling J, van Driel D, Heymans HS, et al. Coumarin during pregnancy: long term effects on growth and development in school age children. *Thromb Haemost.* 2001;**85**:609–13.

29. Wesseling J, van Driel D, Smrkovsky M, et al. Neurological outcome in school-age children after in utero exposure to coumarins. *Early Hum Dev.* 2001;**63**:83–95.

30. Turrentine MA, Braems G, Ramirex MM. Use of thrombolytics for the treatment of thromboembolic disease during pregnancy. *Obstet Gynecol Surv.* 1995;**50**:534–41.

31. Nassar AH, Abdallah ME, Moukarbel GV, et al. Sequential use of thrombolytic agents for thrombosed mitral valve prosthesis during pregnancy. *J Perinat Med.* 2003;**31**:257–60.

32. Anbarasan C, Kumar VS, Latchumanadhas K, Mullasari AS. Successful thrombolysis of

prosthetic mitral valve thrombosis in early pregnancy. *J Heart Valve Dis.* 2001;**10**:393–5.

33. Henrich W, Schmider A, Henrich M, Dudenhausen JW. Acute iliac vein thrombosis in pregnancy treated successfully by streptokinase lysis: a case report. *J Perinat Med.* 2001;**29**:155–7.

34. Kozer E, Nikfar S, Costei A, Boskovic R, Nulman I, Koren G. Aspirin consumption during the first trimester of pregnancy and congenital anomalies: a meta-analysis. *Am J Obstet Gynecol.* 2002;**187**:1623–30.

35. Sugiyama O, Watanabe S, Matsuda K, et al. Teratology study of recombinant human G-CSF (RG-CSF) in rats. *Yakuri to Chiryo.* 1990;**18**:S2355.

36. Kim S, Chung M, Han S, Roh J. Teratogenicity study (segment II) of recombinant granulocyte-macrophage colony stimulating factors (LBD-005) in rats. *J Toxicol Sci.* 1993;**18**:1–17.

37. Calhoun DA, Rosa C, Christensen RD. Transplacental passage of recombinant human granulocyte colony-stimulating factor in women with an imminent preterm delivery. *Am J Obstet Gynecol.* 1996;**174**:1306–11.

38. Azim HA Jr, Pavlidis N, Peccatori FA. Treatment of the pregnant mother with cancer: a systematic review on the use of cytotoxic, endocrine, targeted agents and immunotherapy during pregnancy. Part II. Hematological tumors. *Cancer Treat Rev.* 2010;**36**:110–21.

39. Ohba T, Yoshimura T, Araki M, et al. Aplastic anemia in pregnancy: treatment with cyclosporine and granulocyte-colony stimulating factor. *Acta Obstet Gynecol Scand.* 1999;**78**:458–61.

40. Kaufmann SJ, Sharif K, Sharma V, McVerry BA. Term delivery in a woman with severe congenital neutropenia, treated with growth colony stimulating factor. *Hum Reprod.* 1998;**13**:498–9.

41. Arango HA, Kalter CS, Decesare SL, et al. Management of chemotherapy in a pregnancy complicated by a large neuroblastoma. *Obstet Gynecol.* 1994;**84**:665–8.

42. Cavallaro AM, Lilleby K, Majolino I, et al. Three to six year follow-up of normal donors who received recombinant human granulocyte colony-stimulating factor. *Bone Marrow Transplant.* 2000;**25**:85–9.

43. Sangalli MR, Peek M, McDonald A. Prophylactic granulocyte colony-stimulating factor treatment for acquired chronic severe neutropenia in pregnancy. *Aust N Z J Obstet Gynecol.* 2001;**41**:470–1.

44. Fung YL, Pitcher LA, Taylor K, Minchinton RM. Managing passively acquired autoimmune neonatal neutropenia: a case study. *Transfus Med.* 2005;**15**:151–5.

45. Dale DC, Cottle TE, Fier CJ, et al. Severe chronic neutropenia: treatment and follow-up of patients in the Severe Chronic Neutropenia International Registry. *Am J Hematol.* 2003;**72**:82–93.

46. Scarpellini F, Sbracia M. Use of granulocyte colony-stimulating factor for the treatment of unexplained recurrent miscarriage: a randomized controlled trial. *Hum Reprod.* 2009;**24**:2703–8.

47. Eschbach JW, Egrie JC, Downing MR, Browne JK, Adamson JW. Correction of the anemia of end-stage renal disease with recombinant human erythropoietin: results of a combined phase I and II clinical trial. *N Engl J Med.* 1987;**316**:73–8.

48. Reisenberger K, Egarter C, Kapiotis S, Sternberger B, Gregor H, Husslein P. Transfer of erythropoietin across the placenta perfused in vitro. *Obstet Gynecol.* 1997;**89**:738–42.

49. *Epogen. [Product information].* Thousand Oaks, CA: Amgen; 2000.

50. Briggs GG, Freeman RK, Yaffe SJ. *Drugs in pregnancy and lactation.* 8th ed. Philadelphia: Lippincott Williams and Wilkins; 2008.

51. Fleisch H. Bisphosphonates: pharmacology and use in the treatment of tumor-induced hypercalcemia and metastatic bone disease. *Drugs.* 1991;**42**:919–44.

52. Munns CF, Rauch F, Ward L, Glorieux FH. Maternal and fetal outcome after long-term

pamidronate treatment before conception: a report of two cases. *J Bone Miner Res.* 2004;**19**:1742–5.

53. Graepel P, Bentley P, Fritz H, Miyamoto M, Slater SR. Reproduction toxicity studies with pamidronate. *Arzneimittel-Forschung.* 1992;**42**:654–67.

54. Minsker DH, Manson JM, Peter CP. Effects of the bisphosphonate, alendronate, on parturition in the rat. *Toxicol Appl Pharmacol.* 1993;**121**:217–23.

55. Levy S, Fayez I, Taguchi N, et al. Pregnancy outcome following in utero exposure to bisphosphonates. *Bone.* 2009;**44**:428–30.

56. Djokanovic N, Klieger-Grossmann C, Koren G. Does treatment with bisphosphonates endanger the human pregnancy? *J Obstet Gynaecol Can.* 2008;**30**:1146–8.

57. Ornoy A, Wajnberg R, Diav-Citrin O. The outcome of pregnancy following pre-pregnancy or early pregnancy alendronate treatment. *Reprod Toxicol.* 2006;**22**:578–9.

58. Nahum GG, Uhl K, Kennedy DL. Antibiotic use in pregnancy and lactation. *Obstet Gynecol.* 2006;**107**:1120–38.

59. Buhimschi CS, Weiner CP. Medications in pregnancy and lactation. Part 2. Drugs with minimal or unknown human teratogenic effect. *Obstet Gynecol.* 2009;**113**:417–32.

60. Berkovitch M, Pastuszak A, Gazarian M, Lewis M, Koren G. Safety of the new quinolones in pregnancy. *Obstet Gynecol.* 1994;**84**:535–8.

61. Schaefer C, Amoura-Elefant E, Vial T, et al. Pregnancy outcome after prenatal quinolone exposure. Evaluation of a case registry of the European Network of Teratology Information Services (ENTIS). *Eur J Obstet Gynecol.* 1996;**69**:83–9.

62. Demers P, Fraser D, Goldbloom RB, et al. Effects of tetracyclines on skeletal growth and dentition. A report by the Nutrition Committee of the Canadian Paediatric Society. *Can Med Assoc J.* 1968;**99**:849–54.

63. Czeizel AE, Rockenbauer M, Sorensen HT, Olsen J. The teratogenic risk of trimethoprim-sulfonamides: a population

based case-control study. *Reprod Toxicol.* 2001;**15**:637–46.

64. Hernandez-Diaz S, Werler MM, Walker AM, Mitchell AA. Neural tube defects in relation to use of folic acid antagonists during pregnancy. *Am J Epidemiol.* 2001;**153**:961–8.

65. Dunn PM. The possible relationship between the maternal administration of sulphamethoxypyridazine and hyperbilirubinemia in the newborn. *J Obstet Gynaecol Br Commonw.* 1964;**71**:128–31.

66. Bruel H, Guillemant V, Saladin-Thiron C, Chabrolle JP, Lahary A, Poinsot J. Hemolytic anemia in a newborn after maternal treatment with nitrofurantoin at the end of pregnancy. *Arch Pediatr.* 2000;**7**:745–7.

67. Ryo E, Ikeya M, Suqimoto M. Clinical study of the effectiveness of imipenem/cilastatin sodium as the antibiotics of first choice in the expectant management of patients with preterm premature rupture of membranes. *J Infect Chemother.* 2005;**11**:32–6.

68. Aleck KA, Bartley DL. Multiple malformation syndrome following fluconazole use in pregnancy: report of an additional patient. *Am J Med Genet.* 1997;**72**:253–6.

69. Lopez-Rangel E, Van Allen MI. Prenatal exposure to fluconazole: an identifiable dysmorphic phenotype. *Birth Defects Res A Clin Mol Teratol.* 2005;**73**:919–23.

70. Nørgaard M, Pedersen L, Gislum M, et al. Maternal use of fluconazole and risk of congenital malformations: a Danish population-based cohort study. *J Antimicrob Chemother.* 2008;**62**:172–6.

71. Sporanox [product monograph]. In: Repchinsky C, editor-in-chief. *Compendium of pharmaceuticals and specialties.* Ottawa, ON: Canadian Pharmacists Association; 2010. Ottawa, ON; 2010. p. 2215.

72. Bar-Oz B, Moretti ME, Bishai R, et al. Pregnancy outcome after in utero exposure to itraconazole: a prospective cohort study. *Am J Obstet Gynecol.* 2000;**183**:617–20.

73. De Santis M, Di Gianantonio E, Cesari E, Ambrosini G, Straface G, Clementi M. First-trimester itraconazole exposure and pregnancy outcome: a prospective cohort study of women contacting teratology information services in Italy. *Drug Saf.* 2009;**32**:239–44.

74. Frenkel LM, Brown ZA, Bryson YJ, et al. Pharmacokinetics of acyclovir in the term human pregnancy and neonate. *Am J Obstet Gynecol.* 1991;**164**:569–76.

75. Acyclovir Pregnancy Registry and Valacyclovir Pregnancy Registry. Final study report. 1 June 1984 through 30 April 1999. Glaxo Welcome; 1999.

76. Pasternak B, Hviid A. Use of acyclovir, valacyclovir, and famciclovir in the first trimester of pregnancy and the risk of birth defects. *JAMA.* 2010;**304**:859–66.

77. Tanaka T, Nakajima K, Murashima A, Garcia-Bournissen F, Koren G, Ito S. Safety of neuraminidase inhibitors against novel influenza A (H1N1) in pregnant and breastfeeding women. *CMAJ.* 2009; **181**:55–8.

78. Li DK, Liu L, Odouli R. Exposure to non-steroidal anti-inflammatory drugs during pregnancy and risk of miscarriage: population based cohort study. *BMJ.* 2003;**327**:368.

Chapter

17

Management of nutritional problems in the pregnant cancer patient

Deborah A. Kennedy

Introduction

The nutrition requirements of the pregnant women are increased during pregnancy. The recommended increases are, in calories, 340 kcals per day in the second trimester and 452 kcals per day in the third trimester [1].

New guidelines recently released by the Institute of Medicine for overall weight gain in pregnancy are determined based on pre-pregnancy body mass index (BMI) (Table 1). The placenta, fetus, and amniotic fluid comprise approximately 35% of the gestational weight gain, with the remaining weight accruing to the uterus, mammary glands, blood, and adipose tissue [3–5].

Adequate weight gain in pregnancy is a key determinant in fetal birth weight with fetal survival correlated strongly with a birth weight of 3,000 to 4,000 grams (6.6 to 8.2 lbs) [5,6]. Low birth weight increases the risk for neonatal complications [7]. Several researchers have studied the effects on undernutrition resulting from the Dutch famine, which occurred during World War II. The timing of famine during gestation had an impact on the health of these children in adulthood. Undernutrition during gestation in this cohort of children, born of mothers who experienced the Dutch famine, was associated with glucose intolerance [8]. Obesity and cardiovascular disease is more prevalent in later life for those whose undernutrition occurred early in gestation, whereas hypertension was found in those individuals for whom the famine occurred later in gestation [8,9]. There was no association with an increase in congenital malformations during this time [10]. Although starvation and cancer cachexia are not equivalent states, the outcomes from the famine can provide some insight into the impact on the fetus resulting from undernutrition.

Table 1.

	Pre-pregnancy BMI	Gestational weight gain recommended ranges[2]
Underweight	< 18.5	28–40 lbs (12.5–18 kg)
Normal weight	18.5–24.9	25–35 lbs (11.5–16 kg)
Overweight	25–29.9	15–25 lb (7–11.5 kg)
Obese	>30.0	At least 15 lb (7 kg)

Cancer in Pregnancy and Lactation: The Motherisk Guide ed. Gideon Koren and Michael Lishner. Published by Cambridge University Press. © Cambridge University Press 2011.

Standard laboratory assessments, such as CBC, serum albumin, ferritin, and folate, and thyroid function testing (T3, T4, and TSH) may provide some insight into nutritional reserves during pregnancy. In the absence of hepatic insufficiency, low serum albumin level may reflect insufficient protein intake [5]. Fetal growth can be assessed by symphysis–fundal height and also by serial ultrasongraphic measurements.

General dietary recommendations

Anorexia or the loss of the desire to eat is often a consequence of cancer, resulting from either the cancer itself or as a side effect of treatment [11,12]. Eating full meals can be difficult, however, snacking or eating small amounts of food throughout the day can improve intake [13].

It has been hypothesized that the placenta may act as a nutrient sensor to coordinate fetal growth with the ability of the mother to provide nutrients [14,15]. Glucose, amino acids, and fatty acids are the key nutrients for the fetus [16]. Studies using fetal blood sampling techniques have determined that amino acid concentrations are higher within the fetus during the second half of pregnancy, that the placenta preferentially transfers arachdonic acid (AA) and docosahexaenoic acid (DHA) to the fetus and that glucose concentrations in fetal circulation are lower in the fetus, however, these change in parallel to maternal concentrations [16,17].

Protein requirements in pregnancy are increased. The average recommended daily intake of protein for adults is 0.8 g/kg per day [1,5]. In pregnancy, the suggested increase is an additional 1.3 g, 6.1 g and 10.7g per day in each trimester, respectively [5]. With cancer, protein requirements may be higher. Hypoalbumineria, in the absence of hepatic insufficiency, would be an indicator of protein insufficiency in the diet [5]. Consider referral to a dietitian or doctor of naturopathic medicine to provide more specific guidance regarding food choices and strategies.

Fatty acids

Supplementation with omega-3 fatty acids during pregnancy, DHA in particular, is an area of controversy. The fetus is dependent upon maternal fatty acid nutrition as its source for long chain polyunsaturated fatty acids for structural lipids, and these are not synthesized by the placenta [17]. Supplementation with omega-3 fatty acids does enhance pregnancy duration and, while the evidence is inconclusive, may assist with weight maintenance in cancer patients [17–19]. This may not be as relevant in countries where, historically fish intake in women is high. Suggested dosing of 300 mg of DHA in pregnancy [20] and 1.5 g of omega 3 fatty acids (eicosapentaenoic acid [EPA] and DHA) in cancer patients was found to be effective [18].

Vitamin D

Our understanding of the importance of adequate levels of vitamin D in health is growing, demonstrating a role in not only bone health, but brain development and cardiovascular health [21]. Vitamin D has also been shown to have anticancer and antiinflammatory roles, exhibiting both antiangiogentic and antiproliferative properties [22]. Furthermore, upwards of 80% of pregnant women have been found to be deficient in vitamin D [21].

Most multivitamins contain 400 IU of vitamin D, which is sufficient to raise serum 25(OH)D 2.8 to 4.8 ng/mL, however, this may not resolve a vitamin D deficiency [21,23]. Identification of a deficiency through the laboratory assessment of serum 25 (OH)D levels and supplementation to achieve serum concentrations above 30 ng/mL (75 nmol/L) are suggested [23].

Prenatal vitamins

The determination regarding continuation of prenatal vitamins is best assessed on a case by case basis. There is, however, evidence to suggest that supplementation with micronutrients may be beneficial to offset an inadequate nutritional status in cachexia [24].

Consideration should be given to enteral or parenteral nutrition if the patient is unable to maintain nutrition for an extended period [5].

Strategies to address the side effects of chemotherapy, radiation, and pregnancy

Diarrhea

There are several approaches to reduce the impact of frequent loose stools associated with some cancer treatments. Eating small frequent meals throughout the day, and reducing the intake of greasy, fried, or spicy foods can assist [13]. Dehydration is an important concern, so drinking water, clear broth, or eating foods high in sodium and/or potassium, such as crackers, sports drinks, bananas, and soups are recommended [13]. The probiotics species *Lactobacillus* and *Bifidobacterium* have been found to be safe in pregnancy [25,26] and effective for reducing chemotherapy- and radiation-induced diarrhea [27–29]. Psyllium, a soluble fiber, may also assist with providing bulk to the stool and reduce stool frequency [29].

Constipation

Constipation is often experienced in pregnancy and may also be associated with the use of narcotic medications for pain management. Ensuring adequate hydration, 8–10 glasses of fluids, and 25–35 grams of fiber per day in the diet can provide assistance [30]. Other strategies include the incorporation of prunes or prune juice which may stimulate the bowels to move [13]. Senna, as a laxative, has been found to be safe for use in pregnancy [31].

Nausea and vomiting of pregnancy

Morning sickness is a common occurrence in pregnancy. Ginger has been shown to be effective in improving the nausea and vomiting associated with pregnancy, and postoperative and chemotherapy-induced nausea [20,31–34]. Powdered ginger extract in doses ranging from 125 mg to 250 mg 4 times per day have been found to be safe and effective [34]. Supplementation of pyridoxine (B6) has also shown to be effective in reducing the symptoms of nausea and vomiting of pregnancy. Dosing of vitamin B6 ranges from 25 to 50 mg every 8 hours up to 200 mg per day [34]. Many antiemetic pharmaceutical drugs have also been found to be safe for use in pregnancy, such as Diclectin® a combination of B6 and doxylamine succinate [34,35].

Mucositis

Mucositis can be a treatment side effect of both chemotherapy and radiation. Strategies to reduce the discomfort associated with eating include eating soft foods such as banana, mashed potatoes, puddings, etc., avoiding spicy, hard, or irritating foods such as citrus fruit, toast, and granola and frequent rinsing of the mouth [13]. Honey and glutamine are emerging as having benefits in reducing the severity and healing time associated with mucositis [36–40]. Pasteurized honey at a dose of 20 ml (approximately 1 tablespoon) 15 minutes before and after radiation therapy demonstrated a significant reduction in the severity of mucositis [37].

Acknowledgements

Laura A. Magee, MD, FRCPC, MSc; Fran Berkoff, RD; and Carole Leduc, Pdt, were the authors of this chapter in the first edition.

References

1. Institute of Medicine. *Dietary reference intakes, the essential guide to nutrient requirements*. Washington DC: National Academies Press; 2006.

2. Siega-Riz AM, Deierlein A, Stuebe A. Implementation of the new institute of medicine gestational weight gain guidelines. *J Midwifery Womens Health*. 2010;**55**:512–9.

3. Pitkin RM. Nutritional support in obstetrics and gynecology. *Clin Obstet Gynecol*. 1976;**19**:489–513.

4. Institute of Medicine. Weight gain during pregnancy: reexamining the guidelines. In: Rasmussen KM, Yaktine AL, editors. *Committee to Reexamine IOM Pregnancy Weight Guidelines, Food and Nutrition Board and Board on Children, Youth, and Families*. Washington DC: IOM; 2009.

5. Hamaoui E, Hamaoui M. Nutritional assessment and support during pregnancy. *Gastroenterol Clin North Am*. 2003; **32**:59–121.

6. MacBurney M, Wilmore D. Parenteral nutrition in pregnancy. In: Rombeau JL, Caldwell MD, editors. *Clinical nutrition: parenteral nutrition*. 2nd ed. Philadelphia: WB Saunders; 1993.

7. Osrin D, de L Costello AM. Maternal nutrition and fetal growth: practical issues in international health. *Semin Neonatol*. 2000;**5**:209–19.

8. Roseboom T, de Rooij S, Painter R. The Dutch famine and its long-term consequences for adult health. *Early Hum Dev*. 2006;**82**:485–91.

9. Kyle UG, Pichard C. The Dutch Famine of 1944–1945: a pathophysiological model of long-term consequences of wasting disease. *Curr Opin Clin Nutr Metab Care*. 2006;**9**:388–94.

10. Smith CA. Effects of maternal malnutrition on fetal development. *Am J Dis Child*. 1947;**73**:243.

11. Langstein HN, Norton JA. Mechanisms of cancer cachexia. *Hematol Oncol Clin North Am*. 1991;**5**:103–23.

12. Tisdale MJ. Cancer cachexia. *Anticancer Drugs*. 1993;**4**:115–25.

13. Canadian Cancer Society. Eating well when you have cancer. *A guide to good nutrition*. Toronto: Canadian Cancer Society. 2008.

14. Myatt L, Powell T. Maternal adaptions to pregnancy and the role of the placenta. In: Symonds ME, Ramsay MM, editors. *Maternal-fetal nutrition during pregnancy and lactation*. New York: Cambridge University Press; 2010. p. vii, 208 p.

15. Jansson T, Powell TL. IFPA 2005 Award in Placentology Lecture. Human placental transport in altered fetal growth: does the placenta function as a nutrient sensor? – a review. *Placenta*. 2006;**27**(suppl A):S91–7.

16. Pardi G, Cetin I. Human fetal growth and organ development: 50 years of discoveries. *Am J Obstet Gynecol*. 2006;**194**:1088–99.

17. Brown L, Regnault T, Rozance P, et al. Pregnancy and feto-placental growth: macronutrients. In: Symonds ME, Ramsay MM, editors. *Maternal-fetal nutrition during pregnancy and lactation*. Cambridge; New York: Cambridge University Press; 2010. 208 p.

18. Colomer R, Moreno-Nogueira JM, Garcia-Luna PP, et al. N-3 fatty acids, cancer and cachexia: a systematic review of the literature. *Br J Nutr*. 2007;97:823–31.

19. Mazzotta P, Jeney CM. Anorexia-cachexia syndrome: a systematic review of the role of dietary polyunsaturated fatty acids in the management of symptoms, survival, and quality of life. *J Pain Symptom Manage*. 2009;37:1069–77.

20. Mallory J. Integrative care of the mother-infant dyad. *Prim Care*. 2010;37:149–63.

21. Kaludjerovic J, Vieth R. Relationship between vitamin D during perinatal development and health. *J Midwifery Womens Health*. 2010;55:550–60.

22. Krishnan AV, Feldman D. Mechanisms of the anti-cancer and anti-inflammatory actions of vitamin D. *Annu Rev Pharmacol Toxicol*. 2010;51:311–36.

23. Food and Drug Administration. *Dietary supplement fact sheet*. Vitamin D. Silver Spring, MD: Food and Drug Administration.

24. Strohle A, Zanker K, Hahn A. Nutrition in oncology: the case of micronutrients (review). *Oncol Rep*. 2010;24:815–28.

25. Dugoua JJ, Machado M, Zhu X, Chen X, Koren G, Einarson TR. Probiotic safety in pregnancy: a systematic review and meta-analysis of randomized controlled trials of Lactobacillus, Bifidobacterium, and Saccharomyces spp. *J Obstet Gynaecol Can*. 2009;31:542–52.

26. Luoto R, Laitinen K, Nermes M, Isolauri E. Impact of maternal probiotic-supplemented dietary counselling on pregnancy outcome and prenatal and postnatal growth: a double-blind, placebo-controlled study. *Br J Nutr*. 2010;103:1792–9.

27. Chitapanarux I, Chitapanarux T, Traisathit P, Kudumpee S, Thaaravichitkul E, Lorvidhava V. Randomized controlled trial of live lactobacillus acidophilus plus bifidobacterium bifidum in prophylaxis of diarrhea during radiotherapy in cervical cancer patients. *Radiat Oncol*. 2010;5:31.

28. Urbancsek H, Kazar T, Mezes I, Neumann K. Results of a double-blind, randomized study to evaluate the efficacy and safety of Antibiophilus in patients with radiation-induced diarrhoea. *Eur J Gastroenterol Hepatol*. 2001;13:391–6.

29. Muehlbauer PM, Thorpe D, Davis A, Drabot R, Rawlings BL, Kiker E. Putting evidence into practice: evidence-based interventions to prevent, manage, and treat chemotherapy- and radiotherapy-induced diarrhea. *Clin J Oncol Nurs*. 2009;13:336–41.

30. National Cancer Institute. PDQ® Nutrition in Cancer Care. [cited 2010 October 28]; Available from: http://cancer.gov/cancertopics/pdq/supportivecare/nutrition/HealthProfessional

31. Mills E, Duguoa J-J, Perri D, Koren G. *Herbal medicines in pregnancy & lactation*. New York: Taylor & Francis; 2006.

32. Vutyavanich T, Kraisarin T, Ruangsri R. Ginger for nausea and vomiting in pregnancy: randomized, double-masked, placebo-controlled trial. *Obstet Gynecol*. 2001;97:577–82.

33. Pace JC. Oral ingestion of encapsulated ginger and reported self-care actions for the relief of chemotherapy-associated nausea and vomiting. *Diss Abstr Int*. 1986;47:3297–8.

34. Einarson A, Maltepe C, Boskovic R, Koren G. Treatment of nausea and vomiting in pregnancy: an updated algorithm. *Can Fam Physician*. 2007;53:2109–11.

35. Gill SK, Einarson A. The safety of drugs for the treatment of nausea and vomiting of pregnancy. *Expert Opin Drug Saf*. 2007;6:685–94.

36. Bardy J, Slevin NJ, Mais KL, Molassiotis A. A systematic review of honey uses and its potential value within oncology care. *J Clin Nurs*. 2008;17:2604–23.

37. Motallebnejad M, Akram S, Moghadamnia A, Moulana Z, Omidi S. The effect of topical application of pure honey on radiation-induced mucositis: a randomized clinical trial. *J Contemp Dent Pract.* 2008;**9**:40–7.

38. Khanal B, Baliga M, Uppal N. Effect of topical honey on limitation of radiation-induced oral mucositis: an intervention study. *Int J Oral Maxillofac Surg.* 2010;**39**:1181–5.

39. Rashad UM, Al-Gezawy SM, El-Gezawy E, Azzaz AN. Honey as topical prophylaxis against radiochemotherapy-induced mucositis in head and neck cancer. *J Laryngol Otol.* 2009; **123**:223–8.

40. Noe JE. L-glutamine use in the treatment and prevention of mucositis and cachexia: a naturopathic perspective. *Integr Cancer Ther.* 2009;**8**:409–15.

Chapter

18

Pharmacological and nonpharmacological treatment of chemotherapy-induced nausea and vomiting

Caroline Maltepe

Introduction

The current literature shows that perinatal outcomes on women who were exposed to chemotherapy after their first trimester were not at an increased risk of congenital anomalies, preterm delivery, and growth restriction compared to the general population. However, chemotherapy in first trimester is associated with an increased risk of malformations [1,2].

The most common cause of nausea and vomiting (NV) in patients with cancer is chemotherapy. There are several pharmacological and nonpharmacological treatments available to treat NV and many studies showing their safety in human pregnancy.

Ondansetron seems to be the *5HT3 antagonist* of choice, given reassuring, albeit limited data on teratogenicity. If indicated, concomitant therapy with *corticosteroids* should be regarded as safe for the fetus after 12 weeks gestation; maternal blood pressure and blood sugar should be monitored. The data on *metoclopramide* indicate that it is not teratogenic; however, the doses that have been studied in pregnancy have been substantially lower than those advocated for relief of acute or delayed chemotherapy-induced NV. *Phenothiazines* are not teratogenic, but their use near term may be associated with extrapyramidal side effects in the newborn. If a *benzodiazepine is* used for anticipatory NV, in early gestation of pregnancy, a very small risk of oral clefting has been reported, but not confirmed in other studies. Nonpharmacological treatments such as ginger, vitamin B6, acupuncture, and acupressure may also be beneficial and are not teratogenic if used within the recommended dosages.

Chemotherapy-induced nausea and vomiting (CINV)

Patients with cancer may experience NV for many reasons. NV is usually multifactorial in etiology, resulting from the disease process itself (e.g., gastric involvement, raised intracranial pressure, hypercalcemia, migraine), drug therapy (e.g., opiates, antibiotics, antifungals), and/or radiotherapy, chemotherapy, or surgery [3]. Whereas it is important to identify and treat other causes, the focus of this chapter is specifically on CINV.

Among patients with cancer, NV occurs in up to 80% of those who receive chemotherapy, with 10–44% experiencing anticipatory NV [4]. CINV is very stressful and greatly affects the quality of life of patients. For example, many have difficulty performing their day-to-day

Cancer in Pregnancy and Lactation: The Motherisk Guide ed. Gideon Koren and Michael Lishner.
Published by Cambridge University Press. © Cambridge University Press 2011.

tasks, have poor nutrition, dehydration, weakness, and have reduced ability to tolerate and/or refuse future cycles. Therefore, control of NV remains a priority among oncologists [4–6].

To assess the incidence of CINV, one must look into patient-related risk factors, as well as, emetogenic potential of varying chemotherapy protocols in either acute or delayed phase. The following are some examples of patients with a higher risk of NV: women, younger age (<50), low or no alcohol use, breast cancer patients, history of motion sickness, anxiety, depression, previous CINV, and severe nausea and vomiting of pregnancy [3,4,7–9].

The emetogenic potential of varying chemotherapeutic regimens administered without antiemetics is a risk factor for NV and can be stratified into four groups. The high emetic risk (HEC) affects over 90% of patients and includes agents such as ciplastin, dacarbazine, and carmustine.The moderate emetic risk (MEC) affects 30–90% of patients and includes agents such as oxaliplatin, carboplatin, and irinotecan. The low emetic risk (LEC) affects 10% to 30% of patients and includes agents such as, capecitabine, fluorouracil, and pemetrexed. The minimal emetic risk affects less than 10% of patients and includes agents such as, bleomycin, methotrexate, and fludarabine [4,6,7,10]. Although activation of the chemoreceptor trigger zone (CTZ) is thought to be the most common single mechanism by which chemotherapy causes NV, most agents act at different and/or multiple sites [11].

CINV can be classified by the following [3,6,10,11]:

- *Acute*, nausea and vomiting occurs within 24 hours of chemotherapy
- *Delayed*, nausea and vomiting occurs 24 hours to several days after treatment
- *Anticipatory*, nausea and vomiting occurs before a new cycle of chemotherapy and have developed a conditioned response, such as smells, tastes, sights, thoughts, and anxiety
- *Breakthrough*, nausea and vomiting occurs despite being treated with prevention antiemetic therapy(ies)
- *Refractory*, nausea and vomiting occurs during subsequent cycles when prophylaxis antiemetic therapy(ies) have failed in earlier cycles

Management of emesis in the patient with cancer

A variety of antiemetics have been used for the treatment of various causes of NV associated with cancer and its treatment. Choices have been based on the variety of pathways involved in the pathophysiology of nausea and emesis: CTZ (which is richly innervated with receptors for dopamine, histamine, acetylcholine, and serotonin), vestibular apparatus (where cholinergic and histaminergic fibers are thought to be involved in transmission), visceral afferents (e.g., dopamine receptors mediate motor reflexes in the stomach), and vagal afferents (e.g., serotonin receptors (specifically 5-HT3) located in close proximity to enterochromaffin cells in the intestinal tract [6,11].

The list of effective antiemetic agents has grown beyond only the phenothiazines which were available in the 1970s. This is an area of active research given that no single agent is effective in all patients. The antiemetics used most commonly, especially for acute CINV, are type 3 serotonin (5-HT3) receptor antagonists, such as ondansetron, granisetron, and dolasetron. They appear to be interchangeable and are well-tolerated [10]. Concomitant corticosteroid therapy can also improve the efficacy of 5-HT3 antagonists for acute and delayed NV [4], hyperglycemia may be a side effect [3]. Steroids have also been used as monotherapy for delayed NV, although some experts advocate the addition of metoclopramide.

The efficacy of cannabinoids for CINV have been reported, however, due to concerns in pregnancy we will not discuss this further.

Antihistamines, such as diphenhydramine and hydroxyzine, have not shown to have an antiemetic effect in preventing CINV [10].

Pharmacological treatment for CINV in pregnancy

There are no data on the efficacy of antiemetic therapy for CINV in the pregnant patient with cancer. Therefore, what has been reviewed is the safety data in human pregnancy, as well as, antiemetics used commonly to treat nausea and vomiting of pregnancy (NVP) and hyperemesis gravidarum (HG).

5-HT3 Antagonists

Information about reproductive toxicity was available only for ondansetron and granisetron. Reproductive toxicology studies of ondansetron in rats, at doses of 20–80 times the recommended dose in humans, failed to produce developmental toxicity. However, there was evidence of fetotoxicity, as doses of 10–30 times the recommended dose in humans were associated, in rats and rabbits, with intrauterine fetal growth restriction [12]. A study published in 2006 showed that ondansetron readily crosses the placenta in the first trimester of pregnancy and that its fetal tissue concentration was 41% of the corresponding maternal plasma [13].

Use of ondansetron in human pregnancy is limited, however, case reports and some studies showed no increased risk of birth defects. No malformations were reported in the 3 case reports and also in the randomized controlled trial of 15 patients exposed during the first trimester of pregnancy [14–17]. Two additional studies looked at safety during pregnancy. The first study conducted in Sweden had 45 women exposed to ondansetron throughout pregnancy with 21 exposed in the first trimester and no malformation were reported [18]. The second study conducted in Canada had 176 women exposed to ondansetron during their first trimester with no increased risk of birth defect [19]. The recommended oral dose in pregnancy is 4 to 8 mg every 6 to 8 hours. When given by IV, 8 mg over 15 min every 12 hours or 1 mg/hr continuously up to 24 hours [20,21].

Animal studies in rats and rabbits administered granisetron, in doses up to 200 times that recommended in humans, failed to produce teratogenic or fetotoxic effects. There are no controlled studies in human pregnancies [22]. There is 1 case report published in 1999 with the use of granisetron. It was used in conjunction with ifosfamide and adriamycin for Ewing's sarcoma of the pelvis in the third trimester of pregnancy. A cesarean section was performed and the patient had a small but healthy baby girl. The follow-up conducted 2 years later showed that the mother was disease free and the daughter showed no chemo-related side effects [23].

Metoclopramide

Metoclopramide is a dopamine receptor antagonist, and high doses are given for CINV (20–40 mg orally every 4 to 6 hours or 1–2 mg/kg IV every 3–4 hours) [24]. Metoclopramide seems to be efficacious in preventing delayed NV. However, extrapyramidal symptoms are observed due to high doses given, which may require that diphenhydramine be added to the regimen [24,25].

Several animal studies conducted could not detect malformations in pregnant mice, rats, or rabbits. They were given 250 times the recommended human dose; no teratogenesis was observed [26–28]. Metoclopramide has been commonly used as an antiemetic in pregnancy, as well as, aiding in reducing gastric emptying time. Published studies have reported daily doses up to 40 mg a day [21,26,29].

There are several prospective studies showing no increased risk of birth defects in early pregnancy, in either (1) a study involving 309 women, or (2) a prospective cohort study of 126 women receiving metoclopramide for treatment of hyperemesis gravidarum, or (3) a surveillance study of 192 women [26,28]. Also, the largest study published in 2009 with more than 3,400 women exposed in first trimester did not show an increased risk [30].

Corticosteroids

Corticosteroids that have been commonly used for chemotherapy-induced nausea and vomiting are dexamethasone and prednisone. Preliminary animal data suggested that first-trimester exposure to steroids was associated with an increased risk for cleft palate (CP) [31–33].

A meta-analysis published in 2000 found a trend toward an increased risk of oral cleft following first-trimester exposure to corticosteroids (3.35; 95% confidence interval [CI]: 1.97–5.69) [34]. Subsequent studies have also shown a slight increase of oral clefts. Lastly, a study published in 2007, suggested that there was an increased risk of cleft lip with or without cleft palate (CLP) with corticosteroid use before 12 weeks of pregnancy (CLP 1.7; 95% CI: 1.1–2.6 and CP 0.5; 95% CI: 0.2–1.3) [35].

Prolonged therapy with steroids throughout pregnancy, for prevention of recurrent fetal loss, has been associated with premature delivery, hypertension, and gestational diabetes [36]. However, short-term use (i.e., high-dose dexamethasone) is commonly administered to accelerate fetal pulmonary maturity [26].

Cleft lip and palate generally develops during the sixth to twelfth week of pregnancy [37]. Therefore, it would be expected that similar short courses of steroids for management of chemotherapy-induced NV would not represent a fetal risk if administered after 12 weeks gestation. It would be prudent to monitor maternal blood pressure and blood sugar.

Phenothiazines

Phenothiazines, such as prochlorperazine, promethazine, and chlorpromazine, are commonly used for low emetic risk and breakthrough CINV [7]. Although anecdotal case reports have tried to associate phenothiazines exposure in early pregnancy with major malformations, prospective and retrospective cohort, and record linkage studies of various phenothiazines have failed to demonstrate an increased risk for major malformations. When used late in gestation, the newborn may experience neonatal withdrawal and self-limited extrapyramidal effects [26,28,38,39].

Benzodiazepines

Although several drugs are available in this class, lorazepam is widely used as an antiemetic for CINV. Lorazepam has been very helpful in reducing anticipatory NV and also has been beneficial to patients due to its anxiolytic, amnesic, and sedative properties [3,11,40].

There was a meta-analysis published in 1998, looking at the use of benzodiazapines including lorazepam during the first trimester of pregnancy. There were 23 studies, which included case-control and cohort studies. The pooled data from the case-control studies found a significant increase risk of major malformations (odds ratio = 3.01; 95% CI: 1.32–6.84) and for oral cleft alone (odds ratio = 1.79; 95% CI: 1.13–2.82). However, the pooled data from the cohort studies found no increase in major malformations (odds ratio = 0.90; 95% CI: 0.61–1.35) nor in oral clefts (odds ratio = 1.19; 95% CI: 0.34–4.15) [41].

Other large studies have been published following the meta-analysis, which reported no increased risk of major malformations including oral clefts. One study followed 460 pregnancies exposed to benzodiazepines in early pregnancy and reported no statistical significance in the rates of malformations in the exposed group compared to control (3.1% vs. 2.6%, $P = 0.51$, odds ratio = 1.2; 95% CI: 0.5–2.8) [42].

Another study following over 1,900 women exposed in early pregnancy to benzodiazepines (BZD) and /or hypnotic benzodiazepine receptor antagonists (HBRA) showed rates of malformation (5.3%) was comparable with that of all the births (4.7%) in the registry (n = 873,879) and no increased risk for oral clefts. However, they did conclude that maternal exposure may increase the risk for preterm birth, low birth weight, although this is complicated by the fact that the indication for treatment may have been threatened preterm birth. Also they concluded that there was an increase of neonatal symptoms and a possible association with pyloric stenosis and alimentary tract atresia [43].

In summary, maternal use of BZD and/or HBRA is associated with poor neonatal adaptation symptoms. The data have suggested a possible risk for preterm birth and/or low birth weight. The risk for oral cleft, if it exists, appears to be very low (incidence of oral clefts in the general population is approximately 1 in 1000).

Nonpharmacological treatments for CINV in pregnancy

Nonpharmacological treatments that are commonly used to treat nausea and vomiting of pregnancy have also shown to be beneficial when given in addition to the antiemetic regimen of CINV. These include the following: ginger, vitamin B6, acupressure, and acupuncture [11,20,44]. With increased fear of taking medications in the pregnancy, the latter nonpharmacological treatments have also been studied for safety in pregnancy [20,21,44].

Several studies have focused on the antiemetic properties of ginger (*Zingiber officinale*), a natural remedy [44,45]. There is some mixed evidence of its benefits in treating CINV. A randomized, controlled trial studied 162 cancer patients and the effect of ginger in treating their CINV. In combination with their pharmacological antiemetic therapies, patients received either 1 g or 2 g of ginger, or placebo for 3 days. Researchers concluded that ginger provided no additional benefit in reducing symptoms of acute or delayed CINV [46]. Conversely, other large studies have documented the effectiveness of receiving complementary ginger [47,48] reporting acute and delayed CINV was improved compared to controls.

The safety of ginger up to 1,000 mg/day (root powder equivalent) in treating pregnancy-induced nausea and vomiting is well documented [44,45,49–51] and in some studies, has been reported to be superior to vitamin B6 [52,53].

Vitamin B6 is a water soluble vitamin that is commonly used as an antiemetic agent and could be beneficial in treating CINV in pregnant women. A 2009 study looked at the efficacy of treating CINV with ovarian cancer patients. They were randomized to receive vitamin B6 point PC6 injection (50 mg IM each side) with acupressure, acupressure alone, or vitamin B6 alone (50 mg twice a day IM). These researchers concluded that acupuncture plus vitamin B6 PC6 point injection was beneficial in treating emesis (reducing the number of emesis episodes and increasing the number of emesis-free days) [54].

The usefulness and safety of vitamin B6 in pregnancy has been well researched [55–57]. In 2006, a study of 96 women who took large doses of vitamin B6 in their first trimester of pregnancy did not appear to be associated with an increased risk of major malformations. The dose of vitamin B6 taken ranged from 50 mg up to 510 mg/day (average of 132.3 mg/day) for their NVP symptoms, however, only 11 patients were treated with doses exceeding 200 mg/day [55]. The current recommendation of vitamin B6 that can be safely taken in pregnancy should not exceed 200 mg/day [20,21,55].

Lastly, the use of acupuncture and/or acupressure may be beneficial as complementary therapies in reducing CINV [58,59]. In a 2008 review, 4 of 7 studies found acupressure to be an effective treatment [59]. Acupuncture-point stimulation, specifically electro-acupuncture and needle point stimulation, has been shown to significantly reduce acute CINV symptoms. Manual stimulation has been reported to have no effect and neither type was reported to reduce delayed CINV [60]. The safety of acupressure or acupuncture at acupoint P6 has been reported with varying degrees of effectiveness in pregnancy-induced nausea and vomiting [44,61,62].

In summary, these nonpharmacological treatments such as vitamin B6, ginger, acupuncture, or acupressure may be beneficial when used concurrently with other antiemetic therapies in reducing CINV in pregnant women.

References

1. Pereg D, Koren G, Lishner M. Cancer in pregnancy: gaps, challenges and solutions. *Cancer Treat Rev.* 2008;**34**:302–12.

2. Cardonick E, Usmani A, Ghaffar S. Perinatal outcomes of a pregnancy complicated by cancer, including neonatal follow-up after in utero exposure to chemotherapy: results of an international registry. *Am J Clin Oncol.* 2010;**33**:221–8.

3. Lohr L. Chemotherapy-induced nausea and vomiting. *Cancer J.* 2008;**14**:85–93.

4. Navari RM. Antiemetic control: toward a new standard of care for emetogenic chemotherapy. *Expert Opin Pharmacother.* 2009;**10**:629–44.

5. Feeney K, Cain M, Nowak AK. Chemotherapy induced nausea and vomiting – prevention and treatment. *Aust Fam Physician.* 2007;**36**:702–6.

6. Hawkins R, Grunberg S. Chemotherapy-induced nausea and vomiting: challenges and opportunities for improved patient outcomes. *Clin J Oncol Nurs.* 2009;**13**:54–64.

7. Wickham R. Best practice management of CINV in oncology patients: II. Antiemetic guidelines and rationale for use. *J Support Oncol.* 2010;**8**(2 suppl 1):10–5.

8. Booth CM, Clemons M, Dranitsaris G, et al. Chemotherapy-induced nausea and vomiting in breast cancer patients: a prospective observational study. *J Support Oncol.* 2007;**5**:374–80.

9. Ettinger DS, Bierman PJ, Bradbury B, et al. Antiemesis: clinical practice guidelines in oncology. *J Natl Compr Canc Netw.* 2007;**5**:12–33.

10. Jordan K, Sippel C, Schmoll HJ. Guidelines for antiemetic treatment of chemotherapy-induced nausea and vomiting: past, present, and future recommendations. *Oncologist.* 2007;**12**:1143–50.

11. Mahesh R, Perumal RV, Pandi PV. Cancer chemotherapy-induced nausea and vomiting: role of mediators, development of drugs and treatment methods. *Pharmazie.* 2005;**60**:83–96.

12. Tucker ML, Jackson MR, Scales MD, et al. Ondansetron: pre-clinical safety evaluation. *Eur J Cancer Clin Oncol.* 1989;**25**(Suppl 1): S79–93.

13. Siu SS, Chan MT, Lau TK. Placental transfer of ondansetron during early human pregnancy. *Clin Pharmacokinet.* 2006;**45**:419–23.

14. Guikontes E, Spantideas A, Kiakakis J. Ondansetron and hyperemesis gravidarum. *Lancet.* 1992;**340**:1223.

15. World MJ. Ondansetron and hyperemesis gravidarum. *Lancet.* 1993;**341**:185.

16. Tincello DG, Johnstone MJ. Treatment of hyperemesis gravidarum with the 5-HT3antagonist ondansetron (Zofran). *Postgrad Med J.* 1996; **72**:688–9.

17. Sullivan CA, Johnson CA, Roach H, et al. A pilot study of intravenous ondansetron for hyperemesis gravidarum. *Am J Obstet Gynecol.* 1996;**174**:1565–8.

18. Asker C, Norstedt W, Kallen B. Use of antiemetic drugs during pregnancy in Sweden. *Eur J Clin Pharmacol.* 2005;**61**:899–906.

19. Einarson A, Maltepe C, Navioz Y, et al. The safety of ondansetron for nausea and vomiting of pregnancy: a prospective comparative study. *Br J Obstet Gynaecol.* 2004;**111**:940–3.

20. American College of Obstetrics and Gynecology. ACOG practice bulletin: nausea and vomiting of pregnancy. *Obstet Gynecol.* 2004;**103**:803–14.

21. Einarson A, Maltepe C, Boskovic R, Koren G. Treatment of nausea and vomiting in pregnancy: an updated algorithm. *Can Fam Physician.* 2007;**53**:2109–11.

22. Baldwin JA, Caton FD, Davidson EJ, et al. Toxicity study of granisetron hydrochloride: reproduction studies in rats by oral administration. *Yakuri to Chiryo.* 1993;**21**:1753–69.

23. Merimsky O, Le Chevalier T, Missenard G, et al. Management of cancer in pregnancy: a case of Ewing's sarcoma of the pelvis in the third trimester. *Ann Oncol.* 1999;**10**:345–50.

24. National Comprehensive Cancer Network. Antiemesis. *National Comprehensive Cancer Network.* Jenkintown, PA. 2006. Available from: http://www.nccn.org/professionals/physician_gls/PDF/antiemesis.pdf

25. DeMulder PHM, Seynaeve C, Vermorker JB, et al. Ondansetron compared with high-dose metoclopramide in prophylaxis of acute and delayed cisplatin-induced nausea and vomiting:multicenter, randomized, double-blind, crossover study. *Ann Intern Med* 1990;**113**:834–40.

26. Briggs GG, Freeman RK, Yaffe SJ. *Drugs in pregnancy and lactation.* 8th ed. Lippincott, Baltimore, MD: Williams and Wilkins; 2008.

27. Watanabe N, Iwanami K, Nakahara N. Teratogenicity of metoclopramide. *Jpn J Pharmacy Chem.* 1968;**39**:92–106.

28. Gill SK, Einarson A. The safety of drugs for the treatment of nausea and vomiting of pregnancy. *Expert Opin Drug Saf.* 2007;**6**:685–94.

29. Harrington RA, Hamilton CW, Brogden RN, et al. Metoclopramide: an update review of its pharmacological properties and clinical use. *Drugs.* 1983;**25**:451–94.

30. Matok I, Gorodischer R, Koren G, et al. The safety of metoclopramide use in the first trimester of pregnancy. *N Engl J Med.* 2009;**360**:2528–35.

31. Fainstat T. Cortisone-induced congenital cleft palate in rabbits. *Endocrinology* 1954;**55**:502–8.

32. Jacobson SJ, Pastuszak A, Koren G. Effects of prenatal exposure to prednisone: a prospective study. *Pediatr Res.* 1997;**41** (Pt 2):348.

33. Richards ID. A retrospective enquiry into possible teratogenic effects of drugs in pregnancy. *Adv Exp Med Biol.* 1972;**27**:441–55.

34. Park-Wyllie L, Mazzotta P, Pastuszak A, et al. Birth defects after maternal exposure to corticosteroids: prospective cohort study and meta-analysis of epidemiological studies. *Teratology.* 2000;**62**:385–92.

35. Carmichael SL, Shaw GM, Ma C, et al. Maternal corticosteroid use and orofacial clefts. *Am J Obstet Gynecol.* 2007;**197**:585. e1–7; discussion 683–4, e1–7.

36. Laskin CA, Bombardier C, Hannah ME, et al. Prednisone and aspirin in women with autoantibodies and unexplained recurrent fetal loss. *N Engl J Med.* 1997;**337**:148–53.

37. Mossey PA, Little J, Munger RG, Dixon MJ, Shaw WC. Cleft lip and palate. *Lancet.* 2009;**374**:1773–85.

38. Magee L, Mazzotta P, Koren G. Evidence-based view of safety and effectiveness of pharmacological therapy for nausea and vomiting of pregnancy (NVP). *Am J Obstet Gynecol.* 2002;**186**: S256–61.

39. Moser J, Caldwell J, Rhule F. No more than necessary: safety and efficacy of low-dose promethazine. *Ann Pharmacother.* 2006;**40**:45–8.

40. Rosen R. Management of chemotherapy-induced nausea and vomiting. *J Pharm Pract.* 2002;**15**:32–41.

41. Dolovich LR, Addis A, Vaillancourt JM, et al. Benzodiazepine use in pregnancy and major malformations or oral cleft: meta-analysis of cohort and case-control studies. *BMJ.* 1998;**317**:839–43.

42. Ornoy A, Arnon J, Shechtman S, et al. Is benzodiazepine use during pregnancy really teratogenic? *Reprod Toxicol.* 1998;**12**:511–5.

43. Wikner BN, Stiller CO, Bergman U, et al. Use of benzodiazepines and benzodiazepine receptor agonists during pregnancy: neonatal outcome and congenital malformations. *Pharmacoepidemiol Drug Saf.* 2007;**16**:1203–10.

44. Ebrahimi, N, Maltepe C, Einarson A. Optimal management of nausea and vomiting of pregnancy. *Int J Womens Health.* 2010;**2**:241–8.

45. White B. Ginger: an overview. *Am Fam Physician.* 2007;**75**:1689–91.

46. Zick S, Ruffin M, Lee J, et al. Phase II trial of encapsulated ginger as a treatment for chemotherapy-induced nausea and vomiting. *Support Care Cancer.* 2009;**17**:563–72.

47. Pillai A, Karma K, Gupta Y, Bakhshi S. Anti-emetic effect of ginger powder versus placebo as an add-on therapy in children and young adults receiving high emetogenic chemotherapy. *Pediatr Blood Cancer.* 2010;**56**:234–8.

48. Ryan JL, Heckler C, Sakhil SR, et al. Ginger for chemotherapy-related nausea in cancer patients: a URCC CCOP randomized, double-blind, placebo-controlled clinical

trial of 644 cancer patients. *J Clin Oncol.* 2009;**27**:(suppl; abstr 9511).

49. Borrelli F, Capasso R, Aviello G, et al. Effectiveness and safety of ginger in the treatment of pregnancy-induced nausea and vomiting. *Obstet Gynecol.* 2005;**105**:849–56.

50. Ozgoli G, Goli M, Simbar M. Effects of ginger capsules on pregnancy, nausea and vomiting. *J Altern Complement Med.* 2009;**15**:243–6.

51. Smith C, Crowther C, Willson K, et al. A randomized controlled trial of ginger to treat nausea and vomiting in pregnancy. *Obstet Gynecol.* 2004;**103**:639–45.

52. Chittumma P, Kaewkiattikun P, Wiriyasiriwach B. Comparison of the effectiveness of ginger and vitamin B6 for treatment of nausea and vomiting in early pregnancy: a randomized double-blind controlled trial. *J Med Assoc Thai.* 2007;**90**:15–20.

53. Ensiyeh J, Sakineh MA. Comparing ginger and vitamin B6 for the treatment of nausea and vomiting in pregnancy: a randomized controlled trial. *Midwifery.* 2009;**25**:649–53.

54. You Q, Yu H, Wu D, et al. Vitamin B6 points PC6 injection during acupuncture can relieve nausea and vomiting in patients with ovarian cancer. *Int J Gynecol Cancer.* 2009; **19**:567–71.

55. Shrim R, Boskovic C, Maltepe C, et al. Pregnancy outcome following use of large doses of vitamin B6 in the first trimester. *J Obstet Gynaecol.* 2006; **26**:749–51.

56. Sahakian V, Rouse D, Sipes S, et al. Vitamin B6 is effective therapy for nausea and vomiting of pregnancy: a randomized, double-blind placebo-controlled study. *Obstet Gynecol.* 1991;**78**:33–6.

57. Vutyavanich T, Wongtra-ngan S, Ruangsri R. Pyridoxine for nausea and vomiting of pregnancy: a randomized, double-blind, placebo controlled trial. *Am J Obstet Gynecol.* 1995;**173**:881–4.

58. Ma L. Acupuncture as a complementary therapy in chemotherapy-induced nausea and vomiting. *Proc (Bayl Univ Med Cent)*. 2009;**22**:138–41.

59. Lee J, Dodd M, Dibble S, Abrams D. Review of acupressure studies for chemotherapy-induced nausea and vomiting control. *J Pain Symptom Manage*. 2008;**36**:529–44.

60. Konno R. Cochrane review summary for Cancer nursing: acupuncture-point stimulation for chemotherapy-induced nausea or vomiting. *Cancer Nurs*. 2010;**33**:479–80.

61. Heazell A, Thorneycroft J, Walton V, Etherington I. Acupressure for the in-patient treatment of nausea and vomiting in early pregnancy: a randomized control trial. *Am J Obstet Gynecol*. 2006;**194**:815–20.

62. Jamigorn M, Phupong V. Acupressure and vitamin B6 to relieve nausea and vomiting in pregnancy: a randomized study. *Arch Gynecol Obstet*. 2007;**276**:245–9.

Chapter 19

Fertility considerations and methods of fertility preservation in patients undergoing treatment for cancer

Avi Leader

Introduction

When treating young patients with cancer, one is faced with the task of prolonging survival while limiting toxicity. Even when confronted with life-threatening illness, patients understandably place emphasis on fertility preservation. This is compounded with the fact that a substantial proportion of patients with certain malignancies, such as testicular cancer (TC), acute lymphoblastic leukemia (ALL), and Hodgkin's lymphoma (HL) have pretreatment reproductive potential. This chapter reviews the main effects of cancer treatment on fertility and presents the contemporary approach to fertility preservation. Some aspects of this chapter have been previously reviewed [1–3].

Effect of cancer on pretreatment fertility

The cancer itself may cause impaired fertility, before any gonadotoxic treatment [4]. This effect is mainly documented in males with HL and TC.

There is a significant prevalence of impaired spermatogenesis among patients with testicular germ cell cancers, before treatment [5]. Pretreatment azoospermia has been demonstrated in approximately one quarter of these patients, while another quarter has oligospermia [6].

There is also consistent evidence that only approximately 30% of male HL patients have normal pretreatment sperm samples, while the remainder have varying degrees of dyspermia [7]. There are conflicting reports on the effect of disease stage on sperm quality. A similar phenomenon has been shown in non-Hodgkin's lymphoma (NHL) and other types of cancer, but is supported by less evidence than in HL and TC.

There are several theories on the mechanism of impaired spermatogenesis in cancer. Growth factors, such as β-human chorionic gonadotrophin, produced by some testicular cancers have a detrimental effect on spermatogenesis. In HL and TC pro-inflammatory cytokines, systemic symptoms, such as fever and malnutrition, have all been suggested as possible contributors toward infertility, although these associations are not evidence-based.

Effect of cancer treatment regimens on fertility

In 2008, the practice committee of the American Society for Reproductive Medicine defined infertility as the failure to conceive after one year or more of regular intercourse without taking contraceptive measures.

Cancer in Pregnancy and Lactation: The Motherisk Guide ed. Gideon Koren and Michael Lishner.
Published by Cambridge University Press. © Cambridge University Press 2011.

There are several mechanisms of treatment-induced fertility impairment: primary hypogonadism caused by testicular or ovarian damage as a result of cytotoxic treatment or radiotherapy; secondary hypogonadism due to pituitary or hypothalamic dysfunction after cranial irradiation; structural damage to the uterus or ovaries caused by pelvic irradiation or surgery; damage to pelvic nerves after surgery or irradiation. Depression related to the diagnosis of cancer may also negatively affect the chances of parenting a child. Albeit beyond the scope of our chapter, it is important to note that treatment-related gonadotoxicity may increase the long-term risk of developing other significant health problems, in addition to fertility impairment. For example, both sexes may suffer from osteoporosis, insulin resistance, altered sexual function, and decreased energy, whereas females may also experience symptoms of premature menopause.

Evaluating fertility reserve

Semen analysis is the most reliable noninvasive test for assessing fertility in men. Sperm count should be measured before treatment and re-evaluated 3 months after its completion. In women, acute ovarian failure may occur during or shortly after cancer treatment. In some cases menstrual cycles may resume within months or years; however, resumption of menstrual periods does not necessarily indicate fertility potential. Alternatively, cancer treatment may result in premature ovarian failure (POF), which is defined as amenorrhea for more than 6 months with elevated follicular stimulating hormone (FSH) levels, in women under the age of 40. POF may occur later on in life after resumption of normal menstruation or as a direct continuation of acute ovarian failure.

These are desirable end-points in clinical trials, however, are not always feasible in respect to patient consent and length of follow-up required. Thus, many studies in the field of fertility after cancer treatment rely upon surrogate markers of fertility. One such marker of infertility is elevated FSH, which has debatable reliability in men. A decreased level of Inhibin B, which is produced by Sertoli cells, is another marker of impaired spermatogenesis in patients receiving chemotherapy. Anti-Müllerian hormone (AMH) is considered a sensitive marker of ovarian reserve after chemotherapy, and decreased AMH levels are indicative of decreased reserve. Moreover decreased levels of Inhibin B and elevated FSH are also suggestive of impaired ovarian reserve.

These indirect markers are especially useful in assessing fertility potential before and after cancer treatment in subjects who are prepubertal at the time of treatment and assessment. Baseline measurement of these hormones should be considered. It is also important to note that resumption of menstrual cycles after cancer treatment may still result in POF later in life.

Lastly, regardless of the above-mentioned effort to assess the gonadotoxic effects of cancer treatment, the most important outcome for patients is the ability to father or give birth to a child. Some large trials, mainly observational and retrospective, have provided data on this end-point. However, these data must be interpreted with caution as rates of post-treatment parenthood may be affected by the percentage of patients attempting parenthood. This in turn depends upon interrelated factors such as age, marital status, the number of children before treatment, the patient's perception of fertility potential and the desire to become a parent. In addition, this end-point does not always take into account fertility issues experienced by the patient's partner and the time required achieving parenthood.

General principles

Chemotherapy-induced gonadal failure depends on the type of chemotherapy used. Alkylating agents, especially cyclophosphamide and procarbazine, are the main causes of gonadal dysfunction in men and women [8]. Higher cumulative doses of these agents correlate with a higher risk of treatment-related gonadal failure, although there is no clear cut-off dose above which gonadal damage is inflicted. In addition, males are more susceptible to gonadal damage after chemotherapy incorporating alkylating agents and pelvic radiation than women. Although alkylating agents are the main culprits in chemotherapy-induced gonadal damage, cisplatin is another agent with damaging effects on germinal epithelium [5]. This agent seems to have a less harmful effect than alkylating agents but there is no clear cut-off dose for gonadal damage, although several small studies have proposed a threshold dose of 400–600mg/m^2.

In women receiving chemotherapy, increasing age at first treatment is associated with the risk of POF. This can be explained by a natural age-related decline in oocyte reserve [9]. No such association between age at treatment and incidence of post-treatment fertility impairment has been shown in men. Patients initially rendered azoospermic by cancer treatment may regain gonadal function after a period of months to years.

Pelvic and abdominal irradiation also affects fertility and the combination of radiation with chemotherapy regimens containing alkylating agents has a further harmful effect on gonadal function. Inferior radiation fields carry a higher risk of gonadal dysfunction. Higher cumulative doses of radiation are also associated with more severe gonadal dysfunction. Cumulative testicular doses of 2–3 Gy cause prolonged and often irreversible azoospermia, whereas azoospermia is usually not observed with doses below 0.7 Gy. High-dose pelvic radiation may also contribute to erectile dysfunction [2]. The ovaries are less sensitive to radiation than the testes, although they are also subject to significant damage, especially with direct radiation [9]. The threshold for ovarian radiation injury is approximately 4 Gy. Age at treatment is reversely correlated with the radiation dose needed to cause POF. In addition, high-dose cranial radiation as part of treatment for childhood malignancies is associated with impaired fertility [10].

A large retrospective study of postpubertal cancer patients, demonstrated a 30% and 50% reduction in 10-year postdiagnosis reproduction rates in men and women respectively, compared with the general population. In this study postcancer fertility was positively affected by male sex, younger age, and less children at diagnosis, and was also influenced by the type and extent of the malignancy [11].

Cancer treatment in children results in a favorable probability of survival [3] and carries similar risk factors for fertility impairment as in adults [12]. A large cohort study of 5 year survivors of childhood cancer demonstrated decreased rates of pregnancy in comparison with a sibling cohort [13,14]. Female survivors who received an ovarian/uterine radiation dose greater than 5 Gy, a hypothalamic/pituitary dose $\geq$ 30 Gy, a higher cumulative dose of alkylating agents, or treatment with lomustine or cyclophosphamide were less likely to ever have been pregnant than survivors not receiving such treatment [13]. Factors that resulted in a decreased probability of male survivors siring a child were testicular radiation doses above 7.5 Gy, higher cumulative doses of alkylating agents, and use of cyclophosphamide or procarbazine [14].

There are, however, several unique aspects of treatment-induced fertility impairment among childhood survivors of cancer treatment. First, among boys receiving cancer treatment, there is no evidence that a prepubertal state prevents gonadal damage, and rates of gonadal dysfunction are similar to those in adult males [15]. Younger girls, however, are more likely to maintain normal menses than older girls, which is similar to the age-related associations seen in adult women [16]. Nevertheless, there is still a notable risk of POF later in life. Another important concern is an increased risk of preterm birth, low weight birth or being small for gestational age among offspring of female survivors of childhood cancers. Encouragingly, recent data have demonstrated no increase in genetic disease among children of survivors of childhood cancer [12]. Lastly, because of the lack of satisfactory techniques for preserving fertility among prepubertal patients, efforts should be made to limit the use of gonadotoxic agents in this population.

Disease-specific issues

Lymphoma

The gradual shift of front-line treatment regimens in HL from those containing high doses of alkylating agents, such as MOPP (mechlorethamine, vincristine, prednisone, procarbazine) to regimens devoid of alkylating agents, such as ABVD (doxorubicin, bleomycin, vinblastine, and dacarbazine) affords further insight on the gonadotoxic effect of alkylating agents. Alkylating agent-based treatment results in gonadal dysfunction in approximately 90% of males and premature menopause in around 50% of females surviving HL, whereas ABVD rarely causes permanent azoospermia and poses no documented risk of POF [9,17,18]. Similar rates of gonadal dysfunction occur with the contemporary standard or escalated dose BEACOPP protocol (bleomycin, etoposide, doxorubicin, cyclophosphamide, vincristine, procarbazine, and prednisone) [19]. Male survivors of childhood HL have a comparable 80%–90% incidence of gonadal dysfunction after treatment with alkylating agents but rarely have impaired fertility after ABVD [20]. Lower rates are seen among girls receiving treatment for HL.

It is difficult to quantify the chances of parenthood after treatment for HL with a specific protocol, although treatment with ABVD appears to have little effect on fertility. In one study, 63% of men attempting parenthood after treatment for HL, with various regimens, were successful in fathering a child and 75% of women gave birth without the use of assisted reproductive techniques [21].

There are few data on protocol-specific risks of infertility after treatment for NHL, almost all of which relate to women. Several small studies have shown gonadal dysfunction in less than 15% of women treated with CHOP-based regimens for NHL [22].

Acute leukemia

One of the main factors affecting rates of gonadal dysfunction in leukemia survivors is whether the treatment regimens include hematopoietic stem cell transplantation (HSCT), which poses a significant threat to fertility. On the other hand, standard chemotherapy regimens used to treat ALL and acute myeloid leukemia (AML) have low gonadotoxic potential, in both children and adults [10,23]. Especially in AML, regimens devoid of alkylating agents are commonly used; therefore, treatment-induced infertility is relatively infrequent [24].

The harmful effect of HSCT on gonadal function is a result of pretransplant conditioning, which usually incorporates total body irradiation (TBI), alkylating agents, or both.

TBI-based regimens have a more profound effect on fertility and post-transplant parenthood than conditioning based only on chemotherapy [24–26]. Moreover, both modalities have a dose-related effect on fertility [26]. There is limited but promising evidence that reduced intensity conditioning causes lower rates of POF than myeloablative conditioning regimens [27]. However, there is no evidence that non-myeloablative conditioning spares gonadal function. The effect of both types of conditioning on fertility is currently under investigation. Furthermore, graft versus host disease may play a minor role in post-transplant fertility impairment.

All male survivors of allogeneic HSCT with myeloablative conditioning have some degree of impaired spermatogenesis, whereas at least 70% have azoospermia [25]. This treatment causes comparable rates of gonadal dysfunction in women, who experience POF in 70% to 100% of cases [27]. Recovery of spermatogenesis and menstrual cycles, although rare, may occur years after transplant. Despite a similar incidence of POF and azoospermia, females experience post-transplant parenthood less frequently than men [26], which could be explained by differences in assisted reproductive techniques.

Post-transplant parenthood is uncommon. One retrospective cohort demonstrated a prevalence of 3% among women and 8% in men who survived allogeneic or autologous HSCT [26]. Lower rates of post-transplant parenthood have been shown in men over the age of 30 years at the time of transplant, although conflicting data exist [26]. The risk of gonadal injury in women increases with age at transplant. There are inadequate data on fertility among survivors of childhood HSCT.

Finally, some researchers have reported an increased risk of miscarriage, stillbirth, low weight for gestational age, preterm births, and cesarean sections in pregnant HSCT survivors, although others have shown no such association [26,28,29]. On the other hand, pregnancies conceived spontaneously by male HSCT survivors do not carry an increased risk of miscarriage or stillbirth [26,28,29]. Offspring of male and female survivors of HSCT have a similar proportion of congenital abnormalities as the general population [26,29].

The evidence on fertility impairment after HSCT has several shortcomings: There is a confounding effect of various doses of pretreatment chemotherapy before transplant conditioning; most studies do not clearly differentiate between allogeneic and autologous transplants; no direct comparisons are made between myeloablative, reduced intensity, and non-myeloablative conditioning regimens.

Breast cancer

Breast cancer has the highest incidence among all cancers in young women. The potential effect of treatment on fertility depends on the treatment strategy, which is determined by the disease stage and biologic features of the tumor. The initial treatment for early-stage breast cancer may only entail surgery and irradiation. Postsurgical radiation therapy for breast cancer is typically not associated with significant ovarian toxicity, although internal scatter radiation may still reach the ovaries. Therefore pregnancy or harvesting of oocytes or gonadal tissue should be delayed until after radiation treatment is completed [3]. After initial surgical and radiation treatment, depending on tumor biology, early stage breast cancer patients may require treatment with antiestrogen treatment for at least 5 years, which may be delayed to allow for pregnancy [3]. These patients, provided they receive no chemotherapy, have a minimal risk of impaired fertility.

Patients with a more advanced stage of disease or whose tumor is hormone receptor-negative, require chemotherapy. Chemotherapeutic regimens routinely include the alkylating agent cyclophosphamide, which poses a significant threat to fertility. In contrast, anthracyclines have no clear long-term effect on fertility. Treatment with an anthracycline-based regimen, such as doxorubicin and cyclophosphamide (AC), uses an anthracycline along with a lower dose of the alkylating agent, and thus is associated with a lower risk of POF than older protocols [30]. There are, however, conflicting reports on the effect of taxanes on ovarian function [31,32]. In addition, infertility is also caused by bilateral oophorectomy, which is sometimes advised for young women with hormone receptor-positive disease or as a risk reduction method for carriers BRCA1/2 gene mutations [31].

There is a lack of prospective studies evaluating the effect of contemporary chemotherapeutic regimens on future fertility in this patient population. Adjuvant chemotherapy does not appear to affect the outcome of pregnancy in patients conceiving at least 6 months after diagnosis. Moreover, there is no evidence of an increased incidence of stillbirth, premature birth or congenital malformations in pregnancies conceived by survivors of breast cancer [31]. There is also no hard evidence that subsequent pregnancy has a detrimental effect on survival [31].

Gynecological malignancies

Gynecological malignancies that require surgical intervention can be managed conservatively whenever the type of disease and the stage permit. Patients with stage Ia1, Ia2, and to a lesser extent Ib1 cervical cancer are potentially eligible for conservative fertility-sparing surgery. In a suitable patient, radical hysterectomy can be replaced by fertility-sparing procedures such as excisional cone biopsy or radical vaginal trachelectomy with a staging laparoscopic pelvic lymphadenectomy. Radical abdominal trachelectomy may be an option for patients with more extensive disease. Pregnancies after these procedures carry a higher risk of premature delivery and miscarriage [33].

Hysterectomy may also be avoided in patients with well-differentiated stage Ia endometrial adenocarcinoma, where hormonal therapy with progestagens is a possible alternative. One concern with this approach is uncertainty over the actual disease stage in the absence of a hysterectomy specimen. The extent of disease and, crucially, myometrial invasion may be detected in most but not all cases, by various imaging modalities [33].

Depending on the extent of disease and histological type, appropriate patients with ovarian cancer can be surgically managed in a conservative manner with preservation of the uterus and normal contralateral ovary without compromising survival [34]. Stage Ia epithelial ovarian cancer requires surgery alone, whereas stage II and III disease may necessitate adjuvant chemotherapy [33]. There are few data available on the effects of chemotherapy on fertility in women with ovarian cancer. Moreover, parts of the resected ovary or ovarian biopsy can be cryopreserved for future gamete use.

Testicular cancer

Similar to HL, testicular cancer (TC) carries a favorable probability of long-term survival and therefore fertility is one of the main concerns of survivors. Chemotherapy appears to have a more deleterious effect on testicular function than orchidectomy alone, while local radiotherapy is even more detrimental [5]. Cisplatin is the main perpetrator of chemotherapy-induced gonadal damage and cisplatin-based regimens have more gonadotoxic potential than protocols based on carboplatin [6]. Moreover, erectile dysfunction may occur after certain treatment regimens and may also affect post-treatment fatherhood rates [35]. The type of surgical procedure used can affect fertility in several ways by means of nerve damage by causing decreased seminal fluid volume, retrograde ejaculation, disturbed emission, or absence of ejaculation. Non nerve-sparing retroperitoneal lymph node dissection is most damaging to fertility due to the above reasons, and patients have a low probability of achieving fatherhood without assisted reproductive techniques. This damage may be avoided by nerve-sparing surgery whenever feasible [36].

A cohort study of 170 patients with testicular germ cell cancer receiving chemotherapeutic regimens based on either carboplatin or cisplatin demonstrated azoospermia in 32% and oligospermia in a further 25% of patients. In contrast, only approximately one third of patients who had normal sperm counts before treatment had impaired spermatogenesis at a median of 30 months after chemotherapy [6]. Pregnancy rates of 67% were achieved by survivors of TC attempting fatherhood after orchidectomy ± chemotherapy or radiotherapy [35]. Similar rates have been demonstrated in other studies and are affected by the type of treatment employed [36].

Effect of tyrosine kinase inhibitors and monoclonal antibodies on fertility

Initial animal data suggested impaired spermatogenesis under imatinib treatment, but this has not been supported by clinical experience in humans [37]. Imatinib is also not believed to affect fertility in women, although primary ovarian insufficiency has been reported after imatinib treatment [38]. Several successful pregnancies after female and male use of second-generation tyrosine kinase inhibitors have recently been reported; however, there is still limited experience with these drugs [39]. Importantly, these data are inadequate and based on small studies and case reports, and should be interpreted with caution. Despite significant clinical experience with monoclonal antibodies such as rituximab in hematological malignancies, little is known of their effect on gonadal function.

Methods of fertility preservation

Fertility preservation is an integral component of contemporary treatment plans for patients with cancer. Thus, dialog between the hematologist or oncologist and a fertility preservation expert is of paramount importance, as is counseling patients on options for fertility preservation and fertility risks posed by cancer treatment [40]. Potential benefits of preservation methods should be weighed up against long-term risks. In 2006, Lee *et al.* published general recommendations for fertility preservation in cancer patients, while other disease-specific general management guidelines also relate to fertility preservation [40,41].

The advances in fertility preservation are accompanied by several ethical and legal issues that are especially intricate in children and adolescents. There are several notable aspects: obtaining valid consent for performing preservation procedures; the effect on the patient's expectations of survival and procreation; how to deal with stored reproductive material in the case of the patient's death; the importance of acting in the patient's best interest. The Human Fertilization and Embryology Act (HFEA, 1990) covers only some of the legal aspects that arise during contemporary and investigative fertility preservation. The legal and ethical issues pertaining to tissue harvesting, storage, and subsequent fertilization in children differ between gametes and gonadal tissue and have been discussed in several review articles [1,42,43]. Guidelines and recommendations are needed to ensure adequate regulation of fertility preservation.

Naturally methods of fertility preservation differ between male and females and are, therefore, discussed separately. Furthermore, it is important to distinguish between established, proven methods and those under investigation and to make the patient aware of these differences.

Males
Proven methods

Pubertal males undergoing treatment for cancer should be offered semen cryopreservation and storage before treatment, irrespective of sperm quality and motility, which may be poor due to the effects of malignancy. In the latter case, high success rates can be achieved using intracytoplasmic sperm injection (ICSI) [44]. Semen samples are obtained by masturbation but if necessary may also be attained by penile vibratory stimulation, electro-ejaculation, testicular fine needle aspiration (TEFNA), or testicular tissue aspiration (TESE). Another established technique is external lead shielding of the testes during radiation therapy.

Methods under investigation

There is a lack of proven methods for preserving fertility in prepubertal boys. Therefore different techniques of cryopreserving, thawing, and subsequently transplanting testicular tissue containing spermatogonial stem cells are being explored. There are abundant promising data from animal research, but these techniques are still not viable in humans [45]. Furthermore, suppression of testosterone by gonadotropin releasing hormone (GnRH) analogs has been hypothesized to protect testicular function in patients undergoing gonadotoxic treatment. This suppression does not protect the stem cells; therefore, the mechanism of potential gonado-protection is unclear. The vast majority of clinical trials have shown no protective effect of hormone suppression on male gonadal function [46].

Females
Proven methods

In vitro fertilization (IVF) with cryopreserved embryos is the most established method of female fertility preservation. IVF indicated for fertility preservation achieves similar results as IVF used for male factor infertility, and boasts several decades of experience. There are several important drawbacks to this technique: (1) depending on the timing of the patient's menstrual cycle, the preservation process may enforce treatment delay of between 2 and 6 weeks, which may not be acceptable in urgent or emergent cancer cases; (2) oocyte harvesting is only feasible in pubertal patients; (3) patients without sperm from a partner must use donor sperm to fertilize the oocyte; (4) the reluctance to use a sperm donor or ethical and religious considerations may preclude the use of this technique. The latter 2 limitations may be circumvented by a new option of oocyte vitrification, which may achieve fertilization and pregnancy rates which are comparable to those attained with fresh oocytes [47].

Several types of cancer require radiation therapy that may include the ovaries in the field of radiation. External lead shielding may be used to protect the ovaries during irradiation.

There are also several surgical techniques of ovarian transposition, which may limit or avoid ovarian radiation damage by displacing the ovaries from the radiation field. In some instances, the ovaries may maintain their natural connection with the Fallopian tubes and uterus, thus enabling spontaneous pregnancy. In other cases, subsequent surgical repositioning or IVF may be required.

Methods under investigation

The most promising technique under investigation is ovarian tissue cryopreservation and subsequent transplantation [48]. First, ovarian cortex biopsy or oophorectomy is performed during laparotomy or laparoscopy, and may be combined with other surgical procedures, such as tumor resection, if necessary. Moreover, patients may benefit from concurrent aspiration of follicles. Thereafter, the ovarian cortex is cryopreserved using slow-freezing or vitrification protocols. Subsequently, after cancer remission, the thawed ovarian tissue is auto-transplanted, which may result not only in restoration of fertility but also in resumption of normal hormonal production. Although over a dozen live births have resulted from this procedure, this technique is still not fully established, and the majority of data is on young adults. This technique may be offered to prepubertal girls [49] or pubertal women who cannot be afforded the delay in cancer treatment needed to harvest oocytes for embryo cryopreservation. Moreover, no hormonal stimulation is required, which is advantageous especially in hormone receptor-positive breast cancer. The major concern of this method is reimplantation of malignancy through ovarian grafts contaminated with malignant cells, which has been documented in patients with hematological malignancies [50]. This risk may also exist in other types of cancer. As a result, several methods of reducing this risk are being explored, such as preoperative imaging, histological analysis with immunohistochemical staining, and polymerase chain reaction amplification [51].

The process of embryo or oocyte cryopreservation requires hormonal stimulation of the ovaries, which may be contraindicated in patients with estrogen and progesterone receptor-positive breast cancer. Induction of ovulation incorporating the selective estrogen-receptor modulator tamoxifen or aromatase inhibitors, with or without low-dose FSH, is possibly a safe alternative, but requires further study [31,52]. Another emerging option for such patients is the aspiration of follicles without exposure to exogenous hormone stimulation, but the success rate is low [3].

A different investigational option is treatment with GnRH analogs during chemotherapy, which is hypothesized to protect ovarian follicles by decreasing follicular recruitment and reducing accelerated atresia. There are conflicting results on the efficacy of this treatment and few studies in humans have supported a protective effect of GnRH administration [53]. The efficacy and safety of this treatment is yet to be established in large prospective randomized trials. GnRH analogs have an added value of inducing a hypogonadotrophic state that prevents the uterine bleeding associated with myelosuppression in patients with hematological malignancies.

Planning fertility preservation

If cancer treatment is urgently indicated, no fertility preservation should be offered. If surgery is part of cancer treatment, procedures that conserve fertility should be used when possible. This is particularly relevant in patients with gynecological malignancies and TC. Testicular and ovarian shielding should be used in all patients receiving abdominal or pelvic irradiation, whereas ovarian transposition is an additional proven option. Because of the safety of this technique, all pubertal males undergoing cancer treatment should provide a sperm sample for cryopreservation, whether by masturbation, testicular sperm aspiration, or electro-ejaculation. Pubertal women who are willing or able to use sperm from a partner or donor may undergo the process of embryo cryopreservation. Otherwise, pubertal women should be offered oocyte cryopreservation. In addition GnRH agonists should be offered to all women receiving chemotherapy, because of the added value of preventing uterine bleeding. Prepubertal girls can be offered the investigational method of ovarian tissue cryopreservation, because no proven alternatives exist. This option can also be offered to pubertal women who cannot be afforded the 2 to 6 weeks needed for embryo or oocyte cryopreservation. There are no satisfactory methods of fertility preservation for prepubertal boys.

Because oocyte or embryo cryopreservation requires ovarian stimulation, it is not without risks. Moreover, ovarian cryopreservation is a surgical procedure. Therefore, when choosing one of these methods, the probability of treatment-induced fertility impairment should be weighed up against the potential side effects and efficacy of fertility preservation.

References

1. Brougham MF, Wallace WH. Subfertility in children and young people treated for solid and haematological malignancies. *Br J Haematol.* 2005;**131**:143–55.

2. Nakayama K, Milbourne A, Schover LR, Champlin RE, Ueno NT. Gonadal failure after treatment of hematologic malignancies: from recognition to management for health-care providers. *Nat Clin Pract Oncol.* 2008;**5**:78–89.

3. Jeruss JS, Woodruff TK. Preservation of Fertility in Patients with Cancer. *N Engl J Med.* 2009;**360**:902–11.

4. van Casteren NJ, Boellaard WP, Romijn JC, Dohle GR. Gonadal dysfunction in male cancer patients before cytotoxic treatment. *Int J Androl.* 2010;**33**:73–9.

5. Howell SJ, Shalet SM. Spermatogenesis after cancer treatment: damage and recovery. *J Natl Cancer Monogr Inst.* 2005;**34**:12–7.

6. Lampe H, Horwich A, Norman A, Nicholls J, Dearnaley DP. Fertility after chemotherapy for testicular germ cell cancers. *J Clin Oncol.* 1997;**15**:239–45.

7. Rueffer U, Breuer K, Josting A, et al. Male gonadal dysfunction in patients with Hodgkin's disease prior to treatment. *Ann Oncol.* 2001;**12**:1307–11.

8. Kiserud CE, Fossa A, Bjøro T, Holte H, Cvancarova M, Fossa SD. Gonadal function in male patients after treatment for malignant lymphomas, with emphasis on chemotherapy. *Br J Cancer.* 2009;**100**: 455–63.

9. De Bruin ML, Huisbrink J, Hauptmann M, et al. Treatment-related risk factors for premature menopause following Hodgkin lymphoma. *Blood.* 2008;**111**:101–8.

10. Byrne J, Fears TR, Mills JL, et al. Fertility of long-term male survivors of acute lymphoblastic leukemia diagnosed during childhood. *Pediatr Blood Cancer.* 2004;**42**:364–72.

11. Cvancarova M, Samuelsen SO, Magelssen H, Fossa SD. Reproduction rates after cancer treatment: experience from the Norwegian radium hospital. *J Clin Oncol.* 2009;**27**:334–43.

12. Green DM, Sklar CA, Boice JD Jr, et al. Ovarian failure and reproductive outcomes after childhood cancer treatment: results from the Childhood Cancer Survivor Study. *J Clin Oncol.* 2009;**27**:2374–81.

13. Green DM, Kawashima T, Stovall M, et al. Fertility of female survivors of childhood cancer: a report from the childhood cancer survivor study. *J Clin Oncol.* 2009;**27**: 2677–85.

14. Green DM, Kawashima T, Stovall M, et al. Fertility of male survivors of childhood cancer: a report from the Childhood Cancer Survivor Study. *J Clin Oncol.* 2010;**28**:332–9.

15. Ben Arush MW, Solt I, Lightman A, Lightman A, LinnS, Kuten A. Male gonadal function in survivors of childhood Hodgkin and non-Hodgkin lymphoma. *Pediatr Hematol Oncol.* 2000;**17**:239–45.

16. Chemaitilly W, Mertens AC, Mitby P, et al. Acute ovarian failure in the childhood cancer survivor study. *J Clin Endocrinol Metab.* 2006;**91**:1723–8.

17. Behringer K, Breuer K, Reineke T, et al. Secondary amenorrhea after Hodgkin's lymphoma is influenced by age at treatment, stage of disease, chemotherapy regimen, and the use of oral contraceptives during therapy: a report from the German Hodgkin's Lymphoma Study Group. *J Clin Oncol.* 2005;**23**:7555–64.

18. van der Kaaij MA, Heutte N, Le Stang N, et al. Gonadal function in males after chemotherapy for early-stage Hodgkin's lymphoma treated in four subsequent trials by the European Organisation for Research and Treatment of Cancer: EORTC Lymphoma Group and the Groupe d'Etude des Lymphomes de l'Adulte. *J Clin Oncol.* 2007;**25**:2825–32.

19. Sieniawski M, Reineke T, Nogova L, et al. Fertility in male patients with advanced Hodgkin lymphoma treated with BEACOPP: a report of the German Hodgkin Study Group (GHSG). *Blood.* 2008;**111**:71–6.

20. van den Berg H, Furstner F, van den Bos C, Behrendt H. Decreasing the number of MOPP courses reduces gonadal damage in survivors of childhood Hodgkin disease. *Pediatr Blood Cancer.* 2004;**42**:210–5.

21. Kiserud CE, Fossa A, Holte H, Fossa SD. Post-treatment parenthood in Hodgkin's lymphoma survivors. *Br J Cancer.* 2007;**96**:1442–9.

22. Elis A, Tevet A, Yerushalmi R, et al. Fertility status among women treated for aggressive non-Hodgkin's lymphoma. *Leuk Lymphoma.* 2006;**47**:623–7.

23. Watson M, Wheatley K, Harrison GA, et al. Severe adverse impact on sexual functioning and fertility of bone marrow transplantation, either allogeneic or autologous, compared with consolidation chemotherapy alone: analysis of the MRC AML 10 trial. *Cancer.* 1999;**86**:1231–9.

24. Leung W, Hudson MM, Strickland DK, et al. Late effects of treatment in survivors of childhood acute myeloid leukemia. *J Clin Oncol.* 2000;**18**:3273–9.

25. Anserini P, Chiodi S, Spinelli S, et al. Semen analysis following allogeneic bone marrow transplantation. Additional data for evidence-based counselling. *Bone Marrow Transplant.* 2002; **30**:447–51.

26. Carter A, Robison LL, Francisco L, et al. Prevalence of conception and pregnancy outcomes after hematopoietic cell transplantation: report from the Bone Marrow Transplant Survivor Study. *Bone Marrow Transplant.* 2006;**37**:1023–9.

27. Cheng YC, Saliba RM, Rondón G, et al. Low prevalence of premature ovarian failure in women given reduced-intensity conditioning regimens for hematopoietic stem-cell transplantation. *Haematologica.* 2005;**90**:1725–6.

28. Sanders JE, Hawley J, Levy W, et al. Pregnancies following high-dose cyclophosphamide with or without high-dose busulfan or total-body irradiation and bone marrow transplantation. *Blood.* 1996;**87**:3045–52.

29. Salooja N, Szydlo RM, Socie G, et al. Pregnancy outcomes after peripheral blood or bone marrow transplantation: a retrospective survey. *Lancet.* 2001; **358**:271–6.

30. Sonmezer M, Oktay K. Fertility preservation in female patients. *Hum Reprod Update.* 2004;**10**:251–66.

31. Hickey M, Peate M, Saunders CM, Friedlander M. Breast cancer in young women and its impact on reproductive function. *Hum Reprod Update.* 2009;**15**:323–39.

32. Pérez-Fidalgo JA, Roselló S, García-Garré E, et al. Incidence of chemotherapy-induced amenorrhea in hormone-sensitive breast cancer patients: the impact of addition of taxanes to anthracycline-based regimens. *Breast Cancer Res Treat.* 2010;**120**:245–51.

33. Farthing A. Conserving fertility in the management of gynaecological cancers. *BJOG*. 2006;**113**:129–34.

34. Gershenson DM. Fertility-sparing surgery for malignancies in women. *J Natl Cancer Inst Monogr*. 2005;**34**:43–7.

35. Huyghe E, Matsuda T, Daudin M, et al. Fertility after testicular cancer treatments: results of a large multicenter study. *Cancer*. 2004;**100**:732–7.

36. Matos E, Skrbinc B, Zakotnik B. Fertility in patients treated for testicular cancer. *J Cancer Surviv*. 2010;**4**:274–8.

37. Hensley M, Ford JM. Imatinib treatment: specific issues related to safety, fertility and pregnancy. *Semin Hematol*. 2003;**40**:21–5.

38. Christopoulos C, Dimakopoulou V, Rotas E. Primary ovarian insufficiency associated with imatinib therapy. *N Engl J Med*. 2008;**358**:1079–80.

39. Cortes J, O'Brien S, Ault P, et al. Pregnancy outcomes among patients with chronic myeloid leukemia treated with dasatinib. *Blood*. 2008;**112**: abstract 3230.

40. Lee SJ, Schover LR, Partridge AH, et al. American Society of Clinical Oncology. Recommendations on fertility preservation in cancer patients. *J Clin Oncol*. 2006;**24**:2917–31.

41. Brusamolino E, Bacigalupo A, Barosi G, et al. Classical Hodgkin's lymphoma in adults: guidelines of the Italian Society of Hematology, the Italian Society of Experimental Hematology, and the Italian Group for Bone Marrow Transplantation on initial work-up, management, and follow-up. *Haematologica*. 2009;**94**: 550–65.

42. Grundy R, Gosden RG, Hewitt M, et al. Fertility preservation for children treated for cancer (1): scientific advances and research dilemmas. *Arch Dis Child*. 2001;**84**:355–9.

43. Grundy R, Larcher V, Gosden RG, et al. Fertility preservation for children treated for cancer (2): ethics of consent for gamete storage and experimentation. *Arch Dis Child*. 2001;**84**:360–2.

44. Hourvitz A, Goldschlag DE, Davis OK, Gosden LV, Palermo GD, Rosenwaks Z. Intracytoplasmic sperm injection (ICSI) using cryopreserved sperm from men with malignant neoplasm yields high pregnancy rates. *Fertil Steril*. 2008; **90**:557–63.

45. Wyns C, Curaba M, Vanabelle B, Van Langendonckt A, Donnez J. Options for fertility preservation in prepubertal boys. *Hum Reprod Update*. 2010;**16**: 312–28.

46. Meistrich ML, Shetty G. Hormonal suppression for fertility preservation in males and females. *Reproduction*. 2008;**136**:691–701.

47. Grifo JA, Noyes N. Delivery rate using cryopreserved oocytes is comparable to conventional in vitro fertilization using fresh oocytes: potential fertility preservation for female cancer patients. *Fertil Steril*. 2010;**93**:391–6.

48. Donnez J, Jadoul P, Squifflet J, et al. Ovarian tissue cryopreservation and transplantation in cancer patients. *Best Pract Res Clin Obstet Gynaecol*. 2010; **24**:87–100.

49. Jadoul P, Dolmans MM, Donnez J. Fertility preservation in girls during childhood: is it feasible, efficient and safe and to whom should it be proposed? *Hum Reprod Update*. 2010;**16**:617–30.

50. Dolmans MM, Marinescu C, Saussoy P, Van Langendonckt A, Amorim C, Donnez J. Reimplantation of cryopreserved ovarian tissue from patients with acute lymphoblastic leukemia is potentially unsafe. *Blood*. 2010;**116**: 2908–14.

51. Meirow D, Hardan I, Dor J, et al. Searching for evidence of disease and malignant cell contamination in ovarian tissue stored from hematologic cancer patients. *Hum Reprod*. 2008;**23**:1007–13.

52. Oktay K, Buyuk E, Libertella N, Akar M, Rosenwaks Z. Fertility preservation in

breast cancer patients: a prospective controlled comparison of ovarian stimulation with tamoxifen and letrozole for embryo cryopreservation. *J Clin Oncol.* 2005;**23**:4347–53.

53. Beck-Fruchter R, Weiss A, Shalev E. GnRH agonist therapy as ovarian protectants in female patients undergoing chemotherapy: a review of the clinical data. *Hum Reprod Update.* 2007;**14**:553–61.

Long-term neurodevelopment of children exposed *in utero* to treatment for maternal cancer

Irena Nulman, Claire Tobias, BA, and Elizabeth Uleryk

Cancer complicates 0.01% of all pregnancies. The management of maternal cancer during pregnancy is challenging and complex, as it creates a conflict between optimal maternal therapy and fetal well-being. A significant body of research has focused on immediate pregnancy outcomes following chemotherapy and/or radiation therapy in pregnancy, demonstrating that both treatment modalities may be associated with increased rates of birth defects. Accordingly, the existing guidelines recommend that treatment for maternal cancer be administered after the first trimester. As the central nervous system (CNS) develops throughout pregnancy, its outcomes must be taken into consideration when treatment guidelines are presented. This report will provide a summary of the available knowledge on children's long-term outcomes to assist women and healthcare professionals in making informed, evidence-based decisions for the management of cancer in pregnancy.

Introduction

Cancer is the second most common cause of death among women during the reproductive years, complicating approximately 1/1,000 pregnancies [1–4]. The occurrence of cancer during gestation is likely to increase with women's tendency to delay child-bearing, concurrent with an increase in the diagnosis attributable to better diagnostic procedures. Malignant conditions during pregnancy are believed to be associated with an increase in poor perinatal and fetal outcomes due to maternal disorder and treatment. Physicians should weigh the benefits of treatment against the risks of fetal exposure. To date, the literature has focused mainly on morphologic observations made very close to the time of delivery and suggests that exposure to antineoplastic medications after the first trimester does not pose an increased teratogenic risk. There is a paucity of data collected on children's long-term neurodevelopment following *in utero* exposure to malignancy and treatment. Because the brain differentiates throughout pregnancy and in early postnatal life, damage may occur even after first-trimester exposure. The possible delayed effects of treatment on a child's neurological, intellectual, and behavioral functioning have been insufficiently evaluated.

Maternal cancer

The undesirable effects of maternal cancer in pregnancy on children's neurodevelopmental outcomes must be elucidated. Metastasis to the placenta and/or fetus is very rare [1,4].

Cancer in Pregnancy and Lactation: The Motherisk Guide ed. Gideon Koren and Michael Lishner.
Published by Cambridge University Press. © Cambridge University Press 2011.

Melanoma is the most frequent of the few malignancies that do metastasize to the placenta and fetus [4]. Live-born children exposed to such malignancies tend to die within a 1-day to 10-month period. Comprehensive reports about physical and mental health of the surviving children are not available. Cancer patients have an increased tendency to undergo febrile illnesses due to infections and/or as a result of the tumor itself. The relationship between hyperthermia, fetal brain development, and the incidence of child cognitive and functional impairment in humans has not been addressed. Human studies do support the hypothesis that maternal fever in early pregnancy may be associated with neural tube defects and microphthalmia [5–12]. Malignancies may also be associated with maternal malnutrition and subsequent adverse neonatal outcome [13–16]. Human data obtained during historical periods of starvation (i.e., during World War II) have shown little or no adverse child effects [17]. Some studies have suggested that severe ketoacidosis, due to dehydration or severe weight loss, may pose an additional risk to the developing fetus [18,19]. Conversely, analysis of military screening examinations of all Dutch males at age 19 failed to demonstrate any difference in IQ score between boys whose mothers starved during pregnancy and the general male population [20].

Treatment

Surgery

Surgical interventions may be required for both the diagnosis and treatment of certain malignancies [21,22]. Approximately 0.5–2% of pregnant women in North America undergo surgery for reasons unrelated to their pregnancy [7,8], and approximately 7,000 to 30,000 of these women are in their first trimester [25], which is a critical time for central nervous system (CNS) development [26]. Furthermore, this is the time period when the woman is often unaware that she is pregnant. Surgery during pregnancy may also be associated with hypotension, hypoxia, coagulation, metabolic disturbances [27], and decreased utero-placental perfusion, most secondary to prolonged maintenance in the supine position [28]. In a review of the possible adverse effects of general and/or local anesthetics and occupational exposure to anesthetic agents, a major teratogenic risk in humans was not observed [29]. However, Kallen and Mazze, in a case control study [30], assessed the pregnancy outcome of 2,252 infants born to women who had first-trimester surgery. Six neonates (expected number = 2.5) had neural tube defects (NTDs). Five of the 6 mothers underwent operations during the fourth and fifth weeks of gestation, the time window for the development of the neural tube. However, the authors suggested that the association between anesthetic exposure and NTDs may be random and a subsequent investigation failed to replicate this effect [129]. Sylvester [25] found a strong association between anesthesia exposure, hydrocephalus, and eye defects (odds ratio = 1.7; 95% confidence interval [CI]: 0.8–3.3). However, no information was found addressing the effects of these procedures on later childhood neurodevelopment.

Chemotherapy

Cancer treatment protocols require the use of chemotherapy and/or radiation as well as immunosuppressive agents. Numerous studies have concluded that chemotherapy, administered to women before conception or after the first trimester, results in normal births in the majority of cases [31–39]. Although studies have shown that chemotherapy can be safely delivered after the first trimester and is not associated with increased risk of structural birth defects, these conclusions may not apply to the prolonged development of the CNS.

Insufficient evidence-based information is available with regard to the impact of chemotherapy on neurocognitive fetal development which, in addition to physical development, is a key concern among patients diagnosed with cancer in pregnancy. Some chemicals, such as xenobiotics, alcohol, and heavy metals are known to adversely affect CNS development in the second and third trimester [40,41]. Research specifically addressing the long-term developmental outcome is sparse and mainly consists of small series and case reports [42–47]. Dipaola *et al.* reported results on ABVD exposure (doxorubicin, bleomycin, vinblastine, and decarbazine) after the first trimester. Nine women were prospectively followed up. They found 1 minor malformation (syndactyly), which was unlikely to be associated with the chemotherapy as the drugs were not given during organogenesis. Long-term follow up showed normal development and all children (the oldest of which was 5) were meeting developmental milestones [82]. Two separate case reports on rituximab treatment for non-Hodgkin's lymphoma beginning in the first trimester and docetaxal for metastatic breast cancer beginning at week 21 were published. Both children were followed up and showed normal neuropsychological development [83,84]. Aviles *et al.* followed 84 children born to mothers with hematological malignancies who were exposed to chemotherapeutic agents. Thirty-eight of these mothers received chemotherapy during their first trimester of pregnancy. In a long-term follow up which ranged from 6 to 29 years (with a median of 18.7 years) neurological, psychological, cognitive, cytogenetic, and hematological disorders as well as physical health and growth were examined. Because of the length of the follow-up, some of these patients had themselves become parents and the second-generation children were also assessed. Aviles and Neri reported that none of the children showed physical, neurological, or psychological abnormalities [85]. Table 1 presents the results of 134 children in whom neurodevelopment and school performance, following *in utero* exposure to chemotherapy, was addressed. In 92 children, 5 with occupational exposure, formal cognitive tests were performed and compared with a control group [38–41,85]. Of the remaining 43 children, results relied only on maternal, physician and school reports [48–51,82–84]. The general impression, based on these reports, suggests that chemotherapy does not have a major impact on later neurodevelopment. However, the majority of these reports used a retrospective design, inappropriate control groups, and a cross-sectional rather than longitudinal approach. Most authors did not conduct formal motor, cognitive, or behavioral tests, thereby decreasing the probability of detecting more subtle neurodevelopmental abnormalities. Thus, these studies may not have the power to detect small but clinically significant effects. A lack of evidence-based information on the safety of chemotherapeutic agents for the long-term neurodevelopment of children is a cause for concern among patients, and may in some cases result in the postponement of treatment until after delivery, putting them at high risk for increased morbidity and mortality from cancer. A better understanding of the impact of chemotherapy on the neurocognitive development of the child is critical for those faced with the difficult decision of undertaking chemotherapy during pregnancy.

Interferon-alpha

Interferon alpha (IFN-α) is a biological response modifier cytokine protein that works to increase the function of various components of the body's immune system. It is an approved treatment for a variety of hematological disorders. When used in monotherapy during pregnancy, this drug has not been found to be associated with an increased rate of major malformations. Three pregnant women who were treated with IFN-α for chronic

Table 1. *In utero* exposure to chemotherapeutic agents

Indication	Authors	Time of exposure in pregnancy	Study design	Sample size N = 134	Age assessed	Medications	Tests	Results
Different forms of malignancies	Blatt et al. 1980	Preconceptionally or 1st trimester	Retrospective	4	1 month to 12 years old	Combined chemotherapy	Denver Developmental Screening Test, School reports	Normal development and school performance
Acute leukemia	Dara et al. 1981	Preconception and up to 8 weeks postconception						
Hodgkin's disease	Baisogolov & Shishkin, 1985		Retrospective	19	1 to 14 years old	Combined chemotherapy	Parent and school reports	Normal development
Hodgkin's disease	Balcewicz-Sablinska et al. 1990	1st trimester	Retrospective	3	Up to age 6	MOPP	No formal testing	Normal development
Hodgkin's disease	Aviles et al. 1991	1st and 2nd trimesters	Retrospective, controlled	15	3 to 17 years	MOPP, ABVD	Wechsler and Bender-Gestalt cognitive tests, School report	Not different from controls
Hematological malignancies	Aviles et al. 1991	1st, 2nd, and 3rd trimesters	Retrospective, controlled	43	3 to 19 years	Combined chemotherapy	Wechsler and Benter-Gestalt cognitive tests, School reports	Not different from controls
Acute leukemia	Aviles et al. 1990	1st trimester or sometime during pregnancy	Retrospective, controlled	17	4 to 22 years	Combined chemotherapy	Wechsler and Benter-Gestalt cognitive tests, School reports	Not different from controls

Rheumatic disease	Kozlowski et al. 1990	1st trimester	Retrospective	5	3.7 to 16.7 years	Low-dose methotrexate	Parent reports	Normal development
Occupational exposure	Medkova, 1991	Preconceptionally and/or during pregnancy	Retrospective, controlled	5		Low-dose cytostatics	No formal testing	Normal development
Metastatic breast cancer	De Santis et al. 2000	3rd trimester	Case report	1	20 months	Docetaxel 100 mg/m^2 every 3 weeks	No formal testing	Regular psychophysical development
Hematological malignancies	Aviles and Neri, 2001	38 exposed 1st trimester, 46 exposed sometime after 1st trimester	Prospective study	12	6 to 29 years	Chemotherapy at full dose	Physician assessment	Normal development
Hodgkin's diseases	Dipaola RS et al. 1997	2nd and 3rd trimester	Prospective study	9	Oldest is 5 years	ABVD	No formal testing	Normal development, meeting developmental milestones
Non-Hodgkin's lymphoma	Kimby et al. 2004	1st trimester	Case report	1		Rituximab 375mg/m^2	Pediatrician assessment	Psychomotor development within standard limits

N, number of exposed children in study.

myeloid leukemia (CML) beginning in the first trimester delivered babies with a normal appearance, 1 of whom had mild thrombocytopenia (for 2 weeks duration). The children were followed up at 4, 12, and 30 months, and all showed normal growth and development [86]. Similar neonatal and early childhood results were obtained following the treatment of a pregnant woman with HCV hepatitis who was administered IFN-α between 13 and 33 weeks gestation [123]. Other investigators assessed 21 children exposed to IFN-α at different times in gestation and reported normal outcome, although formal tests were not performed [87–101]. Although no adverse effects in the small number of human pregnancies exposed to this drug have been reported, it should still be used with caution and more research is needed to confirm its reproductive safety profile.

Glucocorticoids

Glucocorticoids are part of the treatment protocol for malignancies, in patients following organ transplantation, and for fetal lung maturation when preterm delivery is suspected. Although there have been several studies on the neurodevelopmental effects of glucocorticoids when administered late in pregnancy [70–74], there are few well-designed studies on the effects when taken early in pregnancy or throughout gestation [75–77]. Animal studies have demonstrated that exposure to high levels of glucocorticoids can cause neurodevelopmental damage during fetal or early postnatal development, although no deficits in learning ability and memory in one progeny were observed [112,113]. Further evidence from animal studies suggests that fetal exposure to glucocorticoids may alter and impede neuronal development and that there may indeed be critical periods in which such effects occur [114,115]. It is unclear as to whether these results may be extrapolated to humans. Table 2 presents the results of 2,022 children, exposed *in utero* to glucocorticoids, in whom neurodevelopment and school performance was addressed [70–77,111,116,119]. Formal cognitive tests were performed in 1,972 children and were contrasted with comparison groups [70–74,77,106–109,111,116,119]. The data on the remaining 50 children were collected from maternal and/or school reports only [75,76]. The pregnancy and long-term outcome of 1,282 children exposed during late pregnancy is presented [70–76,106–108,111,116]. The NIH Consensus Conference [74] data were based on the analysis of all available reports pertaining to corticosteroid exposure in pregnancy and indicated that there was not an increased risk for long-term neurodevelopmental impairments. There is, however, evidence that repeated doses, similar to what is encountered in cancer chemotherapy are associated with microcephaly and low birth weight [110]. Conversely, the prospective randomized control trials of single versus weekly courses of antenatal corticosteroids also found a decrease in birth weight, but did not support the previous finding of reduction in mean head circumference [103–105]. The same studies found a trend to higher rates of severe hemorrhage, chorioamnionitis, and cerebral palsy in children exposed on a weekly basis. In a follow-up study by French *et al.* in 2004, findings in children of 3 and 6 years of age were presented. These authors concluded that, in this cohort (of 541 very preterm infants), repeated antenatal courses of corticosteroids may protect against cerebral palsy. Corticosteroids were not associated with internalizing behavior and intelligence quotient abnormalities but are associated with hyperactivity later in childhood [106]. Conversely, Ward *et al.* [111] reported on the long-term developmental–behavioral outcomes of fetal oral corticosteroid treatment for alloimmune thrombocytopenia and found that this antenatal regimen did not affect children's behavioral outcomes. Of the 71 exposed and unexposed

Table 2. Children exposed *in utero* to glucocorticoids

Indication	Authors	Time of exposure in pregnancy	Study design	Sample size N = 2022	Age assessed	Medications	Tests	Results
Lung maturation *in Hungarian	Veszelovszky et al. 1981	3rd trimester	Retrospective, controlled	125	12–36 months	Dexamethasone	Neurological and psychological	No difference from the control group
Fetal lung maturation	MacArthur et al. 1981 and 1982	3rd trimester	Prospective, controlled	139	Age 4 and 6	Betamethasone	Standford-Binet Intelligence Scale, Frostig Visual Perception Test, Vineland Social Maturity Scale, Illinois Test of Psycholinguistic Abilities, Peabody Vocabulary Test, Raven's Matrices, Bender-Gestalt Test	No difference from the control group
Fetal lung maturation	Collaborative Group on Antenatal Steroid Therapy (1984)	3rd trimester	Prospective, randomized, placebo controlled, double-blind	200	36 months	Dexamethasone	Bayley Scales, McCarthy Scales	No difference from the control group
Fetal lung maturation	NIH Consensus Conference, 1995	3rd trimester	Analysis of available data		Up to age 12	Corticosteroids		No increased risk of long-term neurodevelopmental impairment
Maternal SLE	Tincini et al. 1992	Throughout pregnancy	Prospective	21	1–85 months	Flucocortolone plus aspirin and azathioprine (if needed)	No formal tests	No long-term consequences

Table 2. (cont.)

Indication	Authors	Time of exposure in pregnancy	Study design	Sample size N = 2022	Age assessed	Medications	Tests	Results
Maternal heart transplants	Wagoner et al. 1993	"During pregnancy"	Prospective	29	3 months to 6.5 years	Corticosteroids plus other immunosuppressives	No formal tests	All children reported to be in good health
Fetal congenital adrenal hyperplasia	Trautman et al. 1995	Started from week 1 to 21 weeks of gestation	Prospective, controlled plot study	26	6 months to 5.5 years	Dexamethasone for 2–29 weeks	Denver Developmental Questionnaire, Minnesota Child Development Inventory, Child Behavior Checklist, Temperament Questionnaire, EAS Temperament Survey	More shy, emotional, less sociable, and a trend for greater avoidance than control group. No differences in cognitive abilities.
Cranial abnormalities	Arad et al. 2002		Prospective cohort study	251	6 and 8 years	Corticosteroids	Kauffman Assessment Battery for Children, Wide Range Achievement Test, Achenbach Teacher's Report Form and Child Behavioral Check List	Long-term benefits on cognition of very low birth weight infants with cranial ultrasound abnormalities. Children with normal cranial ultrasounds and normal cognitive function.

Condition	Study	Timing	Study type	N	Age	Treatment	Measures	Findings
Preterm delivery	Thorp et al. 2003	Later pregnancy	Secondary analysis of a double-blind clinical trial	299	7 years	Phenobarbital and Vitamin K with multiple dose antenatal corticosteroids	Wechsler Intelligence Scale for Children, Wide Range Achievement Tests, Achenbach Teacher's Report Form and Child behavioral Checklist	No association with adverse effects on intelligence, achievement, behavior or head circumference
Preterm delivery	French et al. 2004	3rd trimester	Nonrandomized regional cohort	541	3 and 6 years	Repeated antenatal corticosteroids	Standord-Binet Intelligence test, Child behavior Checklist	May protect against cerebral palsy but associate with hyperactivity later in childhood. Measures of internalizing behavior and intelligence quotient were unaffected.
Congenital adrenal hyperplasia as well as without CAH	Heino et al. 2004		Retrospective study	174	Up to 12 years	Dexamethasone	Kent Infant Development Scale, Revised Prescreening Developmental Questionnaire, Child Development Inventory, Child behavior Checklist	No effects on developmental outcome were found.
Alloimmune thrombocytopenia	Ward et al. 2006	3rd trimester	Randomized multicenter study	71	2 to 11 years	Fetal oral corticosteroid	Medical questionnaire, Behavioral Assessment System for Children (BASC)	Antenatal treatment regime did not affect children's behavioral outcomes

Table 2. *(cont.)*

Indication	Authors	Time of exposure in pregnancy	Study design	Sample size N = 2022	Age assessed	Medications	Tests	Results
Congenital adrenal hyperplasia	Hirvikoski *et al.* 2007	Early pregnancy	Retrospective study	26	7 to 17 years	Dexamethasone	Developmental Neuropsychological Assessment (NEPSY), Wechsler Intelligence Scales, Self-Perception Profile for Children, Child Behavior Checklist/4–18 School Scales, Social Anxiety Scale for Children-Revised	Exposed children born at term had persistent impairments in tests of verbal working memory.
Physical growth and neurodevelopment	Peltoniemi *et al.* 2009	3rd trimester	Prospective blinded design following a randomized multicenter trial	120	2 years	Single repeat dose of Betamethasone	Bayley Scales of Infant Development II (BSID-II), Griffiths Developmental Score	Exposed children were no different on measures of physical growth and neurodevelopment

N, number of exposed children in study; SLE, systemic lupus erythematosus; CAH, congenital adrenal hyperplasia.

sibling pairs (aged 2 to 11) assessed using a medical questionnaire and the Behavioral Assessment System for Children (BASC), treated children had better long-term developmental–behavioral outcomes than their untreated siblings.

A report published by Thorp *et al.* analyzed prospectively the effects of phenobarbital and vitamin K associated with multiple dose corticosteroids on the developmental outcome of children at age 7 [107]. Two hundred ninety-nine children who were exposed to these drugs were followed up at age 7 when intelligence, achievement, behavior, and head circumference were assessed. This study concluded that antenatal phenobarbital and repetitive antenatal corticosteroid therapy was not associated with adverse affects on intelligence, achievement, behavior, or head circumference. McArthur *et al.* [71,72] studied a cohort of 139 children at age 4 and age 6. Their results suggested that there were no significant differences in the cognitive or psychosocial development between the betamethasone exposed group and control group. Peltoniemi *et al.* [116] reported similar findings. Using a prospective, blinded design following a randomized multicenter trial, 120 infants prenatally exposed to a single repeat dose of betamethasone and placebo controls underwent neurological and psychometric examinations and a speech evaluation at a corrected age of 2 years. Exposed and unexposed infants were no different on measures of physical growth and neurodevelopment. Arad *et al.* performed neurodevelopmental assessments on 251 children at the ages of 6 and 8 [108]. Antenatal corticosteroids conferred substantial long-term benefits on cognition of very low-birth-weight infants with cranial abnormalities and were positively associated, in a dose–response manner, with IQ scores. In children with normal cranial ultrasound scans, cognitive function was not found to be associated with antenatal corticosteroid exposure. Trautman *et al.* [77] assessed the pregnancy outcomes of 26 children exposed to dexamethasone in early pregnancy and found that those children who were exposed displayed more internalizing and higher avoidance behavior and were more shy and emotional and less sociable than unexposed children. The children from the study group were not found to be different from the control group on cognitive performance. Meyer-Bahlburg *et al.* [109] assessed 487 children between the ages of 1 month and 12 years who had been exposed to early prenatal dexamethasone. Analysis of 4 standardized questionnaires showed no significant difference in motor and cognitive development between these children and the control group. Conflicting results were reported by Hirvikoski *et al.* [119] addressing the long-term neuropsychological functions and scholastic performance of 26 children aged 7 to 17 who had been prenatally treated with dexamethasone in early pregnancy to prevent congenital andrenal hyperplasia. Using standardized neuropsychological tests and both child- and parent-completed questionnaires assessing scholastic competence, exposed children who were born at term had persistent impairments in tests of verbal working memory when compared with sex- and age-matched controls. Shinwell and Eventov-Friedman [117] conducted a meta-analysis on the relationship between postnatal dexamethasone, cerebral palsy, and neurodevelopment, reporting neurotoxic effects of postnatal dexamethasone and the unproven safety of this drug administered in lower doses. The available results regarding the use of glucocorticoids in late pregnancy are reassuring. However, although repeated doses of corticosteroids have not been shown to adversely affect children's IQ, they are associated with behavioral problems.

Cyclosporine

In the cases of leukemia, lymphoma, and multiple myeloma, a bone marrow transplant in conjunction with immunosuppressant therapy may be required. Cyclosporine is an immunosuppressant used to prevent rejection following solid organ and bone marrow transplantation. In addition, the ability of cyclosporine to inhibit T-cell activation has been shown to have a role in the treatment of other diseases such as aplastic anemia. Using a cohort study with matched controls from a prospectively collected database, Nulman *et al.* [118] evaluated the long-term neurodevelopmental outcomes of 39 children following *in utero* cyclosporine exposure after maternal renal transplant. On measures of intelligence, visuomotor abilities, and psychologic adjustment, cyclosporine was not found to be associated with long-term neurocognitive and behavioral development. However, within the cyclosporine group, children born premature achieved significantly lower scores on these measures. Thus, the effects of premature delivery on neurocognitive outcomes should always be carefully considered in management decisions.

Bromocriptine

Pituitary adenomas are not uncommon forms of tumors in women of child-bearing age. Bromocriptine is an alkaloid that functions as a dopamine receptor agonist that suppresses prolactin production. It is the treatment of choice for pituitary tumors during pregnancy. Pregnancy outcome and children's well-being at long-term follow-up (up to age 9) of hundreds of children exposed *in utero* to bromocriptine were reported to be normal [78–81]. However, no formal cognitive and behavioral tests were performed. Although bromocriptine was not found to be associated with an increased risk for neurodevelopmental disorders in children exposed *in utero*, more well-designed studies including formal cognitive and behavioral testing should be performed to detect more subtle effects of this medication.

Radiation

Radiation is widely used for diagnostic and therapeutic purposes in various malignancies. Based on live birth rate statistics in the United States, approximately 33,000 women each year are exposed to diagnostic abdominal radiation in early pregnancy [52]. Presenting various susceptibilities, the developing embryo and fetus are extremely sensitive to ionizing radiation [53]. The CNS maintains its sensitivity to radiation throughout gestation and into the neonatal period, when functional changes may still be observed. Ionizing radiation, a known CNS teratogen, is recognized as a cause of mental retardation and growth restriction, including microcephaly after significant exposure during organogenesis and the early fetal period [122]. It has been suggested that such radiation creates more serious complications and risks than cancer itself [55].

The effects of radiation exposure are dose and time dependent. Animal studies have demonstrated significant variability in radiation effects on the developing brain, such as cell death, disoriented migration, impaired differentiation, disturbed myelin formation, and affected connectivity [54]. The dose–response effects from animal behavioral studies suggest that, although behavioral changes in animals are observed after 1 Gy of radiation, damage to the brain was recorded after as low a dose as 0.2 Gy. However, the generalizability of animal studies to humans is questionable and uncertain.

Available human data demonstrate radiation-induced cellular injury or death above a certain threshold dose. Even in the absence of structural defects, cognitive or behavioral problems may present later in development. For a given dose of radiation, there may be a loss of organ or tissue functionality, leading to pregnancy loss, congenital malformations, neurobehavioral abnormalities, and fetal growth restriction [121]. As the dose increases, so does the incidence of these effects, whereas below a threshold dose, there is no apparent risk of teratogenicity [120]. There is a scarcity of research on the long-term neurodevelopmental and behavioral development of children exposed *in utero* to radiation. Brent [56] stated that radiation doses as low as 50 rad (0.5 Gy) in humans may be harmful to the fetus, especially to the CNS. The experiences at Hiroshima and Nagasaki are the most important sources of information on long-term effects of radiation on the human embryo and fetus. Analysis of the data of survivors in Japan using refined estimates of the absorbed dose in fetal tissues demonstrated that the highest risk of brain damage occurred between 8 and 15 weeks of gestational age [57–60,62,63]. Before week 8 of gestation and after week 25, radiation exposure was not associated with an increased risk of mental retardation. The apparent absence of an effect before the eighth week suggests that neuronal cell migration during weeks 8–15 postconception may be the crucial component of cerebral damage caused by radiation [61]. Smith discussed 2 studies that demonstrated a downward shift in the Gaussian distribution of IQ with an estimated probability coefficient, indicating a loss of 30 IQ points per 1 Gy fetal dose at 8–15 weeks after conception [62]. A similar, but smaller shift toward lower intelligence was detectable following exposure between 16 and 25 weeks of gestation, but not at other periods of pregnancy. Otake *et al.* [63] evaluated the risk of ionizing radiation on the developing human brain and suggested a threshold in the low-dose region to be 0.05 Gy for 8–15 weeks of exposure and 0.25 Gy for 16–25 weeks of exposure. Granroth [64] reported an association between diagnostic x-ray examinations and the occurrence of CNS defects. He observed a significant increase in anencephaly, hydrocephaly, and microcephaly when compared with matched controls. Several studies did not find severe mental retardation in a total of 19 children exposed to 0.015 and 0.1 Gy and in 1,455 children exposed to low doses of radiation [65,66]. However, formal behavioral and cognitive tests were not performed. These results should be considered with caution because of methodological limitations of the study design. Fetal exposure to less than 0.05 Gy does not appear to increase the teratogenic risk [68]. In summary, according to Wilson's criteria, ionizing radiation is a teratogen [69]. Being neurotropic, radiation is capable of producing cognitive and behavioral teratogenic effects, which are demonstrable at doses below those causing visible structural malformations [70].

Summary

Most malignant conditions are not absolute contraindications for pregnancy; however, proper treatment protocols must account for both maternal and fetal well-being. Current research has failed to show neurotoxic effects of exposure to chemotherapy for maternal malignancy after the first trimester; however, more evidence-based information on long-term neurodevelopmental and behavioral outcomes after exposure to radiation and corticosteroids is required. Further research will assist pregnant women and healthcare providers in optimizing the management of cancer in pregnancy.

References

1. Gililland J, Weinstein L. The effects of cancer chemotherapeutic agents on the developing fetus. *Obstet Gynecol Surv*. 1983;**38**:6–13.

2. Silverberg E. Cancer statistics. 1986. *CA Cancer J Clin*. 1986;**36**:9–25.

3. Sutcliffe SB. Treatment of neoplastic disease during pregnancy: maternal and fetal effects. *Clin Invest Med*. 1985; **8**:333–8.

4. Potter JF, Schoeneman M. Metastasis of maternal cancer to the placenta and fetus. *Cancer*. 1970;**25**:380–8.

5. Warkany J. Teratogen update: hyperthermia. *Teratology*. 1986;**33**:365–71.

6. Edwards MJ. Influenza, hyperthermia, and congenital malformation. *Lancet*. 1972;**1**:320–1.

7. Miller P, Smith DW, Spherd TH. Maternal hyperthermia as a possible cause for anencephaly. *Lancet*. 1978;**1**:519–21.

8. Chance PF, Smith DW. Hyperthermia and meningomyelocele and anencphaly. *Lancet*. 1978;**1**:769–70.

9. Layde PM, Edmonds LD, Erickson JD. Maternal fever and neural tube defects. *Teratology*. 1980;**21**:105–8.

10. James WH. Hyperthermia and meningomyelocele and ancephaly. [Letter]. *Lancet*. 1978;**1**:770.

11. Kleinebrecht J, Michaelis H, Michaelis J, et al. Fever in pregnancy and congenital anomalies. [Letter]. *Lancet*. 1979; **1**:1043.

12. Clarren SK, Smith DW, Harvey MA. Hyperthermia: a prospective evaluation of a possible teratogenic agent in man. *J Pediatr*. 1979;**95**:81–3.

13. Metcoff S, Costiloe JP, Crosby W. Maternal nutrition and fetal outcome. *Am J Clin Nutr*. 1981;**34**(suppl 4):708–21.

14. Rosso P. Prenatal nutrition and fetal growth and development. *Pediatr Ann*. 1981;**10**:21–6.

15. Brown JE, Jaconson HN, Askue LH, Pieck MG. Influence of pregnancy weight gain on the size of infants born to underweight women. *Obstet Gynecol*. 1981;**57**:13–7.

16. Edwards LE, Alton IR, Barranda MI, Hakanson EY. Pregnancy in the underweight woman. Course, outcome and growth patterns of infant. *Am J Obstet Gynecol*. 1981;**135**:297–302.

17. Pritchard JA, MacDonald PC, Gant NF. *Williams obstetrics*, 17th ed. Norwalk, CT: Appleton-Century-Crofts; 1985.

18. Churchill JA, Benendes HW. Intelligence of children whose mothers had acetonuria during pregnancy. In: *Perinatal factors affecting human development*. Washington: Pan American Sanitary Bureau; 1969.

19. Naeyl RL, Chez RA. Effects of maternal acetonuria and low pregnancy weight gain on children's psychomotor development. *Am J Obstet Gynecol*. 1981;**139**:189–93.

20. Stein Z, Sussur M, Seanger G, Marolla F. Nutrition and mental performance. *Science*. 1972;**178**:708–13.

21. Duncan PG, Pope WDB, Cohen MM, Greer N. Fetal risk of anesthesia and surgery during pregnancy. *Anesthesiology*. 1986;**64**:790–4.

22. Brodsky JB, Cohen EN, Brown BW Jr, Wu ML, Whitcher C. Surgery during pregnancy and fetal outcome. *Am J Obstet Gynecol*. 1980;**138**:1165–7.

23. Shnider SM, Webster GM. Maternal and fetal hazards of surgery during pregnancy. *Am J Obstet Gynecol*. 1965;**92**:891–900.

24. Smith BE. Fetal prognosis after anesthesia during gestation. *Anesth Analg*. 1963;**42**:521–6.

25. Sylvester G, Khoury MJ, Lu X, Erickson JD. First-trimester anesthesia exposure and the risk of central nervous system defects: a population-based case-control study. *Am J Public Health*. 1994;**84**:1757–60.

26. Webster WS, Lipson AH, Sulik KK. Interference with gastrulation during the third week of pregnancy as a cause of some facial abnormalities and CNS defects. *Am J Med Genet*. 1988;**31**:505–12.

27. Cohen SE. Physiological alterations of pregnancy. *Clin Anesthesiol*. 1986;**4**:NI.

28. Doll DC, Ringenberg OS, Yarbo JW. Management of cancer during pregnancy. *Arch Intern Med*. 1988;**148**:2058–64.

29. Friedman JM. Teratogen update: anesthetic agents. *Teratology*. 1988;**37**: 69–77.

30. Kallen B, Mazze RI. Neural tube defects and first trimester operations. *Teratology*. 1990;**41**:717–20.

31. Nicholson HO. Cytotoxic drugs in pregnancy. *J Obstet Gynecol Br Commonw*. 1968;**75**:307–12.

32. Sokal JE, Lessmann EM. Effects of cancer chemotherapeutic agents on human fetus. *JAMA*. 1960;**172**:1765–71.

33. Greenberg LH, Tanaka KR. Congenital anomalies probably induced by cyclophosphamide. *JAMA*. 1964;**188**:423–6.

34. Hardin JS. Cyclophosphamide treatment of lymphoma during third trimester of pregnancy. *Obstet Gynecol*. 1971;**39**:850–1.

35. Blatt J, Mulvihill JJ, Ziegler JL, Young RC, Poplack DG. Pregnancy outcome following cancer chemotherapy. *Am J Med*. 1980;**69**:828–32.

36. Heino F, Meyer-Bahlburg L, Dolezal C, et al. Cognitive and motor development of children with and without congenital adrenal hyperpasia after early-prenatal dexamethasone. *J Clin Endocrinol Metab*. 2004;**89**:610–4.

37. Sieber SM, Adamson RH. Toxicity of antineoplastic agents in man: chromosomal aberations, antifertility effects, congenital malformations and carcinogenic potential. *Adv Cancer Res*. 1975;**22**:57–155.

38. Gililland J, Weinstein L. The effect of cancer chemotherapeutic agents on the developing fetus. *Obstet Gynecol Surv*. 1983;**38**:6–13.

39. Doll DC, Ringenberg QS, Yarbo JW. Management of cancer during pregnancy. *Arch Intern Med*. 1988;**148**:2058–64.

40. Koren G. Human teratogens. In: Koren G, editor. *Maternal fetal toxicology: clinician's guide*. New York: Marcel Dekker; 1990.

41. Harada M. Congenital minamata disease: intrauterine methylmercury poisoning. *Teratology*. 1978;**18**:285–8.

42. Ortega J. Multiple agent chemotherapy including bleomycin of non-Hodgkin lymphoma during pregnancy. *Cancer*. 1977;**40**:2829–35.

43. Schapira DV, Chudley AE. Successful pregnancy following continuous treatment with combination chemotherapy before conception and throughout pregnancy. *Cancer*. 1984;**54**:800–3.

44. Odom LD, Plouffe L Jr, Butler WJ. 5-Fluorouracil exposure during the period of conception: report on two cases. *Am J Obstet Gynecol*. 1990;**163**(Pt 1):76–7.

45. Jones RT, Weinerman BH. MOPP (Nitrogen mustard, vincristine,

procarbazine and prednisone) given during pregnancy. *Obstet Gynecol*. 1979;**54**:477–8.

46. Reynoso EE, Shepard FA, Messner HA, Farquharson HA, Garvey MB, Baker MA. Acute leukemia during pregnancy: the Toronto Leukemia Study group experience with long-term follow-up of children exposed in utero to chemotherapeutic agents. *J Clin Oncol*. 1987;**5**:1098–106.

47. Cantini E, Yanes B. Acute myelogenous leukemia in pregnancy. *South Med J*. 1984;**77**:1050–2.

48. Woo SY, Fuller LM, Cundiff JH, et al. Radiotherapy during pregnancy for clinical stages IA-IIA Hodgkin's disease. *Int J Radiat Oncol Biol Phys*. 1992;**23**:407–12.

49. Aviles A, Diaz-Maqueo JC, Torras V, Garcia EL, Guzman R. Non-Hodgkin's lymphoma and pregnancy: presentation of 16 cases. *Gynecol Oncol*. 1990;**37**:335–7.

50. Aviles A, Diaz-Maqueo JC, Talavera A, Guzman R, Garcia EL. Growth and development of children of mothers treated with chemotherapy during pregnancy: current status of 43 children. *Am J Hematol*. 1991;**36**:243–8.

51. Catanzarite VA, Ferguson JE Jr. Acute leukemia and pregnancy: a review of management and outcome. *Obstet Gynecol Surv*. 1984;**39**:663–78.

52. US Department of Health and Human Services. *Vital Statistics of the United States*, 1976. Bol. Natality. Hyattsville, MD: National Center for Health Statistics; 1980.

53. Hoffman D, Felten R, Cyr W. *Effects of ionizing radiation on the developing embryo and fetus: a review*. Rockville, MD: US Department of Health and Human Services.

54. Schull WJ, Norton S, Jensh RP. Ionizing radiation and developing brain. *Neurotoxicol Teratol*. 1990;**12**:249–60.

55. Hoel DG. Radiations risk estimation models. *Environ Health Perspect*. 1987;**25**:103–7.

56. Brent RL. Radiation teratogenesis. *Teratology*. 1980;**21**:281–98.

57. Otake M, Schull WJ. In utero exposure to A-bomb radiation and mental retardation:

a reassessment. *Br J Radiol.* 1984;**57**: 409–14.

58. Yoshimaru H, Otake M, Fujikoshi Y, Schull WJ. [Effect on school performance of prenatal exposure to the Hiroshima atomic bomb]. *Nippon Eiseigaku Zasshi.* 1991;**46**:747–54.

59. Otake M, Schull WJ, Yoshimaru H. A review of forty-five years study of Hirishima and Nagasaki atomic bomb survivors. Brain damage among the prenatally exposed. *J Radial Res (Tokyo).* 1991;**32**(suppl):249–64.

60. International Commission on Radiological Protection. Developmental effects of irradiation on the brain of the embryo and fetus. *Annals of the ICRP.* 1986;**16**:1–43.

61. Lione A. Ionizing radiation and human reproduction. *Reprod Toxicol.* 1987;**1**:3–16.

62. Smith H. The detrimental health effects of ionizing radiation. *Nucl Med Commun.* 1992;**13**:4–10.

63. Otake M, Schull WJ, Lee S. Threshold for radiation-related severe mental retardation in prenatally exposed A-bomb survivors: a re-analysis. *Int J Radiat Biol.* 1996;**70**: 755–63.

64. Granroth G. Defects of the central nervous system in Finland. IV. Associations with diagnostic x-ray examinations. *Am J Obstet Gynecol.* 1979;**133**:191–4.

65. Meyer MB, Tonascia JA, Merz T. Long-term of effects of prenatally exposed X-ray on development and fertility of human females. In: *Biological and environmental effects of low-level radiation. II.* Vienna: IAEA; 1976. p. 273–7.

66. Neumeister K. Findings in children after radiation exposure in utero from X-ray examination of mothers. In: *Late biological effects of ionizing radiation.* Vol. I. Vienna: IAEA; 1978. p. 119–34.

67. Koren G. Ionizing and nonionizing radiation in pregnancy. In: Koren G, editor. *Maternal fetal toxicology: a clinician's guide.* New York: Marcel Dekker; 1994. p. 515–72.

68. Wilson JG. Current status of teratology: general principles and mechanisms derived from animal studies. In: Wilson G, Fraser FC, editors. *Handbook of teratology, general principles and etiology.* New York: Plenum Press; 1977.

69. Vorhees CV. Principles of behavioral teratology. In: Riley EP, Vorhees CV, editors. *Handbook of behavioral teratology.* New York: Plenum Press; 1986. p. 23–48.

70. Veszelovszky I, Farkasinszky T, Nagy Z, Bodis L, Szilard J. Psychological and neurosomatic follow-up studies of children of mother treated with dexamethasone. *Orv Hetil.* 1981;**122**:629–31.

71. MacArthur BA, Howie RN, Dezoete JA, Elkins J. Cognitive and psychosocial development of 4-year-old children whose mothers were treated antenatally with betamethasone. *Pediatrics.* 1981;**68**:638–43.

72. MacArthur BA, Howie RN, Dezoete JA, Elkins J. School progress and cognitive development of 6-year old children whose mothers were treated antenatally with betamethasone. *Pediatrics.* 1982;**70**:99–105.

73. Collaborative Group on Antenatal Steroid Therapy. Effects of antenatal dexamethasone administration in the infant: long-term follow-up. *J Pediatr.* 1984;**104**:259–67.

74. NIH Consensus Conference. Effect of corticosteroids for fetal maturation on perinatal outcomes. *JAMA.* 1996;**273**: 413–7.

75. Tincini A, Faden D, Tarantini M, et al. SLE and pregnancy: a prospective study. *Clin Exp Rheumatol.* 1992;**10**:439–46.

76. Wagoner LE, Taylor DO, Olsen SL, et al. Immunosuppressive therapy, management, and outcome of heart transplant recipients during pregnancy. *J Heart Lung Transplant.* 1993;**12**:993–9; discussion 1000.

77. Trautman PD, Meyer-Bahlburg HF, Postelnek J, New MI. Effects of early prenatal dexamethasone on the cognitive and behavioral development of young children: results of a pilot study. *Psychoneuroendocrinology.* 1995;**20**:439–49.

78. Turkalj I, Braun P, Krupp P. Surveillance of bromocriptine in pregnancy. *JAMA.* 1982;**247**:1589–91.

79. Konopka P, Raymon JP, Merceron RE, Seneze J. Continuous administration of bromocriptine in the prevention of neurological complications in pregnant women. *Am J Obstet Gynecol.* 1983;**146**:935–8.

80. Nader S. Pituitary disorders and pregnancy. *Semin Perinatol.* 1990;**14**:24–33.

81. Krupp P, Monka C. Bromocriptine in pregnancy: safety aspects. *Klin Wochenschr.* 1987;**65**:823–7.

82. Dipaola RS, Goodin S, Ratzell M, Florczyk M, Karp G, Ravikumar TS. Chemotherapy for metastatic melanoma during pregnancy. *Gynecol Oncol.* 1997;**66**:526–30.

83. Kimby E, Sverrisdottir A, Elinder G. Safety of rituximab therapy during the first trimester of pregnancy: a case history. *Eur J Haematol.* 2004;**72**:292–5.

84. De Santis M, Lucchese A, De Carolis S, Ferrazzani S, Causo A. Metastatic breast cancer in pregnancy: first case of chemotherapy with docetaxel. *Eur J Cancer Care.* 2000;**9**:235–7.

85. Aviles A, Neri N. Hematological malignancies and pregnancy: a final report of 84 children who received chemotherapy in utero. *Clin Lymphoma.* 2001;**2**:173–7.

86. Mubarak AA, Kakil IR, Awidi A, Al-Homsi U, Fawzi Z, Kelta M, Al-Hassan A. Normal outcome of pregnancy in chronic myeloid leukemia treated with interferon-alpha in 1st trimester: report of 3 cases and review of the literature. *Am J Hematol.* 2002;**69**:115–8.

87. Baer MR. Normal full-term pregnancy in a patient with chronic myelogenous leukemia treated with alpha-interferon. *Am J Hematol.* 1991;**37**:66.

88. Baer MR, Ozer H, Foon KA. Interferon-alpha therapy during pregnancy in chronic myelogenous leukemia and hairy cell leukemia. *Br J Haematol.* 1992;**81**:167–9.

89. Huggstrom J, Adriansson M, Hybbinette T, Harnby E, Thorbert G. Two cases of CML treated with interferon-alpha during second and third trimester of pregnancy, with analysis of the drug in the new-born immediately postpartum. *Eur J Haematol.* 1996;**57**:101–2.

90. Lipton JH, Derzko CM, Curtis J. Alpha-interferon and pregnancy in a patient with CML. *Hematol Oncol.* 1996;**14**:119–22.

91. Kuroiwa M, Gundo H, Ashida K, et al. Interferon-alpha therapy for chronic myelogenous leukemia during pregnancy. *Am J Hematol.* 1998;**59**:101–2.

92. Crump M, Wang XH, Sermer M. Keating A. Successful pregnancy and delivery during alpha-interpheron therapy for chronic myeloid leukemia [letter]. *Am J Hematol.* 1992;**40**:238–9.

93. Delmer A, Rio B, Bauduer F, Ajchenbaum F, Marie JP, Zittoun R. Pregnancy during myelosuppressive treatment for chronic myelogenous leukemia. *Br J Haematol.* 1992;**81**:167–9.

94. Petit JJ, Callis M, Fernandez de Sevilla A. Normal pregnancy in a patient with essential thrombocythaemia treated with interferon-alpha 2b. *Am J Haematol.* 1992;**40**:80.

95. Vianelli N, Gugliotta L, Tura S, Bovicelli L, Rizzo N, Gabrielli A. Interferon-alpha 2a treatment in a pregnant woman with essential thrombocythaemia. *Blood.* 1994;**83**:874–5.

96. Delage R, Demers C, Cantin G, Roy J. Treatment of essential thrombocythaemia during pregnancy with interferon-alpha. *Obstet Gynecol.* 1996;**87**:814–7.

97. Pardini S, Dore F, Murineddu M, et al. Alpha 2b interferon therapy and pregnancy. Report of a case of essential thrombocythaemia [letter]. *Am J Hematol.* 1993;**43**:78–9.

98. Thornley S, Manoharan A. Successful treatment of essential thrombocythaemia with alpha-interferon during pregnancy [letter]. *Eur J Haematol.* 1994;**52**:63–4.

99. Pérez-Encinas M, Bello JL, Pérez-Crespo S, De Miguel R, Tome S. Familial myeloproliferative syndrome. *Am J Hematol.* 1994;**46**:225–9.

100. Sakata H, Karamitsos J, Kundaria B, DiSaia PJ. Case report of interferon alpha therapy for multiple myeloma during pregnancy. *Am J Obstet Gynecol.* 1995;**172**:217–9.

101. Ruggiero G, Andreana A, Zampino R. Normal pregnancy under inadvertent alpha-interferon therapy for chronic hepatitis C. *J Hepatol.* 1996;**24**:646.

102. Huizink AC, Robles de Medina PG, Mulder EJ, Visser GH, Buitelaar JK. Stress during pregnancy is associated with developmental outcome in infancy. *J Child Psychol Psychiatry.* 2003;**44**:810–8.

103. Guinn DA, Atkinson MW, Sullivan L, et al. Single vs weekly courses of antenatal corticosteroids for women at risk of preterm delivery: a randomized controlled trial. *JAMA.* 2001;**286**:1581–7.

104. Aghajafari F, Murphy K, Ohlsson A, Amandwah K, Matthews S, Hannah ME. Multiple versus single courses of antenatal coricosteroids for preterm birth: a pilot study. *J Obstet Gynaecol Can.* 2002; **24**:321–9.

105. McEvoy C, Bowling S, Williamson K, et al. The effect of a single remote course versus weekly courses of antenatal corticosteroids on functional residual capacity in preterm infants: a randomized trial. *Pediatrics.* 2002;**110**:280–4.

106. French NP, Hagan R, Evans SF, Mullan A, Newnham JP. Repeated antenatal corticosteroids: effects on cerebral palsy and childhood behaviour. *Am J Obstet Gynecol.* 2004;**190**:588–95.

107. Thorp JA, O'Connor M, Belden B, Etzenhouser J, Hoffman EL, Jones PG. Effects of phenobarbital and multiple-dose corticosteroids on developmental outcome at age 7 years. *Obstet Gynecol.* 2003;**101**:363–73.

108. Arad I, Durkin MS, Hinton VJ, et al. Long-term cognitive benefits of antenatal corticosteroids for prematurely born children with cranial ultrasound abnormalities. *Am J Obstet Gynecol.* 2002;**186**:818–25.

109. Meyer-Bahlburg HF, Dolezal C, Baker SW, Carlson AD, Obeid JS, New MI. Cognitive and motor development of children with and without congenital adrenal hyperplasia after early-prenatal dexamethasone. *J Clin Endocrinol Metab.* 2004;**89**:610–4.

110. French NP, Hagan R, Evans SF, Godfrey M, Newnham JP. Repeated antenatal corticosteroids: size at birth and subsequent development. *Am J Obstet Gynecol.* 1999;**180**:114–21.

111. Ward MJ, Pauliny J, Lipper EG, Bussel JB. Long-term effects of fetal and neonatal alloimmune thrombocytopenia and its antenatal treatment on the medical and developmental outcomes of affected children. *Am J Perinatol.* 2006;**23**:487–92.

112. Mesquita AR, Wegerich Y, Patchev AV, Oliveira M, Leao P, Sousa N, Almeida OF. Glucocorticoids and neuro- and behavioural development. *Semin Fetal Neonat Med.* 2009;**14**:130–5.

113. Oliveira M, Bessa JM, Mesquita A, et al. Induction of a hyperanxious state by antenatal dexamethasone: a case for less detrimental natural corticosteroids. *Biol Psychiatry.* 2006;**59**:844–52.

114. Fukumoto K, Morita T, Mayanagi T, et al. Detrimental effects of glucocorticoids on neuronal migration during brain development. *Mol Psychiatry.* 2009;**14**:1119–31.

115. Slotkin TA, Kreider ML, Tate CA, Seidler FJ. Critical prenatal and postnatal periods for persistent effects of dexamethasone on serotonergic and dopaminergic systems. *Neuropsychopharmacology.* 2006;**31**:904–11.

116. Peltoniemi OM, Kari MA, Lano A, et al. Two-year follow-up of a randomized trial with repeated antenatal betamethasone. *Arch Dis Child Fetal Neonatal Ed.* 2009;**94**:F402–6.

117. Shinwell ES, Eventov-Friedman S. Impact of perinatal corticosteroids on neuromotor development and outcome: review of the literature and new meta-analysis. *Semin Fetal Neonatal Med.* 2009;**14**:164–70.

118. Nulman I, Sgro M, Barrera M, Chitayat D, Cairney J, Koren G. Long-term neurodevelopmental of children exposed in utero to ciclosporin after maternal renal transplant. *Paediatr Drugs.* 2010;**12**:113–22.

119. Hirvikoski T, Nordenstrom A, Lindhold T, et al. Cognitive functions in children at risk

for congenital adrenal hyperplasia treated prenatally with dexamethasone. *J Clin Endocrinol Metab.* 2007; **92**:542–8.

120. Brent RL. Saving lives and changing family histories: appropriate counseling of pregnant women and men and women of reproductive age, concerning the risk of diagnostic radiation exposures during and before pregnancy. *Am J Obstet Gynecol.* 2009;**200**:4–24.

121. Williams PM, Fletcher S. Health effects of prenatal radiation exposure. *Am Fam Physician.* 2010;**82**:488–93.

122. Streffer C, Shore R, Konermann G, et al. Biological effects after prenatal irradiation (embryo and fetus). A report of the International Commission on Radiological Protection. *Ann ICRP.* 2003;**33**:5–206.

123. Hiratsuka M, Minakami H, Koshizuka S, Sato I. Administration of interferon-alpha during pregnancy: effects on fetus. *J Perinat Med.* 2000;**28**:372–6.

124. Dara P, Slater LM, Armentrout SA. Successful pregnancy during chemotherapy for acute leukemia, *Cancer.* 1981;**47**:845–6.

125. Baisogolov GD, Shishkin IP. Course of pregnancy and condition of infants born to patients treated for lymphogranulomatosis [Russian]. *Med Radiol (Mosk).* 1985;**30**:35–7.

126. Balcewicz-Sablinska K, Ciesluk S, Kopec I, Slomkowski M, Maj S. Analysis of pregnancy, labor, child development and disease course in women with Hodgkin's disease. *Acta Haematol Pol.* 1990;**21**:72–80.

127. Kozlowski RD, Steinbrunner J.V, MacKenzie AH, Clough JD, Wilke WS, Segal AM. Outcome of first-trimester exposure to low-dose methotrexate in eight patients with rheumatic disease. *Am J Med.* 1990;**88**:589–92.

128. Medkova J. Analysis of the health condition of the children born to the personnel exposed to cytostatics at an oncology unit. *Acta Univ Palacki Olomuc Fac Med.* 1991;**130**:323–32.

129. Sylvester GC, Khoury MJ, Lu X, Erickson JD. First trimester anesthesia exposure and the risk of central nervous system defects: a population based case control study. *Am J Public Health.* 1994;**84**:1757–60.

Chapter

21

Fertility of children exposed *in utero* to chemotherapy

Tal Schechter and Ronen Loebstein

Introduction

Concerns regarding gonadal function and reproductive capacity after *in utero* exposure to chemotherapy and radiation are emerging, and their exact full effects are not well defined. There is a lack of large, prospective studies to fully answer this question, and conclusions were made based on a few cohorts, heterogeneous patient populations and chemotherapy regimens, and substantial case report bias [1–5]. It is well known that most drugs reach the fetus in significant concentration after maternal administration as the placenta is not an effective barrier. Although, some authors agree the use of certain chemotherapy regimens (especially in the second or third trimester) is safe as the risk of acute or late complication are low, the risk in the first trimester is yet to be evaluated [1]. Fetal malformations have been reported in children born to mothers who received chemotherapy during the first trimester [1].

Safety guidelines of chemotherapy agents during pregnancy are based on relatively few cohorts and case reports. The effects of chemotherapy on the offsprings' gonadal function stem mainly from different reports of germ cell depletion after administration of alkylating agents in childhood cancer survivors. However, as most of these studies have focused on adults, it was unclear whether exposure to chemotherapy during early childhood and especially *in utero* is associated later with gonadal dysfunction.

Gonadal Function

It has been estimated that the dose of radiation required to destroy 50% of immature oocytes is less than 2 Gy [6]. Destruction of primordial follicles results in impaired ovarian hormone production due to inadequate estrogen exposure [6]. Bath *et al.* studied ovarian function in cancer survivors treated with total-body irradiation. Women with ovarian failure had small uterine volume and undetectable blood flow. Young girls who were exposed to irradiation prepuberty also did not respond well to a sex steroid replacement regimen [7]. In men, administration of alkylating agents with or without radiation to sites below the diaphragm was associated with a fertility deficit of approximately 60% [8]. The use of cyclophosphamide caused azoospermia or aspermia [9,10], and the use of chlorambucil caused permanent azoospermia [9,11]. Recovery of spermatogenesis was found in some patients who received extensive chemotherapy, but it was more likely to occur after 2 years from the last drug therapy [12]. However, antileukemic chemotherapy was found to be compatible with gonadal

Cancer in Pregnancy and Lactation: The Motherisk Guide ed. Gideon Koren and Michael Lishner.
Published by Cambridge University Press. © Cambridge University Press 2011.

development [13]. A retrospective study of more than 2,000 pediatric cancer survivors found them to be less likely to be pregnant compared to healthy controls [14]. However, as these data come from patients exposed to chemotherapy and radiation during childhood, it might not necessarily reflect gonadal function following *in utero* exposure to chemotherapy, especially during the period of gonadal formation (weeks 4–8), and it is not clear whether *in utero* exposure to chemotherapy puts a child at risk for deficits in gonadal function and fertility [15].

Sexual development

The information regarding fertility of adolescents and young adults who have been exposed *in utero* to chemotherapy is scarce [2–4]. This is mainly due to the relative rarity of such cases and the obvious difficulties of a long-term follow-up.

Studies in animals have shown that rats exposed to busulfan *in utero* manifested sex hormone deficiencies and sterility [16].

Recently, Aviles *et al.* reported a cohort of a long-term follow-up of 84 children born to mothers with hematological malignancies who received chemotherapy during pregnancy, including 38 during the first trimester. The follow-up period was 6–29 years (median 18.7 years). Chemotherapy exposure included a combination of cytarabine arabinoside and anthracyclines. All the children, including second-generation children, demonstrated normal growth and development according to height and weight developmental tables. Sexual characteristics demonstrated normal development in the adolescents and young adults, although the authors did not mention how sexual development was evaluated. Sixteen of the 84 patients were married with 12 second-generation children. All were considered to be normal [4].

A different study by Aviles *et al.* reported long-term follow-up of 17 children born to mothers with acute leukemia who received chemotherapy during pregnancy.

Eleven of 17 children received chemotherapy during organogenesis. The children aged 4–22 years have had normal growth and height development.

Two girls (ages 13 and 22) started normal menses. Physical and sexual examination of these individuals was considered normal. The 22-year-old subject gave birth to a normal baby girl [2].

Similar findings were reported by Blatt *et al.* who have reported normal growth and development in 448 children exposed *in utero* to chemotherapy. However, specific evaluation of gonadal function was not done [17].

References

1. Zemlickis D, Lishner M, Degendorfer P, Panzarella T, Sutcliffe SB, Koren G. Fetal outcome after in utero exposure to cancer chemotherapy. *Arch Intern Med.* 1992;**152**:573–6.

2. Aviles A, Niz J. Long-term follow up of children born to mothers with acute leukemia during pregnancy. *Med Pediatr Oncol.* 1988;**16**:3–6.

3. Aviles A, Diaz-Marqueo JC, Talavera A, Gurman R, Garcia EL. Growth and development of children of mothers treated with chemotherapy during pregnancy: current status of 43 children. *Am J Hematol.* 1991;**36**: 243–8.

4. Avila A, Neri N. Hematological malignancies and pregnancy: a final report of 84 children who received chemotherapy in utero. *Clin Lymphoma.* 2001;**2**:173–7.

5. Garber JE. Long-term follow-up of children exposed in utero to anitneoplastic agents. *Semin Oncol.* 1989;**16**:437–44.

6. Critchley HOD, Wallace WHB. Safety of pregnancy during and after cancer treatment: impact of cancer treatment on uterine function. *J Natl Cancer Inst Monogr.* 2005;**34**:64–8.

7. Bath LE, Critchely HO, Chambers SE, Anderson RA, Kelnar CJ, Wallace WH. Ovarian and uterine characteristics after total body irradiation in childhood and adolescence: response to sex steroid replacement. *Br J Obstet Gynacol.* 1999;**106**:1265–72.

8. Chapman RM, Sutcliffe SB, Malpas JS. Cytotoxic-induced ovarian failure in women with Hodgkin's disease I. Hormone function. *JAMA.* 1979;**242**:1877–81.

9. Miller DG. Alkylating agents and human spermatogenesis. *JAMA.* 1971;**217**:1662–5.

10. Fairley KF, Barrie JU, Johnson W. Sterility and testicular atrophy related to cyclophosphamide therapy. *Lancet.* 1972;**1**:568–9.

11. Richter P, Calamera JC, Morgenfeld MC, Kierszenbaum AL, Lavieri JC, Mancini RE. Effect of chlorambucil on spermatogenesis in the human with malignant lymphoma. *Cancer.* 1970;**25**:1026–30.

12. Sherins RJ, DeVita VT Jr. Effects of drug treatment for lymphoma on male reproductive capacity. Studies of men in remission after therapy. *Ann Intern Med.* 1973;**79**:216–20.

13. Blatt J, Poplack DG, Sherins RJ. Testicular function in boys after chemotherapy for acute lymphoblastic leukemia. *N Engl J Med.* 1981;**304**:1121–4.

14. Byrne J, Nulvihill JJ, Myers MH, et al. Effects of treatment on fertility in long-term survivors of childhood or adolescent cancer. *N Engl J Med.* 1987;**317**:1315–21.

15. Patridge AH, Garber JE. Long-term outcomes of children exposed to antineoplastic agents in utero. *Semin Oncol.* 2000;**27**:712–26.

16. Fujii T. Transgenerational effects of maternal exposure to chemicals on the functional development of the brain in the offspring. *Cancer Causes Control.* 1997;**8**:524–8.

17. Blatt J, Mulvihill JJ, Ziegler JL, Young RC, Poplack DG. Pregnancy outcome following cancer chemotherapy. *Am J Med.* 1980;**69**:828–32.

Chapter

22

Lactation and cancer chemotherapy

Taro Kamiya and Shinya Ito

Biological roles of breastfeeding

Compared to formula-fed infants, breastfed infants have reduced rates of bacterial infection. For example, necrotizing enterocolitis is less prevalent in premature infants who receive mother's milk than those who do not. In addition to these short-term benefits, breastfeeding is known to be associated with higher cognitive function in the infants that may be observed years after breastfeeding. The effect size is reportedly approximately 8 points in global IQ and other cognitive tests, which is approximately half of the standard deviation of the indices. This medium-size effect is too large to ignore. However, perception of these benefits varies widely among individual healthcare professionals and patients. Currently, it is recommended that breastfeeding continue for at least 12 months after birth [1].

Determinants of drug excretion into milk

Drug excretion mechanism

Diffusion

If the lactating mother requires drug therapy, safety of breastfed infants is a concern because almost all drugs the mother takes are excreted into milk. Of many factors that determine magnitude of drug excretion into milk, plasma protein binding, ionization characteristics and lipophilicity of drug are the most important. Namely, low plasma protein binding, cationic nature, and higher lipophilicity are often associated with higher degree of drug excretion into milk. This is because unbound drug molecules are subjected to diffusion and other membrane-mediated transfer processes, and milk is more acidic and lipid-rich than maternal plasma.

Carrier-mediated transport

Recently, expression and function of carrier-mediated drug transport in the mammary gland has been elucidated. For example, the lactating mammary gland highly expresses breast cancer resistant protein (BCRP: ABCG2), which carries its substrates from maternal circulation into milk. Initially, its role as a toxin transporter was perplexing as it appeared to actively contaminate mother's milk. However, a later study showed that BCRP in the mammary gland is a major vitamin B2 transporter [2]. Coupled with the fact that some organic cation transporters such as OCTN2 carry both some cationic drugs (i.e., xenobiotics)

Cancer in Pregnancy and Lactation: The Motherisk Guide ed. Gideon Koren and Michael Lishner.
Published by Cambridge University Press. © Cambridge University Press 2011.

and nutrients, main role of mammary gland drug transporters is a nutrient carrier function that is taken over by maternal xenobiotics. In addition to the above-mentioned attributes of drugs, such as protein binding and ionization characteristics, transporter affinity as a substrate is another important factor for defining milk excretion of drugs.

Milk-to-maternal plasma drug concentration ratio (MP Ratio)

Milk-to-maternal plasma ratio of drug concentrations (MP ratio) defines the propensity of drug excretion into milk. Usually, MP ratio is estimated from milk and plasma AUC (area under the curve), and expressed as an average parameter over a time period. Although higher MP ratio indicates a relatively increased level of drug excretion into milk, this index is often misunderstood as the key indicator for drug exposure levels of the infant.

Infant clearance

The MP ratio by itself is not a sole determinant of infant exposure levels for the following reasons. MP ratio is around 1 or less for most drugs, and rarely exceeds 5 [3]. This means that drug concentrations in milk are within the same magnitude as (or less than) those of maternal plasma. Average milk intake of the infant is approximately 150 ml/kg/day or even less. Multiplying this to the average milk drug concentrations gives an estimated daily dose/ kg of drug the infant would ingest through milk, which is invariably in a very low range compared to the therapeutic adult dose of the drug on a body weight basis. Then, the key question is how this estimated (low) dose of the infant through milk compares to the infant therapeutic dose. If the therapeutic plasma concentration of the drug is the same between adults and infants, the relation between the infant milk dose and the infant therapeutic dose (expressed as percentage, and called the Exposure Index) can be given by the following formula [4]:

$$EI(\%) = \text{MP ratio} \times 10/\text{infant clearance (expressed as ml/kg/min)}$$

where the coefficient 10 is derived from the average milk intake (150 ml/kg/day = 0.1 ml/ kg/min) multiplied by 100 to convert it to a percentage parameter. Given that MP ratio is 1 or less, EI becomes > 10% only when infant clearance is < 1 ml/kg/min. To reach therapeutic levels of exposure (i.e., EI = 100%), infant clearance needs to be < 0.1 ml/kg/ min. If MP ratio is 10 (incidentally, this is an extremely rare situation), EI becomes 100% (a therapeutic level) if infant clearance is 1 ml/kg/min. Overall, lower infant clearance is a major factor to push infant exposure levels above the therapeutic level. Thus, infant clearance needs to be taken into account when infant drug exposure through milk is considered.

Cancer chemotherapy in lactating women
Risk assessment

In developed countries, prevalent cancers in women of reproductive age include breast cancer, uterine cervix cancer, malignant melanoma, thyroid cancer, and malignant lymphomas [5,6]. Therefore, cancer chemotherapeutic agents used in these malignant diseases [7] are likely to pose challenges to clinicians treating these women during lactation. Risk assessment of drug therapy during lactation is characterized by several factors that are distinct from those of pregnancy. This also applies to cancer chemotherapy agents. First, average levels of drug exposure in the infant are usually an order of magnitude lower in lactation-mediated exposure than transplacental exposure. Second, the mother has an option to discontinue, or temporarily interrupt, breastfeeding if their risk perception is sufficiently high. Third, cancer chemotherapy schedules may allow breastfeeding women to store their own milk for near-future use. In addition, breastfeeding risk-benefit balance in women on cancer chemotherapy may be different from that of those on noncancer drugs. For example, the mother with cancer may feel more strongly about the precious values of breastfeeding than those without cancer. All these factors play a role in women's decision making.

Excretion of cancer chemotherapeutic agents into milk

Published clinical studies on excretion of cancer chemotherapy agents into milk, and resultant infant plasma levels, are very limited. Table 1 summarizes elimination half-life, oral bioavailability, and approximate plasma/serum concentrations of main chemotherapeutic agents. From these data, one may speculate the likelihood of significant oral absorption by the infant, and the length of time after the dose when milk levels may fall below certain levels. For example, after 5 times half-life, plasma concentrations will decline by > 95% of the initial level. If MP ratio is 1, then, milk levels will be also < 5% of the initial level. Although Table 1 provides some guidance, one must be fully aware of the lack of data on milk excretion and infant outcomes. Breastfeeding-related information is available for the following chemotherapeutic agents in cancer-treatment settings, but levels of evidence are not high enough to make firm recommendations. (Note that information exists for corticosteroids and some immunosuppressants during breastfeeding in noncancer treatment settings; this information is not discussed below.)

Drugs with data during breastfeeding
Cisplatin

There are 3 published case reports on use of cisplatin in lactating women with cancer [8–10]. At various post-dose time points, plasma cisplatin concentrations were measured as platinum. The maternal plasma levels ranged from 0.8 µg/ml to approximately 3 µg/ml, and expressed as platinum, but the MP ratio varied widely, from nearly 0 (milk levels were below the detection limit of platinum) to 1.1. Although these data do not allow us to capture an average pharmacokinetic pattern of cisplatin during lactation, several factors warrant discussion. First, oral absorption of cisplatin is thought to be approximately 30% [11]. But it is not known if this is the case in young infants. Second, whether measured levels of platinum represent cisplatin or other species of platinum is not known. Pharmacological profiles of different species of platinum are not the same. Third, the amount the infant would ingest through milk appears small. Cisplatin pharmacokinetic studies in nonlactating patients indicate that average plasma platinum concentrations after 100 mg/m^2 dosing (a high therapeutic dose) are about 3.91 ± 1.41 µg/ml [12]. Assuming the MP ratio to be the reported highest (i.e., 1.1) the infant would receive 4.3 mg/kg/day of platinum. Taken together, evidence of cisplatin safety/toxicity in breastfeeding is weak. Because of the relatively long half-life of cisplatin, most experts recommend discontinuation of breastfeeding, but emerging data on benefits of breastfeeding and lack of clear toxicity data may require revisiting the current recommendation.

Table 1. Selected pharmacokinetic parameters of cancer chemotherapeutic drugs (27–50)

Drug	Elimination half-life	Oral bioavailability	Peak plasma concentrations (dose)
Aldesleukin*	1.5 hr	Unknown	300 ng/ml (1 million IU/kg intravenously: 60 µg/kg)
Alemtuzumab	12 days	Unknown	26 µg/ml (30 mg/day 3 times weekly)
Amsacrine	5 hr	34%	1.25 µg/ml (100 mg/m^2)
Asparaginase	30 hr (*E. coli*) 16 hr (*Erwinia*) 7 days (PEG)	Unknown	60 IU/ml (5000 IU/kg)
Azacitidine	40 min	17.4%	750 ng/ml (75 mg/m^2 sc)
Bevacizumab	12–22 days	Unknown	280 µg/ml (10 mg/kg dose)
Bleomycin	2 hr	Unknown	2000 micro unit/ml (10-minute infusion of 15–30 unit), decreasing to 200–300 micro unit/ml in 2 hr postdose
Bortezomib	2–8 days	unknown	60–100 ng/ml (1 mg/m^2 twice-weekly)
Busulfan	1–4 hr	80%	1.2–10.4 µmol/L (1 mg/kg)
Carboplatin	5 days (Platinum)	4–12%	Steady-state level: 8–10 nmol/ml (320 mg/m^2)
Capecitabine	1 hr	60%	3–4 µg/ml (1,250 mg/m^2 orally): Concentrations of an active metabolite, fluorouracil, are 0.2–0.3 µg/ml
Carmustine	0.4 hr	Uknown	13 µg/ml (800mg/m^2)
Cetuximab	3–5 days	Unknown	200 µg/ml (400 mg/m^2 initial 250 mg/m^2 weekly)
Chlorambucil	2 hr	80%	1.1 µg/ml (0.6 mg/kg dose)
Cisplatin	5–12 days (Platinum)	30%	4 µg/ml (100 mg/m^2): see text
Cyclophosphamide	5–9 hr	60–90%	37 µg/ml (1,000 mg/m2 iv 1-hr infusion): see text
Cytarabine	2 hr	20%	4 µg/ml (3-hr infusion of 1000 mg/m^2)
Dacarbazine	5 hr	Unknown	1–6 µg/ml (0.5- to 6-hr infusion of 6 mg/kg)
Dasatinib	3–5 hr	Absorbed	40 ng/ml (100 mg/m^2)
Daunorubicin	16 hr	Unknown	360 ng/ml (1–1.5 mg/kg)
Doxetaxel	18 hr	8%**	3.7 µg/L (100mg/m^2 1–2 hr iv infusion)

Table 1. (cont.)

Drug	Elimination half-life	Oral bioavailability	Peak plasma concentrations (dose)
Doxorubicin	17.30 hr***	Unknown	19–35 µg/ml (30–50mg/m² iv every 4weeks): see text
Epirubicin	30 hr***	Unknown	1 µg/ml (intravenous injection of 75 mg/m²)
Erlotinib	10–30 hr	60%	3 µg/ml (200 mg/d)
Etoposide	7 hr	50–80%	20 µg/ml (150 mg/m² over 3.5-hr infusion): see text
Fludarabine	20 hr	60%	1.3 µg/ml# (30-min infusion of 25 mg/m²) 0.3–0.5 µg/ml# (50–90 mg orally)
5-FU	0.4 hr	0–80%	2.8–6.8 µg/ml (315–560 mg/m²:1 hr infusion)
Gefitinib	40 hr	60%	85 ng/ml (250 mg)
Gemcitabine	14 hr	10%	Steady-state level: 43.8 µM (800 mg/m²)
Hydroxyurea	4 hr	80%	130 µg/ml (80 mg/kg orally): see text
Idarubicin	***	20–30%	6–13 ng/ml (40–60 mg/m²)
Imatinib	18 hr	100%	2–4 µg/ml (400–600 mg/day orally): see text
Interferon Alfa	2 hr	Unknown	190 IU/ml (5 x 10⁶ IU/m² intravenously)
Irinotecan	8 hr	9%	1.4 µg/ml (90-min infusion 100 mg/m² weekly x 4)
Lomustine	1.5–75 hr	100%	0.5–2 µg/ml (metabolite) (30–130 mg/m²)
Methotrexate	8–10 hr	50%	0.45–4.5 µg/ml (100 mg/m² iv): see text
Mitoxantrone	215 hr	Unknown	0.6 µg/ml (15-min infusion of 14 mg/m²): see text
6-MP	1.5 hr	16–50%	15–150 ng/ml (75 mg/m² orally)
Oxaliplatin	270 hr (Platinum)	Unknown	1.61 µg/ml (85 mg/m²)
Paclitaxel	10–25 hr	< 6%**	2–12 µg/ml (3-hr infusion of 100–270 mg/m²)
nab-Paclitaxel	24 hr	Unknown	23 µg/ml (260 mg/m²)
Panitumumab	7.5 days	Unknown	200 µg/ml (6 mg/kg every 2 weeks)
Pemetrexed	3.5 hr	Unknown	67–250 ng/ml (600 mg/m² iv)
Porfimer	410–725 hr	Unknown	15–40 µg/ml (2 mg/kg)

Table 1. (*cont.*)

Drug	Elimination half-life	Oral bioavailability	Peak plasma concentrations (dose)
Procarbazine	10 min	100%	0.7 µg/ml (300 mg)
Rituximab	3 to 24 days[##]	Unknown	240–460 µg/ml (375 mg/m^2)
Tamoxifen	5–7 days	100%	65 ng/ml (40 mg)
Temozolomide	1.5 hr	>95%	7–13 µg/ml (100–250 mg/m^2 orally)
Thioguanine	11hr	14–46%	0.03–0.94 µM (100 mg/m^2 orally)
Trastuzmab	4 weeks	Unknown	110 mg/L (4 mg/kg initially followed by 2 mg/kg/wk)
Topotecan	3 hr	30%	140 ng/ml (30-min infusion of 4 mg/m^2)
Tretinoin	0.8 hr	50%	350 ng/ml (45 mg/m^2 orally)
Vinblastine	25 hr	Variable	>100 ng/ml (10-mg injection), declining to 5–40 ng/ml over the following 10 hr
Vincristine	80 hr	Variable	100 ng/ml (2–mg iv bolus)
Vinorelbine	1–2 days	45%	760 ng/ml, declining to 10 ng/ml range in 24 hr postdose (25 mg/m^2 intravenously).
Vorinostat	2 hr	43%	2.5 µmol/L (400 mg)

* : recombinant interleukin-2. Human milk contains physiological levels of endogenous IL-2, which range from 4 pg/ml to >3000 pg/ml, similar to those of maternal levels. Biological activity of IL-2 when ingested by the infant is poorly understood
** : significantly increases if combined with P-glycoprotein inhibitors
*** : terminal half-life
[#] : as an active metabolite (2F-ara-A: 2-fluoro-arabinofuranosyl-adenine)
[##] : longer after repeated doses

Cyclophosphamide

Three case reports of use of this drug during breastfeeding exist. However, there was no quantitative data on cyclophosphamide levels in milk [13–15]. A case exists of a woman with leukemia who received weekly intravenous doses of cyclophosphamide 800 mg and vincristine 2 mg over a 6-week period, in addition to prednisolone (30 mg/day). A 4-month-old infant was breastfed during this treatment cycle and was found to have neutropenia at the end of the treatment, which returned to normal after breastfeeding was discontinued [13]. In another patient with Burkitt lymphoma, who received daily cyclophosphamide 6 mg/kg intravenously for 7 days, the 23-day-old infant developed neutropenia and thrombocytopenia over the 3-day period. The limited information from these reports suggests that cyclophosphamide is not compatible with breastfeeding [14].

Doxorubicin

In milk samples of a woman receiving 70 mg/m^2 doxorubicin (an intravenous dose of 90 mg), the drug and its active metabolite, doxorubicinol, were detected. The peak milk concentration of doxorubicin and doxorubicinol were 128 µg/L (0.24 µM) and 111 µg/L (0.20 µM) 24 hours after the dose, respectively [8]. Anthracyclines may not be absorbed orally, and the dose to the infant, based on the peak levels, may be in the low range of 2% of the weight-adjusted dose. However, safety data are too sketchy to make a firm recommendation at this point.

Etoposide

A 28-year-old woman with acute promyelocytic leukemia received chemotherapy during pregnancy and breastfeeding [16]. She delivered a healthy baby at 34 weeks' gestation. After delivery she received second consolidation therapy. Then she was treated with etoposide (80 mg/m^2/day: days 1–5) and other drugs including mitoxantrone (6 mg/m^2/day: days 1–3) and cytarabine (170 mg/m^2/day: day 1–5) as third consolidation therapy. The post-infusion peak milk concentrations of etoposide ranged from 580 mg/L to 800 mg/L, which quickly declined and became undetectable in 24 hours. Breastfeeding was resumed 3 weeks after the end of the therapy without incident.

Mitoxantrone

In the same woman described above (Etoposide section), the mitoxantrone milk concentration reached 120 µg/ml immediately after the third dose. Mitoxantrone milk concentrations decreased to approximately 20 µg/ml by 7 days after the last (third) dose, and remained at that level 4 weeks after the last dose [16].

Hydroxyurea

A 29-year-old woman with chronic myelocytic leukemia received 500 mg of hydroxyurea orally 3 times a day. Hydroxyurea concentrations in milk obtained 2 hours after the last doses of the day ranged from 3.8 µg/ml to 8.4 µg/ml (mean, 6.1 µg/ml) [17].

Imatinib

After maternal oral doses of imatinib (400 mg/day), milk concentrations are approximately in the range of 0.5 µg/ml – 2.6 µg/ml. Its active metabolite is also in a similar range of concentrations (1µg/ml – 1.5 µg/ml). One infant was breastfed during the maternal imatinib treatment without incident [18–21].

Interferon alpha

A lactating woman with malignant melanoma received 30 million international units of interferon alpha-2B (IFN-α; 20 million IU/m^2) intravenously. A peak milk concentration was 1,551 IU/ml at 4 hours post-dose, which was higher than the average base-line level of 1,072 IU/ml. Given that milk contains various cytokines, it is unclear whether such an increase in milk levels after maternal use is of any significance [22].

Methotrexate

A 25-year-old woman with choriocarcinoma received 22.5 mg of methotrexate orally (15 mg/m^2/day). Peak methotrexate concentrations in milk samples were 2.6 ng/ml on 2 different dosing occasions [23]. In another case of a woman who received a single dose of 65 mg of methotrexate intramuscularly (50 mg/m^2) for an ectopic pregnancy, 6 milk samples over the following 24-hour period did not show detectable levels of the drug [24].

Information resources

To acquire specific information on drugs in breastfeeding, the Web-based data resource, known as LactMed [25], is useful, which is the most updated of all main information resources on the subject [26].

Summary

Studies on excretion of cancer chemotherapeutic agents into human milk are scarce, but accumulating evidence is overwhelmingly supportive of tangible benefit of human milk for infant development in various domains. Given the nature of the maternal diseases in question, risk-benefit assessment of breastfeeding during maternal chemotherapy needs to be carefully individualized.

References

1. Gartner LM, Morton J, Lawrence RA, et al. Breastfeeding and the use of human milk. *Pediatrics.* 2005;**115**:496–506.

2. van Herwaarden AE, Wagenaar E, Merino G, et al. Multidrug transporter ABCG2/breast cancer resistance protein secretion riboflavin (vitamin B2) into milk. *Mol Cell Biol.* 2007;**27**:1247–53.

3. Ito S. Drug therapy for breast-feeding women. *N Engl J Med.* 2000;**343**:118–26.

4. Ito S, Gideon K. A novel index for expressing exposure of the infant to drugs in breast milk. *Br J Clin Pharmacol.* 1994;**38**:99–102.

5. Canadian Cancer Sosiety's Steering Committee. *Canadian Cancer Statistics 2009.* Toronto: Canadian Cancer Society; 2009. April 2009. ISSN 0835-2976.

6. Cancer Care Ontario. *Cancer in Young Adults in Canada*, Toronto, Canada, 2006. May 2006. ISBN 0–921325–10-X (print), ISBN 0–921325–11-8 (pdf).

7. Cancer Care Ontario. 2010. Available from: http://cancercare.on.ca/

8. Egan PC, Costanza ME, Dodion P, Egorin MJ, Bachur NR. Doxorubicin and cisplatin excretion into human milk. *Cancer Treat Rep.* 1985;**69**:1387–9.

9. Ben-Baruch G, Menczer J, Goshen R, Kaufman B, Gorodetsky R. Cisplatin excretion in human milk. *J Natl Cancer Inst.* 1992;**84**:451–2.

10. de Vries EG, van der Zee AG, Uges DR, Sleijfer DT. Excretion of platinum into breast milk. *Lancet.* 1989;**1**:497.

11. Urien S, Brain E, Bugat R, et al. Pharmacokinetics of platinum after oral or intravenous cisplatin; a phase 1 study in 32 adult patients. *Cancer Chemother Pharmacol.* 2005;**55**:55–60.

12. Ostrow S, Egorin M, Aisner M, Bachur N, Wienik PH. High-dose cis-diamminedichloro-platinum therapy in patients with advanced breast cancer: pharmacokinetics, toxicity, and therapeutic efficacy. *Cancer Clin Trials.* 1980;**3**:23–7.

13. Amato D, Niblett JS. Neutropenia from cyclophosphamide in breast milk. *Med J Aust.* 1977;**1**:383–4.

14. Durodola JL. Administration of cyclophosphamide during late pregnancy and early lactation: a case report. *J Natl Med Assoc.* 1979;**71**:165–6.

15. Wiernik PH, Duncan JH. Cyclophosphamide in human milk. *Lancet.* 1971;**1**:912.

16. Azuno Y, Kaku K, Fujita N, Okubo M, Kaneko T, Matsumoto N. Mitoxantrone and etoposide in breast milk. *Am J Hematol.* 1995;**48**:131–2.

17. Sylvester RK, Lobell M, Teresi ME, Brundage D, Bubowy R. Excretion of hydroxyurea into milk. *Cancer.* 1987;**60**:2177–8.

18. Kronenberger R, Schleyer E, Bornhäuser M, Ehninger G, Gattermann N, Blum S. Imatinib in breast milk. *Ann Hematol.* 2009;**88**:1265–6.

19. Ali R, Ozkalemkas F, Kimya Y, et al. Imatinib use during pregnancy and breast feeding: a case report and review of the literature. *Arch Gynecol Obstet.* 2009;**280**:169–75.

20. Russell MA, Garpenter MW, Akhtar MS, Lagattula TF, Egorin MJ. Imatinib mesylate and metabolite concentrations in maternal blood, umbilical cord blood, placenta and breast milk. *J Perinatol.* 2007;**27**:241–3.

21. Gambacorti-Passerini CB, Tornaghi L, Marangon E, et al. Imatinib concentrations in human milk. *Blood.* 2007;**109**:1790.

22. Kumar AR, Hale TW, Mock RE. Transfer of interferon Alfa into human breast milk. *J Hum Lact.* 2000;**16**:226–8.

23. Johns DG, Rutherford LD, Leighton PC, Vogel CL. Secretion of methotrexate into human milk. *Am J Obstet Gynecol.* 1972;**112**:978–80.

24. Tanaka T, Walsh W, Verjee Z, et al. Methotrexate use in a lactating woman with an ectopic pregnancy. *Birth Defects Res A Clin Mol Teratol.* **85**:494.

25. LactMed. Available from: http://toxnet. nlm.nih.gov/cgi-bin/sis/htmlgen?LACT

26. Akus M, Bartick M. Lactation safety recommendations and reliability compared in 10 medication resources. *Ann Pharmacother.* 2007;**41**:1352–60.

27. Lyseng-Williamson K, Jarvis B. *Imatinib. Drugs.* 2001;**61**:1765–73.

28. Konrad MW, Hemstreet G, Hersh EM, et al. Pharmacokinetics of recombinant interleukin-2 in humans. *Cancer Res.* 1990;**50**:2009–17.

29. Nagar S. Pharmacokinetics of anti-cancer drugs used in cancer chemotherapy. *Adv Exp Biol.* 2010;**678**:124–32.

30. Malingre MM, Beijnen JH, Schellens JH. Oral delivery of taxanes. *Invest New Drugs.* 2001;**19**:155–63.

31. DeMario MD, Ratain MJ. Oral chemotherapy: rationale and future directions. *J Clin Oncol.* 1998;**16**:2557–67.

32. Weibe VJ, Benz CC, DeGregorio MW. Clinical pharmacokinetics of drugs used in the treatment of breast cancer. *Clin Pharmacokinet.* 1988;**15**:180–93.

33. Morello KC, Wurz GT, DeGregorio MW. Pharmacokinetics of selective estrogen receptor modulators. *Clin Pharmacokinet.* 2003;**42**:361–72.

34. McKeage K, Perry CM. Trastuzumab: a review of its use in the treatment of metastatic breast cancer overexpressing HER2. *Drugs.* 2002;**62**:209–43.

35. Anderson VR, Perry CM. Fludarabine: a review of its use in non-Hodgkin's lymphoma. *Drugs.* 2007;**67**:1633–55.

36. Robert J. Clinical pharmacokinetics of epirubicin. *Clin Pharmacokinet.* 1994;**26**:428–38.

37. Braess J, Freud M, Hanauske A, et al. Oral cytarabine ocfosate in acute myeloid leukemia and non-Hodgkin's lymphoma-phase I/II studies and pharmacokinetics. *Leukemia.* 1998;**12**:1618–26.

38. Cartron G, Blasco H, Paintaud G, Watier H, Le Guellec C. Pharmacokinetics of rituximab and its clinical use: thought for the best use? *Crit Rev Oncol Hematol.* 2007;**62**:43–52.

39. Gwilt PR, Tracewell WG. Pharmacokinetics and pharmacodynamics of hydroxyurea. *Clin Pharmacokinet.* 1998;**34**:347–58.

40. Dhodapkar M, Rubin J, Reid JM, et al. Phase I trial of temozolomide (NSC 362856) in patients with advanced cancer. *Clin Cancer Res.* 1997;**3**: 1093–100.

41. Loo TL, Housholder GE, Gerulath AH, Saunders PH, Farquhar D. Mechanism of action and pharmacology studies with DTIC (NSC-45388). *Cancer Treat Rep.* 1976;**60**:149–52.

42. Ostrow S, Egorin M, Aisner J, Bachur N, Wienik PH. High-does cis-diamminedichloroplatinum therapy in patients with advanced breast cancer: Pharmacokinetics, toxicity, and therapeutic efficacy. *Cancer Clin Trials.* 1980;**3**:23–7.

43. Muindi JR, Frankel SR, Huselton C, et al. Clinical pharmacology of oral all-trans

retinoic acid in patients with acute promyelocytic leukemia. *Cancer Res.* 1992;**52**:2138–42.

44. Siddiqui MA, Scott LJ. Azacitidine: in myelodysplastic syndromes. *Drugs.* 2005;**65**:1781–9.

45. Linssen P, Brons P, Knops G, Wessels H, de Witte T. Plasma and cellular pharmacokinetics of m-AMSA related to in vitro toxicity towards normal and leukemic clonogenic bone marrow cells (CFU-GM, CFU-L). *Eur J Haematol.* 1993;**50**:149–54.

46. Frampton JE, Wagstaff AJ. Alemtuzumab. *Drugs.* 2003;**63**:1229–43.

47. Reynolds NA, Wagstaff AJ. Cetuximab: in the treatment of metastatic colorectal cancer. *Drugs.* 2004;**64**: 109–18.

48. Burz C, Berindan-Neagoe IB, Balacescu O, et al. Clinical and Pharmacokinetics study of oxaliplatin in colon cancer patients. *J Gastrointestin Liver Dis.* 2009;**18**:39–43.

49. Grochow LB, Jones RJ, Brundrett RB, et al. Pharmacokinetics of busulfan: correlation with veno-occlusive disease in patients undergoing bone marrow transplantation. *Cancer Chemother Pharmacol.* 1989; **25**:55–61.

50. Preiss R, Baumann F, Regenthal R, Matthias M. Plasma kinetics of procarbazine and azo-procarbazine in humans. *Anticancer Drugs.* 2006;**17**: 75–80.

Breast cancer and pregnancy: critical review of the effects of prior and subsequent pregnancy on the prognosis of young women with breast tumor

Nava Siegelmann-Danieli and Ronen Loebstein

Introduction

Pregnancy-associated breast cancer (PABC) is defined as breast malignancy diagnosed during pregnancy, within a year to delivery, or at any time during lactation. Those tumors present a challenging clinical situation, and recommendations for staging workup and local and systemic therapy require the consideration of the welfare of both the mother and her fetus. Whereas patients with PABC often present with poorer survival rates as compared with affected young nonpregnant individuals, there is a debate whether pregnancy per se is a poor prognostic factor or mediates dismal outcome due to association with advanced stage at diagnosis and frequent treatment delays. Similar dismal tumors may occur also in young women susceptible to develop breast tumors in association with ovarian stimulation by fertility drugs, suggesting a common mechanism for breast cancer development in a subgroup of susceptible young women exposed to high levels of endogenous estrogens.

The effect of subsequent pregnancy on the outcome of a premenopausal woman with a history of breast cancer has been suggested to be "protective" in several series mostly in otherwise "healthy mothers" with early breast tumors. At the current time, no solid conclusions can be made with regard to safety in estrogen receptor (ER) -positive disease, especially node-positive disease.

Breast cancer is the most common female malignancy worldwide, expected to affect 207,090 women in the United States in the year 2010 with a median age at diagnosis of 61 years [1]. Although disease occurrence is linked to female sex hormones and reproductive factors [2–5], most patients are diagnosed during their postmenopausal years when potent estrogens are no longer produced by the ovaries. Only 1.9% of tumors occur in women aged 20–34 years, and 10.5% in those aged 35–44 years. Molecular profiling of breast tumors suggests that several disease subtypes exist, each with distinct pathogenesis mechanisms, biological phenotypes, and clinical outcomes. They include the luminal A and B subtypes characterized by expression of estrogen receptors (ER) and genes related to their effect; the Her2 subtype with negative ER expression and overexpression of genes located at the Her2 amplicon; normal breast-like tumors; and the basal-like subtype associated with lack of

Cancer in Pregnancy and Lactation: The Motherisk Guide ed. Gideon Koren and Michael Lishner.
Published by Cambridge University Press. © Cambridge University Press 2011.

expression of ER, progesterone receptors (PR), and Her2 proto-oncogene (also named "triple negative") and frequent expression of cytokeratins 5/6 [6,7]. At the current time, no specific subtype has been assigned specifically to cases developing during pregnancy and lactation. Still, tumors occurring at younger ages (<35 years of age) are more often ER and PR negative, with high histological grade, and with vascular and lymphatic invasion [8] compared with tumors of women 35–50 years old. In addition, cases associated with germ line mutation at the *BRCA1* gene [9] and tumors developing in African Americans 20–34 years old [10] show a higher proportion of "triple negative" phenotypes.

PABC is one of the most common cancers associated with pregnancy. Still, it is a relatively uncommon event complicating 1 in 3,000 pregnancies; only 0.2–2.8% of premenopausal tumors occur during pregnancy, while 10–20% of those developing in women aged 30 and younger occur in association with pregnancy and lactation [11–13]. The incidence of PABC is expected to rise as more women delay child-bearing; it reflects the increased incidence of breast tumors with advancing age [14]. The effect of pregnancy on breast cancer risk is thought to be bi-directional and time dependent, with early increased risk and subsequent later protection [15]; epidemiology data suggest protective effect of young age at first full-term pregnancy, multiple pregnancies (mostly in Western series but not in some Middle East populations) [16,17], and lactation. Potential biological explanations, which include transient immune alternation during pregnancy [18], genetic susceptibility with absence of insulin-like growth factor-1 19 allele repeat [19], changes in the number of breast stem cells [20], and maturation of mammary buds during first pregnancy [21], are beyond the scope of current review.

The literature on the prognostic significance of PABC is far from being consistent. In addition, the topic of subsequent pregnancy in young patients who remain fertile following therapy for nonmetastatic disease is of major importance for recovering women who wish to conceive. Herein we review those two topics.

Methods

Updated literature reviews of the MEDLINE database on those 2 topics from 1966 to December 31, 2010 were conducted. We focused on series of at least 50 patients with PABC, which analyzed data after adjusting for known prognostic confounders. We assessed separately the effect of prior and subsequent pregnancies on the prognosis of breast cancer.

Effects of prior pregnancy on the prognosis of women with breast cancer

Older series suggested pregnancy as a poor prognostic indicator. In a multicenter study, 407 women aged 20–29 who were pregnant before the diagnosis of breast cancer, were followed at 1 of 9 cancer centers between 1978 and 1988 [22]. After adjusting for tumor size, axillary nodal status, and ER expression, the calculated 5-year survival rates of patients who were pregnant at the time of breast cancer diagnosis were significantly lower than that of patients with remote pregnancies (40% vs. 65%; $P = 0.0005$). These differences became even more pronounced when PABC patients were compared to patients who had not conceived before (5-year survival rates of 40% vs. 74%; $P = 0.0001$). Adjusted analysis considering tumor size and lymph node status suggested that shorter time elapsed since last pregnancy has inverse correlation with survival.

A population-based analysis [23] following close to 5,000 young women, reported reduced survival in women diagnosed in the first 2 years following the last childbirth, compared with patients who gave birth 5 or more years previously (relative risk = 1.58, 95% confidence interval [CI]: 1.24–2.02). Findings persisted after adjusting for tumor characteristics (tumor size, number of positive axillary nodes, and histology grade) and adjuvant chemotherapy use. The worse outcome was assigned to women diagnosed within a year to delivery with hazards ratio of 2.1 for death; it was 1.3 for women diagnosed within the second year to delivery.

The prognostic significance of time interval elapsed since last pregnancy and breast cancer diagnosis was further emphasized by different independent reports including together 411 patients with PABC, all of which have demonstrated significantly lower 5-year survival rates compared with age- and stage-matched controls [24–29]. Worthy to note, however, a consistent tendency for a more advanced disease in women with PABC compared to those who had remote pregnancies [25,28,30] reflecting possible delays in diagnosis and managements of women with PABC. Still, however, after correcting for this confounder, recent pregnancy seemed a poor prognostic indicator.

More recent series (mostly after the 90th), where patients are exposed to modern systemic therapy, suggest that while patients with PABC still present with poor prognostic features and advanced stages, the significance of pregnancy per se may be either lost or attenuated. A Canadian series reported the outcome of 118 women with PABC and compared them with 269 nonpregnant patients matched for stage of disease, age, and therapeutic protocol [31]. Although tumors of PABC patients presented with more advanced disease, the 5-, 10-, and 25-year survival rates did not significantly differ between the pregnant and nonpregnant groups after correction for known prognostic factors ($P = 0.6$). An Israeli series compared 22 patients diagnosed with 23 tumors during pregnancy or lactation, 38 patients with 40 breast carcinomas diagnosed subsequent to ovarian stimulation with fertility drug therapy (FDT), with 192 "controls" diagnosed with 201 tumors; groups were matched for patient age and treatment period and modern systemic treatment approach was assigned to all patients [32]. Compared with tumors of "controls," those diagnosed in association with recent pregnancy or recent (<2 years) FDT, tended to occur more frequent in non-Ashkenazi and non-Jewish populations, present with higher tumor stages, lack the expression of the female sex hormone receptors, and display poor histological grade. In multivariate analysis considering patients approached with curative intent, only tumor stage correlated with outcome. An American series [33] compared outcome of 104 young women (<35 years of age) with localized non-inflammatory breast tumors diagnosed in association of pregnancy and lactation, with those of 546 nonpregnant young women. Again, pregnancy was associated with more advanced stages at diagnosis and delays in treatment initiation. Still, it was not an independent prognostic factor. The California Cancer Registry [34] (1991–1999) identified 797 PABC cases and compared them with 4,177 controls. Women with PABC were significantly more likely to present with advanced, larger tumors and ER-negative disease. In survival analysis, PABC had higher death rates as compared with controls (39% vs. 33%, respectively, $P = 0.002$). When controlled for stage, race, and ER status, PABC had only slightly higher (hazard ratio = 1.14) higher risk of death.

Three independent reports including 304 PABC patients also suggested that pregnancy is not an independent prognostic factor [35–37]. However, it is important to recognize the significant limitations of these reports, some of which did not include a control group [36], while others [35,37] suffered from a limited sample size; therefore, subanalysis to determine the influence of important confounders as an independent prognostic factor was not possible.

Overall dismal prognostic features are associated with tumors categorized as PABC, including advanced stages, larger tumors, increased proportions of Grade III histology, and ER-negative disease. The prognostic significance of pregnancy *per se* is suggestive but not conclusive, and its effect is mostly lost in modern series with contemporary treatment approaches.

Effects of subsequent pregnancy on prognosis of women with breast cancer

Concerns that subsequent pregnancy will adversely influence the survival of patients previously suffering from breast carcinoma is based on the hypothesis that gestational hormonal changes may stimulate the growth of residual tumor cells.

A meta-analysis considering retrospective control-matched population-based and hospital-based studies [38] recently published statistics aimed to evaluate the impact of pregnancy on the overall survival of women with a history of breast cancer. The search considered a literature review of complete reports between 1970 and up to September 2009 and identified 1,244 women who became pregnant following breast cancer diagnosis and a "control" group of 18,145 patients. Of the 14 studies included, 7 were case-controls matched for stage, age, and year of diagnosis; 4 requested that controls survived at least to the period up to time of pregnancy of matched cases; and 3 requested that controls were cancer free at least to the time to pregnancy of their matched cases. None of the studies controlled for ER and Her2 expression. Although the pooled relative risk (RR) for death was 0.59, suggesting a "protective" effect of subsequent pregnancy, significant heterogeneity was evident. Correcting for patients who were relapse-free at time of inclusion (and therefore limiting the selection bias of "healthy mothers" who became pregnant) revealed RR for death of 0.85 (15% nonsignificant risk reduction); the risk reduction was evident mostly with node-negative tumors (RR = 0.63) but not in node-positive tumors (RR = 0.96). A subgroup analysis to address the optimal time to become pregnant used data from 5 studies and included 187 and 352 patients who became pregnant within 6–24 months and after 2 years of breast cancer diagnosis, respectively. Findings were similar in both groups, although heterogeneity was significant in the earlier group. The major limitations include the lack of information regarding ER status in the studies analyzed, which hampers solid conclusions in patients with ER-positive tumors; analysis based on published reports rather than original patients' data; and lack of matching for the ER PR and Her2 proto-oncogene.

Another large series [39] collected information from population-based registries in Singapore (n = 319,437) and Sweden (n = 11 million) and identified 492 patients who became pregnant over a year from diagnosis. With a median follow-up of 14 years, women with subsequent child birth had a lower 15-year cumulative mortality rate than other women (16.8 vs. 40.7%, respectively), although their chances of dying were 14 times higher compared with healthy population. Mortality was associated with time elapsed since breast cancer diagnosis, and it was 3-fold higher in women who gave birth within 1–2 years to diagnosis compared with those who delivered 4 or more years from diagnosis. Another recently published large series from a Northern California prepaid healthcare program on 107 women with 1 or more subsequent pregnancies and 344 controls without pregnancy matched for stage at diagnosis, months of survival, and recurrence status at conception.

Results with median follow-up periods of 11–12 years suggested that, while neither risk of recurrence nor death differed significantly by subsequent pregnancy, in a subgroup of women conceiving within 12 months to diagnosis, a nonsignificant adverse effect was seen (RR for recurrence = 1.5) [40].

In conclusion, most data suggest a noninferior outcome in women who subsequently became pregnant, as long as pregnancy was delayed 1–2 years from diagnosis, and possible "protective" effect if tumors were node-negative. Solid conclusions for ER-positive tumors, especially regional advanced, cannot be concluded.

References

1. Altekruse SF, Kosary CL, Krapcho M, et al. editors. *SEER Cancer Statistics Review, 1975–2007*. Bethesda, MD: National Cancer Institute. Available from: http://seer.cancer.gov/csr/1975_2007/, based on November 2009 SEER data submission, posted to the SEER web site, 2010.

2. Zemlickis D, Lishner M, Degendorfer P, Panzarella T, Sutcliffe SB, Koren G. Maternal and fetal outcome following breast cancer in pregnancy. In: Koren G, Lishner M, Farine D, editors. *Cancer in pregnancy*. New York: Cambridge University Press; pp. 95–106.

3. Bergqvist L, Adami HO, Persson I, Hoover R, Schairer C. The risk of breast cancer after estrogen and estrogen-progestin replacement. *N Engl J Med.* 1989;**321**:293–7.

4. Ewertz M, Duffy SW, Adami HO, et al. Age at first birth, parity and risk of breast cancer: a meta-analysis of 8 studies from the nordic countries. *Int J Cancer.* 1990;**46**:597–603.

5. Kelsey JL, Gammon MD, John EM. Reproductive factors and breast cancer. *Epidemiol Rev.* 1993;**15**:36–47.

6. Sørlie T, Perou CM, Tibshirani R, et al. Gene expression patterns of breast carcinomas distinguish tumor subclasses with clinical implications. *Proc Natl Acad Sci U S A.* 2001;**98**:10869–74.

7. Perou CM, Sørlie T, Eisen MB, et al. Molecular portraits of human breast tumours. *Nature.* 2000;**406**:747–52.

8. Colleoni M, Rotmensz N, Robertson C, et al. Very young women (<35 years) with operable breast cancer: features of disease at presentation. *Ann Oncol.* 2002;**13**:273–9.

9. Hedenfalk I, Duggan D, Chen Y, et al. Gene expression profiles in hereditary breast cancer. *N Engl J Med.* 2001;**344**:539–48.

10. Lund MJ, Trivers KF, Porter PL, et al. Race and triple negative threat to breast cancer survival: a population-based study in Atlanta, GA. *Breast Cancer Res Treat.* 2009;**113**:357–70.

11. Reis, L, Hankey, BF, Miller, BA et al. *Cancer statistics review 1973–1988.* Bethesda, MD: National Cancer Institute. NIH publication 91–2789, III.39, 1991.

12. Saunders CM, Baum M. Breast cancer and pregnancy: a review. *J R Soc Med.* 1993;**86**:162–5.

13. Stensheim H, Møller B, van Dijk T, Fossa SD Cause-specific survival for women diagnosed with cancer during pregnancy or lactation: a registry-based cohort study. *J Clin Oncol.* 2009;**27**:45–51.

14. Andersson TM, Joansson AL, Hsieh CC, Cnattingius S, Lambe M. Increasing incidence of pregnancy associated breast cancer in Sweden. *Ostet Gynecol.* 2009;**114**:568–72.

15. Lyons TR, Schedin PJ, Borges VF. Pregnancy and breast cancer: when they collide. *J Mammary Gland Biol Neoplasia.* 2009;**14**:87–98.

16. Labidi SI, Mrad K, Mezlini A, et al. Inflammatory breast cancer in Tunisia in the era of multimodality therapy. *Ann Oncol.* 2008;**19**:473–80.

17. Majid RA, Mohammed HA, Saeed HM, Safar BM, Rashid RM, Hughson MD. Breast cancer in Kurdish women of Northern Iraq: incidence, clinical stage, and case control analysis of parity and family risk. *BMC Womens Health.* 2009;**9**:33.

18. Shakhar K, Valdimarsdottir HB, Bovbjerg DH. Heightened risk of breast cancer following pregnancy: could lasting immune alterations contribute? *Cancer Epidemiol Boimarkers Prev.* 2007;**16**:1082–6.

19. Bageman E, Ingvar C, Rose C, Jernstrom H. Absence of the common insulin-like growth factor-1 19 repeat allele is associated with early age at breast cancer diagnosis in multiparous women. *Br J Cancer.* 2007;**96**:712–7.

20. Sjwko SK, Dong J, Lewis MT, Hilsenbeck SG, Li Y. Evidence that an early pregnancy causes a persistent decrease in the number of functional mammary epithelial stem cells – implications for pregnancy-induced protection against breast cancer. *Stem Cells.* 2008;**26**:3205–9.

21. Russo J, Russo IH. Breast development, hormones and cancer. *Adv Exp Med Biol.* 2008;**630**:52–6.

22. Guinee VF, Olsson H, Moller T, et al. Effect of pregnancy on prognosis for young women with breast cancer. *Lancet.* 1994;**343**:1587–9.

23. Kroman N, Wohlfahrt J, Andersen KW, Mouridsen HT, Westergaard T, Melbye M. Time since childbirth and prognosis in primary breast cancer: population-based study. *BMJ.* 1997;**315**:851–5.

24. Tretli S, Kvalheim G, Thoresen S, Host H. Survival of breast cancer patients diagnosed during pregnancy or lactation. *Br J Cancer.* 1988;**58**:382–4.

25. Anderson BO, Petrek JA, Byrd DR, Senie RT, Borgen PI. Pregnancy influences breast cancer stage at diagnosis in women 30 years of age and younger. *Ann Surg Oncol.* 1996;**3**:204–11.

26. Clark RM, Chua T. Breast cancer and pregnancy: the ultimate challenge. *Clin Oncol (R Coll Radiol).* 1989;**1**:11–8.

27. Makita M, Sakamoto G, Namba K, et al. [Study of breast cancer during pregnancy and lactation]. *Gan No Rinsho.* 1990;**36**:39–44.

28. Bonnier P, Romain S, Dilhuydy JM, et al. Influence of pregnancy on the outcome of breast cancer: a case-control study. *Int J Cancer.* 1997;**72**:720–7.

29. Ishida T, Yokoe T, Kasumi F, et al. Clinicopathologic characteristics and prognosis of breast cancer patients associated with pregnancy and lactation: analysis of case-control study in Japan. *Jpn J Cancer Res.* 1992;**83**:1143–9.

30. Petrek JA, Dukoff R, Rogatko A. Prognosis of pregnancy-associated breast cancer. *Cancer.* 1991;**67**:869–72.

31. Zemlickis D, Lishner M, Degendorfer P, et al. Maternal and fetal outcome after breast cancer in pregnancy. *Am J Obstet Gynecol.* 1992;**166**:781–7.

32. Siegelmann-Danieli N, Tamir A, Zohar H, et al. Breast cancer in women with recent exposure to fertility medications is associated with poor prognostic features. *Ann Surg Oncol.* 2003;**10**:1031–8.

33. Beadle BM, Woodward WA, Middleton LP, et al. The impact of pregnancy on breast cancer outcome in women<or=35 years. *Cancer.* 2009;**115**:1174–84.

34. Rodriguez AO, Chew H, Cress R, et al. Evidence of poorer survival in pregnancy-associated breast cancer. *Obstet Gynecol.* 2008;**112**:71–8.

35. von Schoultz E, Johansson H, Wilking N, Rutqvist LE. Influence of prior and subsequent pregnancy on breast cancer prognosis. *J Clin Oncol.* 1995;**13**:430–4.

36. Ribeiro G, Jones DA, Jones M. Carcinoma of the breast associated with pregnancy. *Br J Surg.* 1986;**73**:607–9.

37. King RM, Welch JS, Martin JK Jr, Coulam CB. Carcinoma of the breast associated with pregnancy. *Surg Gynecol Obstet.* 1985;**160**:228–32.

38. Azim HA Jr, Santoro L, Pavlidis N, et al. Safety of pregnancy following breast cancer diagnosis: a meta-analysis of 14 studies. *Eur J Cancer.* 2011;**47**:74–83.

39. Verkooijen HM, Lim GH, Czene K, et al. Effect of childbirth after treatment on long-term survival from breast cancer. *Br J Surg.* 2010;**97**:1253–9.

40. Kranick JA, Schaefer C, Rowell S, et al. Is pregnancy after breast cancer safe? *Breast J.* 2010;**16**:404–11.

Chapter

24

Effects of the placenta on metastatic breast cancer

Shelly Tartakover-Matalon, Liat Drucker, and Michael Lishner

Controversies regarding breast cancer during pregnancy

Cancer and pregnancy coincide relatively rarely, approximately 1 in 1,000 pregnancies [1,2]. However, the current trend of delaying pregnancy, accompanied by age-related increases in the incidence of many malignancies is expected to increase the incidence of pregnancy-associated cancer [1]. The most common malignancies associated with pregnancy are breast (PABC), cervical cancer, melanoma, and hematological cancers (Table 1) [3–5]. Most malignancies diagnosed during pregnancy and/or lactation do not carry an increased risk of mortality, except for patients diagnosed with PABC or with ovarian cancer during lactation [3]. Women with PABC have a 2.5-fold higher likelihood of being diagnosed with metastatic disease than do nonpregnant women [6]. Furthermore, PABC biopsy specimens exhibit poor histologic and prognostic features [1]. These histological parameters do not differ significantly from those of age-matched, nonpregnant women with breast cancer [6], nevertheless, a higher incidence of estrogen receptor (ER) -negative cancer is observed in pregnant compared to nonpregnant women [7].

The reason for this is not clear. ER levels are regulated by estrogen [8], and breast cancer cells that are exposed to estrogen have reduced ER expression [9]. Thus, the reduced ER expression may reflect the unique hormonal environment of pregnancy. Knowledge of the critical effect of estrogen on breast cancer biology may suggest that it is an additional reason for the advanced stage of cancer often diagnosed during pregnancy [10]. Such observations indicate that pregnancy may affect breast cancer prognosis. However, controversies exist regarding this issue. Some researchers have reported that women diagnosed during pregnancy have worse maternal outcomes, while others did not find such an affect [11]. These differences may be related to variations in research design, as some studies included women diagnosed during pregnancy, and others included women who were postpartum, lactating, or within one year of parturition [11]. Furthermore, controversy exists regarding the cause of advanced PABC, which may be due to delayed diagnosis because of changes in breast morphology during pregnancy and/or to alterations in body physiology and to the unique hormonal and cytokine microenvironment during that period [11]. Alternatively, Schedin *et al.* suggested that mammary gland involution is responsible for accelerating breast cancer postpartum.

Mammary gland involution uses some of the same tissue-remodeling programs that are activated during wound healing and inflammation [11]. These similarities include macrophage cell influx, elevated levels of tumor growth factor beta (TGF-β), matrix

Cancer in Pregnancy and Lactation: The Motherisk Guide ed. Gideon Koren and Michael Lishner. Published by Cambridge University Press. © Cambridge University Press 2011.

Table 1. Most frequent cancer diseases during pregnancy

Reference	Source of data	Years	Number of patients	Most common malignancies
Ref 2	California (100%) Population-based study. Computer linkage of maternal/neonatal hospital discharge and birth/death records with case files in the California Cancer Registry	1991–1999	Pregnancy + Post partum N=4539	Melanoma (9.3%) Thyroid (15.3%) Cervix (12.7%) **Breast (20.3%)**
Ref 3	Norway (100%) Population-based cohort study Cancer Registry and the Medical Birth Registry of Norway	1967–2002	Pregnancy + Lactation N=1047	Melanoma (27.3%) Cervix (18.2%) **Breast (10.3%)** Hematologic malignancies (9.5%)
Ref 4	Belgium (68.4%), Czech (6.0%), Netherland (25.6%) International collaborative between the Hospitals: Leuven Belgium Nijmegen the Netherlands Prague, Czech Republic	1998–2008	Pregnancy N=215	Invasive cancers: **Breast (46%)** Hematologic malignancies (18%) Cervix (8%) Melanoma (5.1%)

metalloproteinases (MMPs), bioactive proteolytic fragments of the extracellular matrix (ECM) proteins, fibronectin, and laminin. Such a microenvironment may accelerate and support tumor progression [11]. Whatever the explanation is, the interactions between pregnancy and breast cancer are extremely complex and varied [11]. Pregnancy before the mid-20s reduces the risk of future breast cancer. However, pregnancy at any age is followed by a transient increase in breast cancer risk for a few years [12,13]. Delay in diagnosis cannot be responsible for these effects and the biological mechanisms underlying the role of pregnancy in breast cancer etiology are not yet clear. In summary, opinions about the effects of pregnancy on breast cancer etiology are variable and controversial. Clarification of these issues requires systematic experimentation that will analyze the effects of each chosen parameter on a well-controlled biological system.

Placental metastasis from maternal primary cancer

A major concern associated with PABC is the possibility that the malignancy will affect the fetus. However, metastasis to the products of conception (placenta and embryo) is rare [14]. Over the past few years, several published reviews have described almost 100 cases of maternal tumor metastasis to the placenta and/or fetus [15–19]. Although breast cancer is one of the most common malignancy in pregnancy, melanoma is by far the most frequent malignancy to involve the placenta [5,14,15], accounting for 31% of cases [15], followed by lung 12–17% [15,16–19], hematological 14.5–17%) [15,16–19] and breast cancers (12–17%) [15] The number of reports in the literature is increasing, with more than 20% of the patient cases being reported in the last decade [15]. Placental metastasis almost always occurs in the presence of widespread hematogenous dissemination of disease and usually indicates poor maternal outcome [14]. Similarly, fetuses that develop maternally derived metastases have an exceptionally poor prognosis, with death typically occurring within 3 months of diagnosis [15]. Only 16 cases of metastatic maternal tumor to the fetus have been published [15,16]. Most authors have reported maternal origin of the fetal tumor on the basis of circumstantial evidence [15].

Interestingly, male infants seem to be at higher risk than females (75% vs. 25%) for developing metastasis from any maternal cancer [15]. Of 16 reported cases, 43% were diagnosed in melanoma patients, followed by hematopoietic malignancies (37%) and lung cancer (18%) [14,15].

No fetus was ever found with breast cancer metastasis from maternal origin. The rarity of metastasis to the fetus is probably due to the placenta, which acts as a physical barrier that prevents cancer cell invasion [16]. Most of the reported cases in which the placenta was examined showed only microscopic deposits of malignant cells in the intervillous space [16], and a true invasion into the placental tissue (villous invasion) was very rare [14]. However, of the 18 cases of villous invasion reviewed by Al-Adnani *et al.*, only 5 metastasized to the fetus (3 melanoma, 1 lymphoma, 1 lung) [16]. Thus, the placental physical barrier is not sufficient for eliminating fetal metastasis. It might be that the rarity of this event is also a consequence of the fetal ability to eliminate metastatic cells. In that case, fetal metastasis can probably occur only following failure of the fetal immune system to recognize maternal cancer cells [14,15]. However, can the placenta provide a suitable environment for cancer cells to settle? The placenta grows rapidly, and must supply the increasing metabolic needs of the growing fetus. Thus, trophoblast tissues establish a plastic functional circulation that promotes maternal–fetal exchange to fulfill embryonic needs at every gestational stage [20,21]. To alter maternal blood vessels, extravillous trophoblast cells (EVT cells) invade the uterine wall, causing complete remodeling of the distal parts of maternal spiral arteries. Trophoblastic cell invasion causes increased dilation of the spiral arteries. At the end of this process, the endometrium of the spiral arteries becomes lined by extravillous trophoblast cells. This process leads to vasodilatation in the terminal portions of the spiral arteries and intervillous inflow tract, and the diameter of the spiral arteries increases 4- to 6-fold. This transformation slows the blood flow and maternal arterial blood pressure falls to that of the intervillous blood pressure. The slow exchange of a generous blood flow in the intervillous space over a large surface area presents a favorable biologic environment for cell growth and is ideal for creating metastasis [14]. Therefore, the limited number of placental metastases suggests that unknown placental factors eliminate the growth of cancer cells. The spiral arteries link the mother with the placenta and fetus. The fact that they are lined by extravillous trophoblast cells suggests that these cells may be involved in metastatic inhibition.

Although breast cancer is the most common malignancy found in pregnancy, and is usually discovered at an advanced stage, no case of fetal or even villous invasion has ever been found in breast cancer patients. Questions arise regarding this interesting phenomenon. Is the placenta indeed a nonsupportive microenvironment for cancer cells and especially for breast cancer cells?

The pregnancy and the placenta as a cancer microenvironment

It is well accepted that tumors arise from normal cells through genetic changes that affect the growth control system [22]. However, the tumor cell-centric view of cancer does not take into account the context in which malignant cells subsist. The English surgeon Stephen Paget (1855–1926) was the first to postulate the important role played by the microenvironment in cancer formation. He originated the "seed and soil" theory, which suggested that a cancer cell (the seed) may be implanted randomly, yet a tumor can grow only in a supportive microenvironment (the soil) [23]. During cancer progression, the surrounding microenvironment co-evolves into an activated state through continuous communication with the malignant cells, thereby promoting tumor growth [22].

Such an aberrant tumor-promoting microenvironment is composed of altered ECM, soluble factors (growth factors, hormones, and cytokines), and various nontransformed cells (fibroblasts, myofibroblasts, leukocytes, myoepithelial and endothelial cells) [24]. Conversely, a normal microenvironment can inhibit cancer formation. Certain epithelial cancers can be induced to "reboot" and regenerate normal tissue morphology when combined with embryonic or exogenous ECM scaffolds [25,26]. Metastatic location and tumor growth is also dependent on interactions between the tumor and the microenvironment. Tumor cells do not metastasize to distant organs randomly [24]. Distinct groups of secreted and membranous proteins are associated with organ preference for metastatic colonization [27].

To form a tumor, cancer cells must acquire unique characteristics. Ten years ago, Hanahan and Weinberg enumerated 6 hallmarks of cancer that are essential for a normal cell to become malignant and for cancer to progress [28]. These hallmarks include self-sufficiency in growth signals, insensitivity to growth-inhibitory signals, evasion of programmed cell death (apoptosis), limitless replicative potential, sustained angiogenesis, and tissue invasion and metastasis [28]. Researchers suggested adding the ability to evade the immune system as the seventh hallmark [29]. Many of these needs are provided by neighboring cells and the ECM [22]. The unique ECM composition contributes to the establishment of a microenvironment that supports tumor dormancy or its switch to metastatic growth [30].

To invade and attach to a new area, ECM remodeling by proteases and expression of molecules that facilitate adhesive interactions such as fibronectin are needed [22,30]. In most tumors, proteases and ECM proteins are expressed not only by tumor cells, but also by normal cells such as fibroblasts, vascular endothelial cells, myofibroblasts, or inflammatory cells [30,31]. Following attachment, cells require mitogenic growth signals to move from a quiescent state into an active, proliferative state. Cancer cell characteristics largely contribute to the increased proliferation; however, they are also being instructed to grow by actively responding growth signals originating from paracrine signaling by the neighboring cells [28]. These signals include various growth factors, such as hepatocyte growth factor (HGF), epidermal growth factor (EGF), hormones (such as estrogen), and cytokines (such as interleukin-6 [IL-6]) [22]. While some factors stimulate, others, such as IL-18, interferons (IFNs), and human chorionic gonadotropin (β-hCG), may inhibit cancer promotion [32].

The ability of a tumor cell population to expand into a new area is also determined by the rate of cell attrition. Programmed cell death represents a major source of this attrition and should be avoided by the cancer cells. Although cancer cells delay apoptosis by altering their death pathways, their survival also depends on the level and types of apoptotic triggering molecules and survival factors in their microenvironment, such as tumor necrosis-related apoptosis-inducing ligand (TRAIL), FAS ligand (FASL), and insulin-like

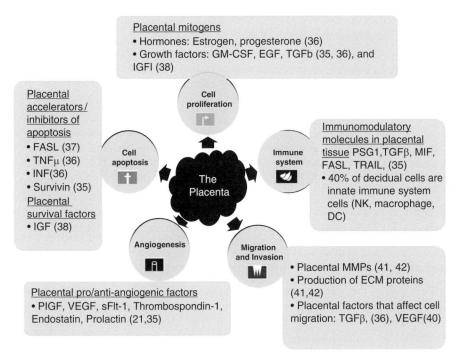

Figure 1. The placenta as a microenvironment that may affect cancer cell fate.

growth factors (IGF-I/II) [33]. Even in the presence of growth factors and eliminated death, to grow beyond a few millimeters, an effective tumor neovasculature needs to be formed [34]. Many angiogenic inducers, such as vascular endothelial growth factor (VEGF), fibroblast growth factor (FGF), and stromal cell-derived factor-1 (SDF-1), are produced by the stromal cells [22]. A microenvironment that does not provide these supporting signals will not allow metastatic growth.

Human placenta as a cancer microenvironment

Human placenta secretes variegated factors, including hormones (such as β-hCG, progesterone, and estrogen), growth factors (such as granulocyte macrophage colony-stimulating factor [GM-CSF], EGF, TGF-β, VEGF and IGF), cytokines (such as IL-6, LIF), heat shock proteins (HSP27), and proteases (such as MMP2 and 9) [35–38]. These factors may play an important role in breast cancer progression, as they are involved in cell proliferation and motility (Figure 1). Furthermore, placental cells synthesize several apoptosis-triggering molecules, such as TNF-α, FasL, and IFN and may induce the death of neighboring cells [36,39]. On the other hand, elevated levels of placental survivin and IGF-I may protect the placenta and its surrounding areas from apoptosis [35,40] (Figure 1). The placenta is a highly vascular organ and vasculogenesis and angiogenesis are involved in its vascular formation [21]. During early pregnancy, Flt-1 (VEGF receptor), placental growth factor (PIGF), and VEGF are expressed by the invading cytotrophoblast cells and may contribute to their invasion and differentiation. Toward the end of pregnancy, the expression of anti-angiogenic factors (such as sFlt-1, thrombospondin-1, endostatin, and prolactin) increases, possibly in preparation for delivery [21,35]. This altered balance from pro- to anti-angiogenic factors may modify tumor growth (Figure 1).

During pregnancy, the placenta actively modulates the host immune response [35]. Many maternal and placental immunomodulatory factors are required for adequate placental invasion. Indeed, around 40% of decidual cells are NK cells, macrophages, and dendritic cells of the innate immune system and immunomodulatory molecules such as pregnancy-specific beta-1-glycoprotein 1 (PSG1), glycodelin, TGF-β2, and MIF are found in conditioned media of placental tissue [35]. Like the placenta, cancer cells engage immune cells for their needs [29]. Thus, interactions between them and the placental immune cells and immunomodulators may alter their fate (Figure 1). The placenta alters not only the soluble factors milieu, but also manipulates its surroundings by altering the ECM composition [41]. EVT cells invade the uterine wall while secreting proteinases that degrade the maternal matrix and concomitantly produce ECM proteins [42]. The altered ECM may also affect migration, invasion, proliferation, and death of breast cancer cells (Figure 1).

The effect of placental-derived hormones on breast cancer progression

As mentioned earlier, the role of pregnancy in breast cancer etiology and the biological mechanisms underlying this role are not clear yet. Several hypotheses have been proposed, most of which posit a role for placental hormones [13]. The contribution of pregnancy-related hormones to tumor promotion/inhibition is complex and as yet, not completely understood [43]. Elevated serum levels of estrogen, progesterone, and prolactin have been proposed as potential contributory factors, whereas other pregnancy-related hormones (β-hCG, relaxin) have been suggested as inhibitors of tumor growth [13,43]. Because it is difficult to directly investigate the maternal hormonal environment during pregnancy and subsequent breast cancer, some authors suggested that insight into biological mechanisms may be gained by correlating between breast cancer risk and certain pregnancy characteristics, which may be associated with specific pregnancy hormones [13]. A systematic review that summarized studies on pregnancy characteristics and maternal breast cancer risk concluded that the most consistent findings were that multiple births and preeclampsia modestly reduce breast cancer risk. Women who deliver twins as well as pre-eclamptic pregnancies, had increased levels of progesterone and HCG during pregnancy compared to healthy women who delivered singletons [13]. These results may suggest a protective effect of β-hCG and progesterone. However, some studies found no such effects [13]. Similarly, two studies have examined placental characteristics and their association with breast cancer risk [13]. The biological rationale was that placental characteristics (e.g., placental weight) may represent placental functionality, which in turn could reflect altered exposure to hormonal factors produced by the placenta [13]. Both studies found an association between breast cancer risks and placental size, suggesting hormonal involvement in breast cancer risk and/or prognosis.

It has long been recognized that hormones have a decisive role in the development and progression of breast cancer. Common therapy for breast cancer that expresses ER incorporates drugs that target the estrogen pathway. Paradoxically, one of the strongest and most extensively documented protective factors for breast cancer in both humans and in rodent models is an early full-term pregnancy [44]. The protective effect of a full-term pregnancy can be mimicked in the laboratory by exposing genetically engineered rodents or carcinogen-exposed rodents to estrogen, estrogen + progesterone, or β-hCG [45,46]. Interestingly, these studies showed that a long duration of estrogen and progesterone exposure is associated with increased breast cancer risk, and a short duration is associated with a reduced breast cancer risk [46]. The underlying mechanism mediating the protective effect is not entirely known. It has been proposed that exposure to hormones down-regulates pituitary hormones and then limits the proliferative stimulus to preneoplastic cells. Others suggested that pregnancy/estrogen + progesterone cause differentiation of the normal mammary gland thereby creating a less carcinogen responsive cell population. Although the mechanism is still unknown, it has been established that the protective effect of pregnancy is accompanied by permanent changes in the stroma of the mammary gland, suggesting the involvement of altered breast epithelial cells microenvironment in this protection [46]. Indeed, in addition to their direct effect on breast cancer cells, estrogen and progesterone can alter ECM composition and integrin expression [47] and thus remodel the microenvironment. Thus, the sum effect of hormones on breast cancer is determined by timing of exposure (women's age), duration of exposure, and their influence on breast epithelial cells and their microenvironment.

The effect of placental explants on breast cancer cells: *in vitro* study

Mechanisms of placental cell implantation are similar to that of malignant tumor cells [48]. Although tumoric and trophoblastic cell invasion share the same biochemical mediators, only trophoblastic invasion is stringently controlled. Our group hypothesized that the same mechanisms that affect and restrain trophoblast cell implantation into maternal tissue may also be responsible for inhibiting metastatic growth in the placental area. To analyze the effect of the placenta on breast cancer cells, we co-cultured human first-trimester placental explants with breast cancer cells. We used the placental explant model where trophoblast cells differentiate into EVT cells, are released from the anchoring villi into the matrigel substrate and implanted there. We co-cultured breast cancer cells (MCF-7/T47D cells) with placental explants during EVT cell differentiation and invasion. MCF-7/T47D cells are breast cancer cell lines that express estrogen and progesterone receptors (ER and PgR). Interestingly, we found reduced breast cancer cell numbers near the placental explant (50% reduction) in comparison to breast cancer cells cultured alone on matrigel [49]. Additional studies with MCF-7 cells demonstrated their absence, especially from regions located near EVT releasing villi[49] (Figure 2). The decreased number of breast cancer cells near the placental area could have been due to reduced proliferation, increased apoptosis, and/or cell detachment/migration from the placental area. Thus, we evaluated these parameters further. We found that the placental explants did not affect the MCF7 cell-cycle, except for modestly elevating their sub-G1 phase by approximately 20%, indicating an elevated cell death rate [49]. Indeed, a similar increase in cell death (~17%) was found in breast cancer cells located near placental explants [49]. Interestingly, increased apoptosis was observed in cells located near EVT cells, again suggesting the special effect of these cells on breast cancer cells. The increased death rate of MCF-7/T47D cells co-cultured with placental explants afforded only a partial explanation for their absence from the placental area. Therefore, we theorized that other mechanisms such as cell migration or detachment were responsible for this phenomenon. Indeed, microscopic observation of the placental-breast cancer co-culture showed that breast cancer cells located near the placenta changed their morphology to one that characterizes motile cells [49] (Figure 2). T47D cells metamorphosed to spindle-like cells and MCF-7 cells formed elongated aggregates. This process was followed by the elimination of these cells from the placental area and by elevated MMPs levels, facilitators of cell invasion/migration, in

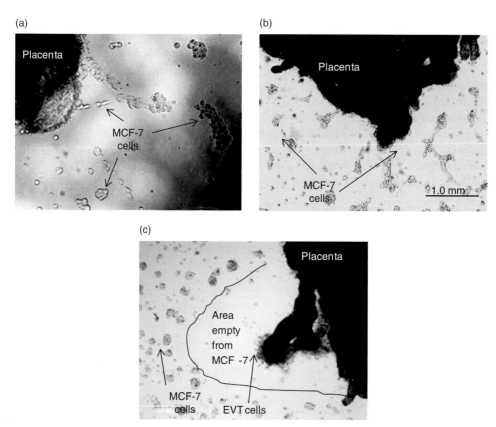

Figure 2. The effect of placental explants on MCF-7 breast cancer cells. MCF-7 cells located near the placental explants generated elongated aggregates (a,b), which eventually (24-60 hours) disappeared (c). This happened especially near placental extravillous trophoblast (EVT) cells.

the co-culture. Furthermore, placental soluble factors contributed to the breast cancer cells' enhanced motility. Increased detachment (from plastic substrate) [50], migration, and invasion (Transwell and scratch assays, respectively) of MCF-7 cells were determined following their exposure to media collected from placental cultures compared to cells exposed to media collected from breast cancer cell culture (unpublished data).

Breast cancer cells that express ERα have lower motility than ERα-negative cells [50]. Furthermore, breast cancer cells of pregnant women have decreased ERα expression [7]. Thus, we analyzed the effect of first trimester human placental explants on MCF-7/T47D ERα levels. As expected, decreased ERα expression was found in MCF-7/T47D cells co-cultured with placental explants compared to MCF-7/T47D cells cultured alone. These results suggest the involvement of hormonal pathways in modulating the placental effect on breast cancer cells. Nevertheless, breast cancer cells were eliminated, especially from areas located near EVT cells, whereas the reduced ERα expression was found in cancer cells around all areas of placental explants. Thus, additional placental factors located near the EVT cells (probably in the ECM) must have been involved in eliminating the breast cancer cells. In the future, we intend to characterize the effect of a placenta-breast cancer cell co-culture on hormone concentrations and ECM composition and the contribution of these factors to the elimination of breast cancer cells.

In summary, opinions about the influence of pregnancy on the etiology of breast cancer are variable and controversial. Whereas the effect of pregnancy on existing breast cancer is still unknown, convincing evidence suggests that a first full term pregnancy at a young age reduces breast cancer risk. Hormones and an altered microenvironment are probably involved in this protection. Similarly, epidemiological data support a role for the placenta in eliminating breast cancer metastasis in its area. Our study, demonstrated for the first time that the placenta inhibits breast cancer cell growth in its area. We showed that breast cancer cells migrated from the implantation site of the placenta that contained EVT cells, suggesting it is a non-supportive microenvironment for breast cancer cells. Our data also suggest the involvement of hormonal pathways and matrix manipulation in mediating this effect. The molecular pathways responsible for the altered breast cancer phenotype are now being explored.

References

1. Pereg D, Koren G, Lishner M. Cancer in pregnancy: gaps, challenges and solutions. *Cancer Treat Rev.* 2008;**34**:302–12.

2. Smith LH, Danielsen B, Allen ME, Cress R. Cancer associated with obstetric delivery: results of linkage with the California cancer registry. *Am J Obstet Gynecol.* 2003;**189**:1128–35.

3. Stensheim H, Moller B, van Dijk T, Fossa SD. Cause-specific survival for women diagnosed with cancer during pregnancy or lactation: a registry-based cohort study. *J Clin Oncol.* 2009;**27**:45–51.

4. Van Calsteren K, Heyns L, De Smet F, et al. Cancer during pregnancy: an analysis of 215 patients emphasizing the obstetrical and the neonatal outcomes. *J Clin Oncol.* 2010;**28**:683–9.

5. Pavlidis NA. Coexistence of pregnancy and malignancy. *Oncologist.* 2002;**7**:279–87.

6. Middleton LP, Amin M, Gwyn K, Theriault R, Sahin A. Breast carcinoma in pregnant women: assessment of clinicopathologic and immunohistochemical features. *Cancer.* 2003;**98**:1055–60.

7. Shousha S. Breast carcinoma presenting during or shortly after pregnancy and lactation. *Arch Pathol Lab Med.* 2000;**124**:1053–60.

8. Smyth CM, Benn DE, Reeve TS. Influence of the menstrual cycle on the concentrations of estrogen and progesterone receptors in primary breast cancer biopsies. *Breast Cancer Res Treat.* 1988;**11**:45–50.

9. Duong V, Boulle N, Daujat S, et al. Differential regulation of estrogen receptor alpha turnover and transactivation by Mdm2 and stress-inducing agents. *Cancer Res.* 2007;**67**:5513–21.

10. Ulery M, Carter L, McFarlin BL, Giurgescu C. Pregnancy-associated breast cancer: significance of early detection. *J Midwifery Womens Health.* 2009;**54**:357–63.

11. Lyons TR, Schedin PJ, Borges VF. Pregnancy and breast cancer: when they collide. *J Mammary Gland Biol Neoplasia.* 2009;**14**:87–98.

12. Dodds L, Fell DB, Joseph KS, et al. Relationship of time since childbirth and other pregnancy factors to premenopausal breast cancer prognosis. *Obstet Gynecol.* 2008;**111**:1167–73.

13. Nechuta S, Paneth N, Velie EM. Pregnancy characteristics and maternal breast cancer risk: a review of the epidemiologic literature. *Cancer Causes Control.* 2010;**21**:967–89.

14. Jackisch C, Louwen F, Schwenkhagen A, et al. Lung cancer during pregnancy involving the products of conception and a review of the literature. *Arch Gynecol Obstet.* 2003;**268**:69–77.

15. Alexander A, Samlowski WE, Grossman D, et al. Metastatic melanoma in pregnancy: risk of transplacental metastases in the infant. *J Clin Oncol.* 2003;**21**:2179–86.

16. Al-Adnani M, Kiho L, Scheimberg I. Maternal pancreatic carcinoma metastatic to the placenta: a case report and literature review. *Pediatr Dev Pathol.* 2007;**10**:61–5.

17. Thelmo MC, Shen EP, Shertukde S. Metastatic pulmonary adenocarcinoma to placenta and pleural fluid: clinicopathologic findings. *Fetal Pediatr Pathol.* 2010;29:45–56.

18. Pages C, Robert C, Thomas L, et al. Management and outcome of metastatic melanoma during pregnancy. *Br J Dermatol.* 2010;162:274–81.

19. Shuhaila A, Rohaizak M, Phang KS, Mahdy ZA. Maternal melanoma with placental metastasis. *Singapore Med J.* 2008;49:e71–2.

20. Charnock-Jones DS, Kaufmann P, Mayhew TM. Aspects of human fetoplacental vasculogenesis and angiogenesis. I. Molecular regulation. *Placenta.* 2004;25 (2–3):103–13.

21. Khankin EV, Royle C, Karumanchi SA. Placental vasculature in health and disease. *Semin Thromb Hemost.* 2010;36:309–20.

22. Pietras K, Ostman A. Hallmarks of cancer: interactions with the tumor stroma. *Exp Cell Res.* 2010;316:1324–31.

23. Ribatti D, Mangialardi G, Vacca A. Stephen Paget and the 'seed and soil' theory of metastatic dissemination. *Clin Exp Med.* 2006;6:145–9.

24. Hu M, Polyak K. Microenvironmental regulation of cancer development. *Curr Opin Genet Dev.* 2008;18:27–34.

25. Ingber DE. Can cancer be reversed by engineering the tumor microenvironment? *Semin Cancer Biol.* 2008;18:356–64.

26. Postovit LM, Margaryan NV, Seftor EA, et al. Human embryonic stem cell microenvironment suppresses the tumorigenic phenotype of aggressive cancer cells. *Proc Natl Acad Sci U S A.* 2008;105:4329–34.

27. Gupta GP, Massague J. Cancer metastasis: building a framework. *Cell.* 2006;127: 679–95.

28. Hanahan D, Weinberg RA. The hallmarks of cancer. *Cell.* 2000;100:57–70.

29. Zitvogel L, Tesniere A, Kroemer G. Cancer despite immunosurveillance: immunoselection and immunosubversion. *Nat Rev Immunol.* 2006;6:715–27.

30. Barkan D, Green JE, Chambers AF. Extracellular matrix: a gatekeeper in the transition from dormancy to metastatic growth. *Eur J Cancer.* 2010;46:1181–8.

31. Jodele S, Blavier L, Yoon JM, DeClerck YA. Modifying the soil to affect the seed: role of stromal-derived matrix metalloproteinases in cancer progression. *Cancer Metastasis Rev.* 2006;25:35–43.

32. Carpi A, Nicolini A, Antonelli A, Ferrari P, Rossi G. Cytokines in the management of high risk or advanced breast cancer: an update and expectation. *Curr Cancer Drug Targets.* 2009;9:888–903.

33. LoPiccolo J, Granville CA, Gills JJ, Dennis PA. Targeting Akt in cancer therapy. *Anticancer Drugs.* 2007;18:861–74.

34. Isayeva T, Kumar S, Ponnazhagan S. Anti-angiogenic gene therapy for cancer [review]. *Int J Oncol.* 2004;25:335–43.

35. Holtan SG, Creedon DJ, Haluska P, Markovic SN. Cancer and pregnancy: parallels in growth, invasion, and immune modulation and implications for cancer therapeutic agents. *Mayo Clin Proc.* 2009;84:985–1000.

36. Bowen JM, Chamley L, Mitchell MD, Keelan JA. Cytokines of the placenta and extra-placental membranes: biosynthesis, secretion and roles in establishment of pregnancy in women. *Placenta.* 2002;23:239–56.

37. Guo S, Colbert LS, Fuller M, Zhang Y, Gonzalez-Perez RR. Vascular endothelial growth factor receptor-2 in breast cancer. *Biochim Biophys Acta.* 2010;1806:108–21.

38. Timoshenko AV, Rastogi S, Lala PK. Migration-promoting role of VEGF-C and VEGF-C binding receptors in human breast cancer cells. *Br J Cancer.* 2007;97:1090–8.

39. Sokolov DI, Kolobov AV, Lesnichija MV, et al. Regulatory mechanisms for apoptosis in placental tissue during normal pregnancy and gestosis-complicated pregnancy. *Bull Exp Biol Med.* 2009;148:766–70.

40. Iniguez G, Gonzalez CA, Argandona F, Kakarieka E, Johnson MC, Cassorla F. Expression and protein content of IGF-I

and IGF-I receptor in placentas from small, adequate and large for gestational age newborns. *Horm Res Paediatr.* 2010;**73**:320–7.

41. McEwan M, Lins RJ, Munro SK, Vincent ZL, Ponnampalam AP, Mitchell MD. Cytokine regulation during the formation of the fetal-maternal interface: focus on cell-cell adhesion and remodelling of the extra-cellular matrix. *Cytokine Growth Factor Rev.* 2009;**20**:241–9.

42. Huppertz B, Kertschanska S, Frank HG, Gaus G, Funayama H, Kaufmann P. Extracellular matrix components of the placental extravillous trophoblast: immunocytochemistry and ultrastructural distribution. *Histochem Cell Biol.* 1996;**106**:291–301.

43. Doyle S, Messiou C, Rutherford JM, Dineen RA. Cancer presenting during pregnancy: radiological perspectives. *Clin Radiol.* 2009;**64**:857–71.

44. Rajkumar L, Kittrell FS, Guzman RC, Brown PH, Nandi S, Medina D. Hormone-induced protection of mammary tumorigenesis in genetically engineered mouse models. *Breast Cancer Res.* 2007; **9**:R12.

45. Sivaraman L, Medina D. Hormone-induced protection against breast cancer. *J Mammary Gland Biol Neoplasia.* 2002;**7**:77–92.

46. Medina D, Kittrell FS, Tsimelzon A, Fuqua SA. Inhibition of mammary tumorigenesis by estrogen and progesterone in genetically engineered mice. *Ernst Schering Found Symp Proc.* 2007:109–26.

47. Helleman J, Jansen MP, Ruigrok-Ritstier K, et al. Association of an extracellular matrix gene cluster with breast cancer prognosis and endocrine therapy response. *Clin Cancer Res.* 2008;**14**:5555–64.

48. Soundararajan R, Rao AJ. Trophoblast 'pseudo-tumorigenesis': significance and contributory factors. *Reprod Biol Endocrinol.* 2004;**2**:15.

49. Tartakover-Matalon S, Mizrahi A, Epstein G, et al. Breast cancer characteristics are modified by first trimester human placenta: in vitro coculture study. *Hum Reprod.* 2010;**18**:2411–54.

50. Platet N, Cathiard AM, Gleizes M, Garcia M. Estrogens and their receptors in breast cancer progression: a dual role in cancer proliferation and invasion. *Crit Rev Oncol Hematol.* 2004;**51**:55–67.

Index